Gastroenterology

POCKET CONSULTANT

Gastroenterology

SIMON P.L. TRAVIS

DPhil, FRCP
Consultant Gastroenterologist
John Radcliffe Hospital
Oxford, UK

TARIQ AHMAD

DPhil, MRCP
Specialist Registrar
John Radcliffe Hospital
Oxford, UK

JANE COLLIER

MD, MRCP
Consultant Hepatologist
John Radcliffe Hospital
Oxford, UK

A. HILLARY STEINHART

MD, FRCP(C)
Head, Combined Division of Gastroenterology
Mount Sinai Hospital
Toronto, Canada

THIRD EDITION

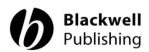 **Blackwell**
Publishing

© 2005 Simon Travis, Tariq Ahmad, Jane Collier, Hillary Steinhart

Published by Blackwell Publishing Ltd

Blackwell Publishing, Inc., 350 Main Street, Malden, Massachusetts 02148-5020, USA

Blackwell Publishing Ltd, 9600 Garsington Road, Oxford OX4 2DQ, UK

Blackwell Publishing Asia Pty Ltd, 550 Swanston Street, Carlton, Victoria 3053, Australia

First published 1991
Second edition 1998
Third edition 2005
Reprinted 2005

Library of Congress Cataloging-in-Publication Data
Gastroenterology / Simon P.L. Travis ... [et al.].– 3rd ed.
    p. ; cm. – (Pocket consultant)
  Rev. ed. of: Gastroenterology / S.P.L. Travis. 2nd ed. 1998.
  Includes bibliographical references and index.
  ISBN 1-4051-1192-5 (alk. paper)
    1. Gastrointestinal system–Diseases–Handbooks, manuals, etc.
  [DNLM: 1. Digestive System Diseases– diagnosis–Handbooks. 2. Digestive System Diseases–therapy–Handbooks. WI 39 G2562 2005] I. Travis, S. P. L. II. Series.
  RC802.T73 2005
  616.3′3–dc22

                                                                2004023181

ISBN-13:978-1-4051-11928
ISBN 1-4051-11925

A catalogue record for this title is available from the British Library

Set in 9.5/11 Ehrhardt by Kolam Information Services Pvt. Ltd, Pondicherry, India
Printed and bound in Great Britain by TJ International Ltd, Padstow, Cornwall

Commissioning Editor: Alison Brown
Development Editor: Claire Bonnett
Production Controller: Kate Charman

For further information on Blackwell Publishing, visit our website:
http://www.blackwellpublishing.com

Contents

Appendices

Preface to the third edition

The field of gastroenterology continues its rapid pace of growth in the understanding of disease processes and the discovery of new diagnostic and treatment strategies. The success of the first and second editions of *Pocket Consultant in Gastroenterology* published in 1991 and 1998, in concert with significant advances in gastroenterology and hepatology over the past 5–6 years, has led to this third edition. The book's enduring appeal is a tribute to the original co-authors, Dr George Misiewicz and Rodney Taylor. Dr. Simon Travis is the leading force in this very useful book, and he has enlisted the fresh perspective of new authors, including Drs. Jane Collier, Tariq Ahmad and Hillary Steinhart. This third edition very effectively captures advances in new knowledge regarding the pathophysiology of gastrointestinal and hepatobiliary diseases and the management of patients with these disorders that has developed since the second edition. The authors continue to use the user-friendly format of short, focused paragraphs, and bulleted lists, supplemented by tables and figures where appropriate. The authors have struck the balance of remaining concise, yet being thorough in their discussions of all major disease entities. The whole story is provided in an economical format that makes this handbook so useful to busy clinicians seeking information in the fast pace of contemporary practice. This remarkable little book should be of value to primary care physicians, trainees in internal medicine and gastroenterology, as well as busy gastroenterology consultants, by providing a rapid and efficient way of refreshing themselves on specific topics. The font and layout of this book makes it particularly easy to seek out specific information. This third edition of *Pocket Consultant in Gastroenterology* is a goldmine of current information distilled into a terse and didactic style, making it indispensable in the clinic and office of the generalist and specialist gastroenterologist.

Emmet B Keeffe, MD
Professor of Medicine
Stanford University School of Medicine
President of the American Gastroenterology
Association 2003-4

Acknowledgements

It is a pleasure to acknowledge the generous support and advice from colleagues. In particular, images from Dr Simon Jackson (Plymouth, UK), Dr Giles Maskell (Truro, UK), Professor Nick Gourtsoyiannis (Crete), Drs Fergus Gleeson, Jane Phillips-Hughes, Helen Bungay, Horace DeCosta, Juan Piris, Markus Frenz and Bryan Warren (all from Oxford, UK), were greatly appreciated. Clementine Travis redrafted the height and weight tables to allow immediate cross-referencing between different countries (kilograms, imperial and US pounds) and Louise Edge kindly updated the useful addresses. Janeane Dart, (Chief Dietitian, John Radcliffe Hospital, Oxford, UK) extensively reviewed and revised nutritional aspects of several chapters, while Sister Smilgin-Humphries (Clinical Physiologist, Oxford, UK) kindly provided illustrations of oesophageal manometry. Professor Derek Jewell (Oxford, UK) deserves special mention, for forebearance as first one (during the first edition) and then another research fellow (this edition) were distracted by authorship from the real business of research. So too do the book's previous authors, George Misiewicz and Rodney Taylor. On the other side of the Atlantic (from Oxford, that is!), Dr David Wong in Toronto kindly reviewed the chapter on liver disease, to correct differences in emphasis between UK and North American practice. Thanks also go to many unnamed colleagues at work, be they clinical, students, clerical, nursing or ancillary staff, who have provided the educational environment that has contributed to this book. Alison Brown at Blackwell Publishing was instrumental in bringing the authors together and creating a most constructive collaboration as well as being a most tolerant commissioning editor. Finally, in place of precedence as the last to be mentioned, are our families, without whose unstinting tolerance and support this book would never have been written.

Simon Travis
Tariq Ahmad
Jane Collier
Hillary Steinhart

1 Alimentary Emergencies

1

1.1 Swallowed foreign body

Toddlers, the mentally disturbed and the elderly most commonly swallow foreign bodies. If no history is available, look for excessive salivation, regurgitation, choking or distress. Objects impact in the pharynx, lower end of the oesophagus, or pylorus. Pain or fever suggests perforation. Once through the pylorus, spontaneous passage is the rule, but perforation can occur in the ileocaecal region.

All cases
- Look in the mouth
- If the object is impacted in the fauces, call the ENT surgeon
- X-ray the chest and abdomen, but failure to visualise an object does not exclude its presence
- Look for surgical emphysema, mediastinal and subdiaphragmatic gas on X-ray
- Barium or Gastrografin examination is not indicated and may hinder endoscopy
- Address the underlying issues to avoid repeated ingestion, especially in prisoners or the mentally disturbed who may have ingested foreign bodies for individual gain

Bones, pins, glass and batteries
- Chest pain suggests perforation, and a small haematemesis may herald perforation of a major vessel. In either case, contact the thoracic surgeon urgently
- Sharp objects should be removed by an experienced endoscopist, unless they have passed the duodenum. A plastic sleeve over the endoscope helps prevent trauma during withdrawal. If possible, the endoscopist should practice snaring or grasping a similar object before starting the procedure in order to determine the best means of retrieval
- After endoscopic removal, further chest pain may indicate delayed perforation
- Batteries, especially small alkaline batteries ingested by toddlers, should be retrieved immediately if in the oesophagus. Corrosive perforation or heavy metal intoxication has been reported. Once in the small intestine, safe passage is the rule

Coins, beads and blunt objects
- Almost always pass spontaneously unless more than 5 cm long or 3 cm in diameter
- Reassure the patient or parents and advise them to check stools for 3 days
- Repeat abdominal X-ray after 36 h if there is doubt about progress. Documented arrest by X-rays for 72 h is an indication for surgical exploration

Body-packing (ingested packets of drugs)
- Smuggled packets of drugs may be swallowed, or secreted per rectum
- Intact packets can cause intestinal obstruction and if packets do not pass within 72 h, surgical removal is advisable

- Endoscopic removal is contraindicated because of the risk of rupturing the bags
- Packets may burst spontaneously and cause life-threatening overdose
- Heroin overdose causes constricted pupils, bradypnoea or coma. Hypoglycaemia or non-cardiogenic pulmonary oedema may occur later. Give intravenous naloxone 0.8 mg rapidly, to a maximum of 2.4 mg if necessary
- Cocaine causes dilated pupils, tachycardia and agitation. Convulsions, metabolic acidosis or coma may occur. Sedate with intravenous midazolam 5–10 mg and give oral propranolol 40 mg three times daily for a few days
- Severe overdose of any narcotic is an indication for ventilation and surgical removal of the packets, to stop drug absorption
- The doctor's immediate duty is the treatment of the patient if body-packing is discovered. Once treatment has been initiated, the appropriate authorities should be notified according to local legal regulations
- Questioning of the patient must wait until the patient is fit, and be sanctioned by the most responsible physician

1.2 Complete oesophageal obstruction

Bolus obstruction causes sudden, complete dysphagia for solids and liquids, with inability to swallow saliva. Food impacted against a benign or malignant stricture is the usual cause. Occasionally the presentation is delayed for a few days in the mentally handicapped or severely debilitated. The obstruction must be relieved urgently.

Clinical features
Ask about and look for:
- Duration of symptoms preceding obstruction
- Predisposing disease (stricture, carcinoma, Schatzki's ring)
- Triggering factors (steak, toast, fibrous foods, tablets)
- Dehydration
- Weight loss (suggests malignant obstruction)
- Supraclavicular nodes (from a carcinoma of the cardia)
- Complications (aspiration pneumonia, perforation)

Investigations
The endoscopist should be contacted as a priority.
- Full blood count—anaemia suggests carcinoma
- Serum electrolytes—high urea indicates dehydration
- Chest X-ray—look for a mediastinal fluid level (obstruction), absent gastric air bubble (obstruction) or right lower lobe consolidation (aspiration)
- Urgent endoscopy—must be performed by an experienced endoscopist
- A barium swallow risks aspiration and is inappropriate, unless the diagnosis is in doubt. This is *not* the same as in dysphagia without obstruction (Section 2.1, p. 51)

Management
- Intravenous fluids
- Endoscopic removal of the obstructing bolus

- Endoscopic dilatation can be done immediately after disimpaction
- Carbonated drinks occasionally disimpact fibrous debris, but endoscopy is needed when a food bolus is stuck for a few hours
- Fine-bore nasogastric feeding, or nutritional supplements are needed (Section 12.2, p. 378) if dilatation is delayed after removal of the bolus. Endoscopic placement of the tube is awkward, but indicated if it cannot be inserted in the normal way (p. 413)
- Intravenous metronidazole 500 mg and cefuroxime 750 mg three times daily for 5 days, if aspiration pneumonia is present

Prevention
Simple measures decrease the risk of acute obstruction in patients with oesophageal strictures or prosthetic oesophageal tubes (pp. 59 and 65):
- Avoid fibrous food (apples, oranges), steak and toast
- Wear dentures if edentulous
- Chew all solids well
- Carbonated drinks with meals
- Avoid oral potassium supplements, salicylates and large tablets>
- A proton-pump inhibitor (PPI; e.g. omeprazole 20–40 mg, lansoprazole 30 mg or rabeprazole 20 mg daily) delays or prevents restricturing in most patients and heals associated oesophagitis. PPIs should be continued indefinitely

1.3 Oesophageal rupture

Sudden chest pain after forceful vomiting is the cardinal symptom when the distal posterior oesophageal wall tears longitudinally in spontaneous perforation (Boerhaave's syndrome). Traumatic perforation after instrumentation or chest injury is more common than spontaneous rupture.

Differential diagnosis
Perforation presents with chest pain, respiratory distress, painful swallowing or subcutaneous emphysema. Early diagnosis is crucial to survival. Failure to consider the possibility is the commonest reason for misdiagnosis.
- Myocardial infarction (ECG, cardiac enzymes)
- Dissecting aneurysm (pulses, chest X-ray, urgent CT scan)
- Perforated peptic ulcer (rigid, silent abdomen, erect chest X-ray)
- Acute pancreatitis (amylase more than fourfold elevated)
- Spontaneous pneumothorax (chest X-ray in expiration)

Investigations
Confirm the diagnosis and site of perforation.
- Chest X-ray—look for mediastinal or subdiaphragmatic gas, or a hydro/pneumothorax (Fig. 1.1)
- Gastrografin swallow—in spontaneous rupture, tears are usually large and leak contrast; after instrumental rupture, tears are often small and do not leak contrast. Upper oesophageal perforations tend to leak into the mediastinum; mid-oesophageal perfo-

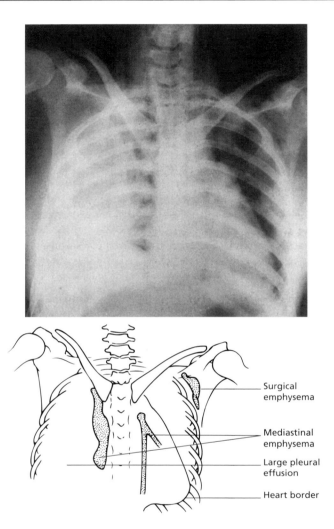

Surgical
emphysema

Mediastinal
emphysema

Large pleural
effusion

Heart border

Fig. 1.1 Chest X-ray in oesophageal rupture showing consequences of oesophageal perforation. There is a large right pleural effusion, mediastinal emphysema and gross surgical emphysema in the neck and upper chest wall.

rations into the mediastinum and right pleura; and distal oesophageal perforations into the mediastinum, left pleural cavity or abdomen

Management

Oesophageal perforation is a potentially lethal condition. Conservative management is confined to highly specific situations. If the perforation has involved the pleural cavity, or has been contaminated by saliva, gastric contents or food, then surgery is mandatory.

Resuscitation
• Intravenous fluids

- Analgesia—intravenous morphine 2.5–5 mg every hour until pain is relieved, then every 4 h
- Involve thoracic surgical colleagues at an early stage

Spontaneous rupture
- Nil by mouth
- Surgical repair and drainage is almost always needed and should occur within 24 h
- Antibiotics (intravenous metronidazole 500 mg and cefuroxime 750 mg three times daily for 5 days)
- Enteral nutrition through a jejunostomy fashioned at the time of surgery is best

Instrumental rupture
- Small tears (with minor symptoms and no leakage of contrast) may be managed conservatively in conjunction with the surgeons. Large tears that leak contrast are managed as for spontaneous rupture
- Nil by mouth
- Nasogastric aspiration for 3 days
- Intravenous fluids
- Antibiotics as above
- Indications for surgery are a persistent fever, or pneumothorax after 48 h
- When perforation complicates palliative treatment of a malignant stricture, patients who are unfit for surgery may be managed by endoscopic insertion of a cuffed oesophageal tube

1.4 Caustic oesophageal injury

Ingestion of caustic cleaning fluids can cause progressive and devastating injury to the oesophagus and stomach. Most occur as accidents in children under 5 years. Symptoms and the appearance of the pharynx do not correlate with the extent of oesophageal or gastric injury.

Clinical features
- There may be no symptoms initially, but diagnosis is not difficult if an accurate history is obtained
- Identify the specific fluid ingested
- Hoarseness and stridor indicate pharyngeal or laryngeal injury
- Painful dysphagia or haematemesis indicate oesophageal oedema and ulceration. This may occur rapidly or be delayed for several hours
- Respiratory distress and shock occur when mediastinitis develops due to oesophageal necrosis
- Acute symptoms may resolve, to be followed by dysphagia after several weeks or months as scar tissue causes an oesophageal stricture

Investigations
- Chest X-ray—look for mediastinal air or oedema
- Direct laryngoscopy and endoscopy—to record the extent of injury. This should be performed under general anaesthetic, since sedation is unsatisfactory in children and

does not allow adequate views of the larynx or hypopharynx. Circumferential burns lead to strictures

Management

Resuscitation
- Nil by mouth
- Establish the airway by intubation or tracheostomy if respiratory symptoms or stridor are present
- Intravenous fluids
- Do *not* give neutralising agents

Minor, non-circumferential burns
- Allow liquids and then a light diet if tolerated
- Arrange psychiatric assessment if ingestion was a suicide attempt

Deep ulcers or circumferential burns
- Remain nil by mouth for 48 h
- Monitor for chest pain or fever, indicating delayed perforation or mediastinitis. If these occur, give intravenous antibiotics, liaise with thoracic surgical colleagues and start nasojejunal feeding
- Allow liquids and a light diet if asymptomatic after 48 h
- Omeprazole 40 mg daily, lansoprazole 30 mg daily, rabeprazole 20 mg daily or equivalent PPI for 4 weeks may reduce the rate of late stricturing, but steroids have no effect

Late complications
- Oesophagogastric strictures occur in about 25%, but almost invariably in those with deep ulcers or circumferential burns
- Review patient after 4 weeks and at 3, 6 and 12 months
- Arrange a barium swallow if dysphagia occurs, before oesophageal dilatation
- Repeated dilatation is frequently necessary. Shortening of the oesophagus may promote gastro–oesophageal reflux, so omeprazole 40 mg daily, lansoprazole 30 mg daily or equivalent PPI is reasonable to reduce restricturing
- Attention to nutrition is vital
- Surgery is indicated if patients cannot tolerate repeated dilatation
- The risk of carcinoma of the oesophagus is substantially increased

1.5 Acute bleeding: upper gastrointestinal tract

The aims of management in upper gastrointestinal bleeding are to stabilise the patient, stop active bleeding and prevent recurrent bleeding. There are about 90 admissions per 100 000 adults annually in the UK, with an overall mortality of 14% unless patients are admitted to a specialised bleeding unit, where a mortality of about 5% can be expected. Most bleeds from peptic ulcers stop spontaneously and about 25% can be identified who have no risk of rebleeding and can be rapidly discharged. The task is to distinguish the 20% who rebleed in hospital and who may need surgical intervention. A standard clinical approach is recommended for every patient, so that patients at highest risk of rebleeding and death are identified early.

Clinical approach
- Assess severity
- Resuscitate
- Establish the site of bleeding
- Liaise with the surgical and intensive care teams on call
- Medical intervention
- Early surgery when appropriate

Assessment
The aim is to identify patients at high risk of rebleeding and death, by clinical and endoscopic examination. The Rockall score is an independently validated risk assessment score that is simple to apply and recommended. All patients with haematemesis or melaena must be treated actively until a stable baseline has been established. There is no room for complacency.

Rockall score
- The Rockall score is applied in two stages. First, there is a clinical score to be performed upon arrivals that estimates mortality:

Criterion		Score	Initial mortality risk score (pre-endoscopy)
• *Age*	<60 years	0	0 = 0.2%
	60–79 years	1	1 = 2.4%
	> 80 years	2	2 = 5.6%
• *Shock*	None	0	3 = 11.0%
	Pulse & sBP > 100	1	4 = 24.6%
	sPB < 100	2	5 = 39.6%
• *Comorbidity*	None	0	6 = 48.9%
	Cardiac/any major	2	7 = 50.0%
	Renal/liver/malig.	3	
• *Total initial score*		(max = 7)	

- Then, after endoscopy the mortality score is updated to produce a final score:

Criterion	Score	Final mortality score (after endoscopy)
• *Endoscopic diagnosis*		0 = 0.0%
No lesion, or M–W tear	0	1 = 0.0%
All other diagnoses	1	2 = 0.2%
Malignancy of upper GI tract	2	3 = 2.9%
• *Stigmata of recent haemorrhage*		4 = 5.3%
None/haematin	0	5 = 10.8%
Clot, visible vessel, blood in stomach	2	6 = 17.3%
• *Final score after endoscopy*	(max = 11)	7 = 27.0%
		8 = 41.1%

Document the following
In addition to a record of the assessment of the patient:
- Preceding symptoms (dyspepsia, vomiting, weight loss)
- Drug and alcohol ingestion
- Presence or absence of melaena on rectal examination
- Signs of chronic liver disease (Table 5.2, p. 137)

Causes
See Table 1.1.

Investigations and management

Resuscitation on arrival
- Ensure a patent airway
- Insert one 14- or two 18-gauge intravenous cannula
- If pulse > 100 b.p.m., give 500–1000 mL colloid (such as Haemaccel, Gelofusin, Pentaspan or pentastarch) over 30–60 min and repeat if necessary whilst waiting for blood
- Transfuse blood until haemodynamically stable in the first few hours, because initial haemoglobin is a poor indicator of the severity of the bleed. Subsequently transfuse up to haemoglobin of 10 g/dL
- Synthetic colloid or crystalloid will cause haemodilution: 1000 mL decreases the pre-transfusion haemoglobin by about 10%
- Reserve group O rhesus negative blood for dire emergencies (such as continuing massive bleeding and systolic BP < 80 mmHg despite 1000 mL intravenous colloid), when the risk from hypotension exceeds that from uncrossmatched blood
- Insert a urinary catheter in patients who need a central venous line (p. 11), to monitor urine output for information regarding fluid balance
- Ensure that the patient remains nil by mouth until endoscopy
- Do not insert a nasogastric tube, because this increases the risk of haemorrhage from gastric and oesophageal lesions
- Admission to a designated specialised unit for gastrointestinal bleeding reduces mortality to 5% or less. If this is not available, consider admission of patients with a predicted mortality > 10% (initial Rockall score ≥ 3) to a critical care unit and contact surgical colleagues as soon as the patient is resuscitated

Table 1.1 Differential diagnosis of haematemesis or melaena

Common	Less common (<5%)	Rare (1%)
Duodenal ulcer (35%)	Duodenitis	Hereditary telangiectasia
Gastric ulcer (20%)	Oesophageal varices	Aortoenteric fistula
Gastric erosion (6%)	Oesophagitis	Haemostatic defect
Mallory–Weiss tear (6%)	Tumours	Pseudoxanthoma elasticum
No lesion found (20%)		Haemobilia
		Pancreatitis
		Angiodysplasia
		Portal hypertensive gastropathy

Initial investigations

- Full blood count, crossmatch, coagulation studies and electrolytes
- Crossmatch 4 units of blood for patients with > 10% mortality risk (Rockall ≥ 3), but group and save alone for lower risk patients. Note that this is a practical application of the Rockall score, but it has not been validated for this purpose
- Haemodynamic status is a better guide to transfusion requirements than measured haemoglobin
- Arterial gases in those with cardiorespiratory disease
- ECG in high-risk patients
- Chest X-ray in high-risk patients (abdominal films rarely help)

Indications for a central venous line

- Signs of major haemorrhage (pulse > 100 b.p.m., systolic BP < 100 mmHg). Reasons for not inserting a central line in patients with a high (> 10%) predicted mortality (p. 9) must be carefully considered
- Rebleed during the same admission
- Inadequate peripheral venous access
- If a central venous line is needed, monitoring in a critical care area is advisable

Establish site of bleeding

- Arrange endoscopy after resuscitation, ideally within 12–24 h. Mucosal lesions and stigmata for rebleeding are otherwise missed. Ensure that the presence or absence of stigmata (p. 11) is recorded
- Indications for emergency endoscopy are continued bleeding, a rebleed in hospital, or if the patient is being considered for surgery
- Profuse haemorrhage may obscure the bleeding site. Gastric lavage to remove clots rarely alters management and can be hazardous. Repeat endoscopy after a further 12 h resuscitation is recommended. Immediate surgery should be a joint decision between surgeons and physicians
- Table 1.1 (p. 10) shows the differential diagnosis
- Interpret the endoscopy report intelligently: it should identify stigmata of recent haemorrhage (predicts risk of rebleeding), state whether there has been intervention (e.g. sclerotherapy of ulcers) and describe the position of ulcers (posterior duodenal ulcers overly a branch of the gastroduodenal artery that can rebleed vigorously)
- Stigmata of recent haemorrhage in the base of an ulcer and risk of rebleeding are:

Stigma	Risk of rebleeding
None	< 1%
Haematin (black spots)	5%
Adherent clot	30%
Visible vessel	50%
Bleeding vessel	80%

- Endoscopic intervention (below) halves, but does not abolish, the risk of rebleeding

Monitoring and discharge
- Pulse, BP, central venous pressure and urine output hourly, until stable
- Re-examine after 4 h
- Coagulation studies if > 4 units transfused
- Daily full blood count, urea and electrolytes for patients being transfused and for 2 days after
- Keep 2 units in the blood bank for 48 h after bleeding has stopped
- Patients who do not have endoscopic stigmata of high rebleeding risk (p. 11) and who have not had endoscopic intervention can safely start eating and drinking immediately after endoscopy and be discharged at any time thereafter, as long as there is adequate support at home
- Patients who have had endoscopic intervention (p. 11) should be kept in hospital for 72 h after bleeding has stopped

Medical intervention
These measures are not an alternative to surgery if an operation is indicated (p. 15), but may help stop bleeding or reduce the risk of rebleeding. Endoscopic intervention is indicated for patients with a peptic ulcer and active bleeding or non-bleeding visible vessel.
- Endoscopic intervention: all techniques halve the risk of rebleeding, but depend on local expertise and may not be available. Injection of adrenaline (up to 10 mL 1 : 10 000) around peptic ulcers, thermocoagulation and laser photocoagulation all have similar efficacy. Sclerosant (ethanolamine) is best avoided as necrosis and perforation have been reported. A combination of adrenaline (1 : 10 000) and thrombin (1000 U/mL) may be more efficacious at preventing rebleeding
- Intravenous omeprazole or pantoprazole (20–80 mg in 250 mL saline infused over 1 h, then 8 mg/h for 72 h) is only indicated after endoscopic intervention for bleeding peptic ulcers. It halves the risk of rebleeding and surgery and reduces mortality by one-third
- Ranitidine, oral omeprazole or other acid-suppressing drugs have **no** place in the initial treatment of bleeding. They should be reserved for treatment once a peptic ulcer has been diagnosed
- Tranexamic acid (1 g intravenously, three times daily for 72 h) has been shown on meta-analysis to reduce rebleeding and mortality. In the absence of a previous thromboembolic event, it is a reasonable adjunct in the treatment of high-risk patients until further trials are available. It also reduces the risk of recurrent bleeding from angiodysplasia
- Determination of *Helicobacter pylori* status should be done at the time of emergency endoscopy, using a biopsy urease (*Campylobacter*-like organism, CLO) test in patients with a bleeding ulcer (p. 87). Eradication therapy for *H. pylori*-positive patients (table 3.2, p. 89) is indicated as soon as oral feeding is restarted
- Terlipressin (Glypressin) 2 mg bolus, then 2 mg every 4 h is indicated for varices (below); Glypressin may not be available in all countries
- Other drugs (octreotide, vasopressin) do not have a proven role in the management of acute non-variceal gastrointestinal bleeding. A combination of ethinyloestradiol (50 μg) and norethisterone (1 mg/day) may decrease episodes of recurrent acute bleeding from angiodysplasia (such as hereditary telangiectasia)

Rebleeding

Rebleeding greatly increases mortality. Patients at high risk of rebleeding (based on endoscopic stigmata, p. 11) need to be recognised and the surgeons told of their admission. Patients are best admitted to a critical care area, where signs of rebleeding should be detected early. Signs of rebleeding are:
- Rise in pulse rate (a sensitive and early sign)
- Fall in central venous pressure
- Decrease in hourly urine output
- Haematemesis or continued melaena
- Looking at the patient (pallor, pulse, postural pressure drop and poor peripheral circulation) is as important as looking at the charts

Indications for surgery

Contact surgical colleagues at the outset, before an operation is necessary rather than when it is inevitable. Delay increases mortality. When the following criteria are met, surgery may be appropriate. Any decision not to operate should only be taken after discussion with the consulting surgeon.
- Age > 60 years and
  - > 4 units transfused in 24 h, or
  - one rebleed in hospital, or
  - continued bleeding, or
  - spurting vessel at endoscopy
- Age < 60 years and
  - > 8 units transfused in 24 h, or
  - one rebleed in hospital, or
  - continued bleeding, or
  - spurting vessel at endoscopy

The differential diagnosis of upper gastrointestinal bleeding is shown in Table 1.1 (p. 10). Individual topics are discussed below.

Oesophageal varices

Cirrhosis is the commonest cause of portal hypertension (p. 152) and oesophageal varices in the UK and North America. Whilst oesophageal varices can be found at endoscopy in almost 50% of patients with cirrhosis, less than one-third of these will bleed from their varices. Mortality during an acute bleed depends on the severity of liver disease on admission. Mortality according to Child's grade A is 10%, grade B is 25% and grade C is 50% (Table 5.5, p. 144), but 60–80% of all patients who bleed from varices will be dead within 4 years.

Assessment
- Bleeding from oesophageal varices is a complex clinical emergency for which control of bleeding is only one aspect
- Attention to infection, control of ascites (p. 147), encephalopathy (p. 144), alcohol withdrawal (Fig. 5.8, p. 177) and nutrition (p. 371) are vital for a successful outcome

Acute bleeding
- Resuscitate and monitor (p. 11). Colloids (synthetic, albumin or blood) are indicated and saline can be used in the acute situation. Avoid 5% dextrose if hyponatraemic

- 30% with known varices have another source of haemorrhage
- During active bleeding, correct disordered coagulation to international normalized ratio (INR) < 1.5 or prothrombin time < 22 s with fresh frozen plasma (FFP). However, FFP is contraindicated in the absence of bleeding, because this increases intravascular volume and variceal pressure, which may precipitate haemorrhage. Platelet transfusion may be necessary for thrombocytopenia (platelet count < 60 × 10^9/L). Discuss with the haematologists
- Arrange urgent endoscopy for banding or sclerotherapy by an experienced endoscopist
- Control of the airway, with endotracheal intubation if necessary, is extremely important when carrying out emergency endoscopy in a patient with an active variceal bleeding
- Give oral lactulose, starting at 90 mL/day or phosphate enemas if nil by mouth to prevent/treat hepatic encephalopathy (p. 145), intravenous vitamins (p. 393) and benzodiazepine, as necessary, for alcohol withdrawal (p. 177).

If endoscopic therapy is not available, or massive bleeding continues:

- Insert a Sengstaken tube until sclerotherapy/banding can be performed or repeated after 12 h
- Start splanchnic vasoconstrictors such as Glypressin (2 mg bolus, then 2 mg every 4 h, for up to 96 h). Glypressin rarely can be associated with ischaemic complications
- For recurrent bleeding after two attempts at endoscopic therapy the alternatives are transjugular intrahepatic portosystemic shunt (TIPSS) or oesophageal transection (see below)
- Where a stent is inserted between the hepatic and portal vein under radiological control, TIPSS can only be performed by experienced interventional radiologists, but is probably the procedure of choice where bleeding is not controlled by other means (Section 5.4, p. 153). Control of bleeding is excellent (approaching 100%), but 1 month mortality is still high (30–40%) owing to liver failure. Late complications (blocked stent, encephalopathy) are common
- Oesophageal transection has a mortality of 50% and should only be considered for patients without other organ failure, who were admitted in Child's group A or B (Table 5.5, p. 144). Splenectomy and proximal gastric devascularisation are needed to prevent subsequent bleeding from gastric varices
- Bleeding gastric varices are one cause of failed endoscopic haemostasis. TIPSS should be considered (Section 5.4, p 153), but preliminary reports suggest that endoscopic injection of bovine thrombin (2–10 mL of 1000 U/mL) or histoacryl (mixed with 1 : 1 lipiodal, 1–2 mL injected) controls active bleeding, although varices are not eradicated. Histoacryl has the potential to glue up the endoscope and should only be used by experienced endoscopists

Balloon tamponade
- Indicated for uncontrolled variceal bleeding, or recurrent haemorrhage despite sclerotherapy or banding
- To be inserted by experienced operators only
- Sedation, or a general anaesthetic to insert an endotracheal tube and secure the airway, may be necessary
- Insert a cooled, lubricated Sengstaken or Minnesota tube beyond 45 cm. The tube can usually be stiffened by inserting a well-lubricated pair of paediatric endoscopic biopsy forceps down the central lumen

- Inflate the gastric balloon with 300 mL tap water containing 50 mL of any intravenous X-ray contrast medium or 300 mL of air. Ensure gastric balloon channel is double-clamped
- Tie a 250 mL bag of saline to the tube to provide traction at the gastro-oesophageal junction, but be very careful to protect the mouth to prevent pressure necrosis
- Aspirate gastric and oesophageal ports (if present) hourly, and connect to a bag for continuous drainage
- It is rarely necessary to inflate the oesophageal balloon. If necessary because of persistent bleeding, inflate the oesophageal balloon to 30 mmHg with air, measured by manometer. Deflate for 5 min every hour.
- X-ray to check position (Fig. 1.2)
- Active bleeding is arrested in 90%. Continued bleeding usually means that the tube is misplaced or that there are gastric varices
- Deflate the oesophageal balloon after 6 h and the gastric balloon after 12–24 h to allow further endoscopic sclerotherapy or banding
- Complications include tracheal intubation, oesophageal rupture from inflating the gastric balloon in the oesophagus, or mucosal necrosis from leaving the balloon inflated for too long

Prevention of rebleeding from varices
- The highest risk of rebleeding is in the first 6 weeks
- Most gastroenterologists repeat endoscopic therapy at 1–2-week intervals until varices are obliterated
- Varices recur after obliteration in 40%, usually within 1 year
- Propranolol 40 mg three times daily decreases the risk of bleeding, can be used following initial endoscopic therapy and in this situation is as effective as repeated endoscopic therapy.
- Portal hypertensive gastropathy may cause bleeding after variceal obliteration. The gastric mucosa (usually fundal) has a characteristic 'snakeskin' appearance at endoscopy. Propranolol is the treatment of choice (p. 153)
- Surgical or percutaneous TIPSS are indicated for recurrent bleeding, especially in non-cirrhotic portal hypertension (p. 153)

Mallory–Weiss tears
A mucosal tear at the oesophagogastric junction due to forceful vomiting results in haematemesis. The typical features are:
- Initial vomitus does not contain blood
- Vomiting has often been provoked by alcohol
- 90% settle with conservative treatment
- Acid-suppressing drugs are unnecessary
- Continued bleeding can be controlled by endoscopic injection or thermocoagulation. Surgery is very rarely needed
- Bleeding after forceful vomiting may also be caused by prolapse of the gastric mucosa resulting in a focal area of haemorrhagic gastropathy ('hernia gastropathy') opposite the gastro-oesophageal junction

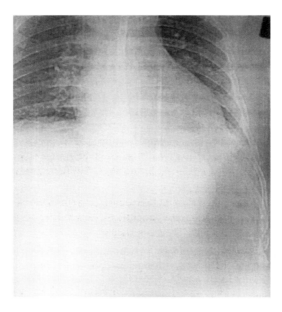

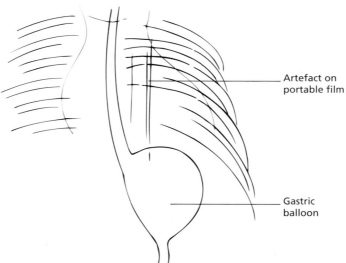

Artefact on portable film

Gastric balloon

Fig. 1.2 X-ray showing Minnesota tube in correct position. Gastric balloon has been inflated with 300 mL water mixed with 50 mL contrast medium.

Acute gastric erosions and haemorrhagic gastropathy

Erosions are diagnosed endoscopically, but may be obscured by oozing from haemorrhagic gastropathy (gastritis is a misleading term that should be reserved for a histological diagnosis). Major haemorrhage from superficial gastric injury is unusual and the cause is often readily apparent.

Causes
- Non-steroidal anti-inflammatory drugs (NSAIDs)
- Alcohol
- Stress (trauma, major surgery or patients in intensive care)

Specific treatment
- A PPI (any) is usually given for 1–4 weeks, depending on the cause
- Persistent bleeding is treated with intravenous tranexamic acid 1 g three times daily, in addition to a PPI (e.g. omeprazole or pantoprazole), which can be given intravenously
- Total gastrectomy is the last resort for continued bleeding after all medical treatment has been vigorously applied for 24–48 h, and should only be performed by an experienced surgeon
- It should be noted that despite the fact that antacids, ranitidine or sucralfate may prevent stress erosions in intensive care patients, there is almost no evidence that they reduce clinically significant bleeding or mortality

Gastric ulcer (Section 3.5, p. 92)
- Consider provoking causes (such as NSAIDs)
- Appropriate endoscopic haemostasis (p. 12) reduces rebleeding and mortality
- Give a PPI (lansoprazole 30 mg, omeprazole 20 mg, pantoprazole 40 mg, rabeprazole 20 mg daily) for 4 weeks once bleeding has stopped, together with *H. pylori* eradication therapy if endoscopic biopsies confirm infection
- For patients with NSAID-associated ulcers who cannot stop NSAIDs (p. 109), concomitant PPI therapy (lansoprazole or omeprazole) has replaced misoprostol in healing ulcers and preventing recurrence
- Arrange a repeat endoscopy after 8–12 weeks, to biopsy and take brushings for cytology from the ulcer site
- If surgery is needed for continued bleeding, a Billroth 1 gastrectomy is usually performed. Undersewing with a vagotomy and pyloroplasty is a simpler operation, but the ulcer cannot be examined histologically to exclude cancer. Wedge resection removes the ulcer and has the lowest morbidity in high-risk elderly patients, but long-term acid suppression is then necessary because it does not prevent recurrent ulceration

Duodenal ulcer (Section 3.9, p. 102)
- Combine ulcer healing with eradication of *H. pylori*
- The optimum treatment is triple, or quadruple eradication therapy (Table 3.2, p. 89)
- Repeat endoscopy is unnecessary, except in special circumstances (e.g. patients needing warfarin)
- Always confirm that eradication of *H. pylori* has been successful after an ulcer has bled, preferably by an isotope breath test (p. 86)
- Successful eradication of *H. pylori* significantly reduces the risk of rebleeding and the risk of bleeding from another ulcer to an extent similar to acid suppression. It is also cheaper in the long term and provides a cure
- Risk of repeat haemorrhage without eradication or maintenance therapy is 20% over 5–10 years, but is higher if associated with NSAIDs
- NSAID-associated ulcers heal with PPIs even if NSAIDs have to be continued, but are not directly associated with *H. pylori* (p. 110)

- Maintenance acid suppression (lansoprazole 15 mg, omeprazole 10 mg daily) is only indicated for patients at high risk of dying from the complications of recurrent ulceration (p. 110) when eradication therapy has been unsuccessful, or when NSAIDs have to be continued

'No source of bleeding found'

This is common (up to 20% acute bleeding) and can produce difficult management problems. Possible causes are:

- Lesion missed on endoscopy
- Mucosal lesion healed before patient endoscoped:
  - erosions
  - Mallory–Weiss tear
  - Dieulafoy's lesion (bleeding vessel with no surrounding ulceration, usually high on the greater curve)
- Bleeding from third part of the duodenum, or beyond:
  - jejunum (ulcerative jejunitis)
  - Meckel's diverticulum
  - colon
- Other:
  - nose bleed
  - rare causes of bleeding (Table 1.1, p. 10)

Management

The management of gastrointestinal bleeding from obscure and occult sources is discussed in more detail on p. 8 and Section 9.7 (p. 329; Fig. 9.9, p. 330).

- Reassess the patient—no further action is necessary for low-risk patients (p. 9)
- Repeat endoscopy in patients with a predicted mortality > 10% (p. 9)
- Investigate rare causes of bleeding (recheck coagulation, discuss small bowel radiology, endoscopic retrograde cholangiopancreatography (ERCP), ^{99}Tc sulphur colloid red cell scan (p. 20) or ^{99}Tc pertechnate scan with radiologists)
- Selective angiography during active bleeding (which must be at a rate of 1 U/4 h) is indicated after two negative endoscopies, preferably in a specialist unit
- Small bowel enteroscopy, including video capsule endoscopy (Section 9.7, p. 329) may be available in specialist units, but referral is necessary, and other procedures (mesenteric angiography, small bowel enema) will normally be repeated in the specialist unit
- Laparotomy, careful examination of the whole bowel with a bright light (e.g. sigmoidoscopy light source) and peroperative endoscopy is the ultimate procedure for recurrent episodes of active bleeding from obscure origin, but may still not identify the source and it is usually wise to refer to a specialist unit if this is contemplated

Aortoenteric fistula

Consider this rare diagnosis in *every* patient with an aortic graft and gastrointestinal bleeding. Exsanguination at the first bleed is uncommon. Small 'herald' bleeds occur for up to 2 weeks. Urgent abdominal CT scan, the diagnostic procedure of choice, may show haematoma around the graft. Endoscopy, if performed, should be to the fourth part of the duodenum, but surgery should not be delayed if hypotension has occurred. Aggressive surgery is needed as soon as the diagnosis is made, preferably in a specialist unit.

Acute bleeding: lower gastrointestinal tract

Bleeding from the colon is recognised by the passage of fresh red or reddish-brown altered blood per rectum. It is usually readily differentiated from upper gastrointestinal bleeding, because it has neither the smell, nor the tarry-black appearance of melaena. Upper tract bleeding rapid enough to cause red rectal bleeding is uncommon, and invariably associated with haemodynamic disturbance.

Clinical approach

- Resuscitate
- First episode, or recurrent (obscure) bleeding? See p. 329
- Establish the site of bleeding
- Specific treatment

Causes

See Table 1.2.

Investigations—first episode

Severe bleeding

- Full blood count, coagulation studies, crossmatch and check electrolytes
- Urgent colonoscopy after full bowel preparation (within 24–48 h) is safe and effective, although some prefer flexible sigmoidoscopy after phosphate enema preparation
- Gastroscopy—particularly in those with haemodynamic disturbance, to exclude brisk upper gastrointestinal haemorrhage
- Mesenteric angiography—if bleeding continues in excess of 1 U/4 h (Fig. 1.3; see Fig. 9.9, p. 330)

Slight/moderate bleeding

- Blood tests as above
- Colonoscopy once the bleeding has stopped

Investigations—obscure (recurrent) bleeding

Bleeding of obscure origin is defined as recurrent bouts of acute or chronic bleeding for which no source has been found after initial upper and lower gastrointestinal endoscopy. The topic is complex and further addressed in Section 9.7 (p. 329) and Fig. 9.9 (p. 330). Consider:

- Repeat colonoscopy—by an experienced operator, since angiodysplasia can be missed

Table 1.2 Causes of rectal bleeding

Common	Less common	Rare
Perianal conditions	Ischaemic colitis	Angiodysplasia
haemorrhoids	Crohn's disease	Anorectal varices
fissures, prolapse	Diverticular disease	Small intestinal
Colorectal polyps		diverticula
Colorectal carcinoma		lymphoma
Ulcerative colitis		Solitary rectal ulcer
		Vasculitis

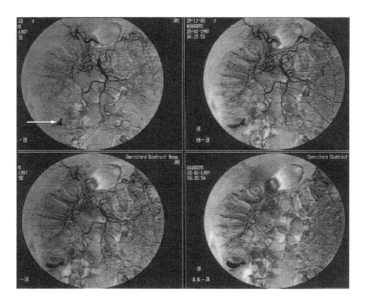

Fig. 1.3 Serial films from mesenteric angiography in a 63-year-old man with continuous bleeding (8 units transfusion in 24 h) and a normal upper gastrointestinal endoscopy. The bleeding vessel in the caecum (→) could not be embolised and laparotomy was necessary.

- Small bowel enema—better than a follow-through for identifying mucosal lesions (p. 423)
- Video capsule endoscopy (p. 329)
- ^{99}Tc sulphur colloid red scan—care must be taken not to overinterpret the scans, which may indicate the wrong area because blood accumulates in the colonic lumen. Early phase scans are the most helpful in localising the site of bleeding
- ^{99}Tc pertechnate Meckel's scan—at an early stage in young patients, but sensitivity is < 80%
- Angiography—during a subsequent episode of brisk bleeding (1 U/4 h)
- Self-induced rectal trauma is a rare cause of recurrent bleeding

Management
Severe bleeding stops spontaneously in 80% of cases after adequate blood replacement. Treatment of the cause (Table 1.2, p. 19) is then needed. In the remainder, bleeding is continuous or recurs, sometimes frequently, over many months. Identifying the site of persistent or recurrent bleeding is one of the most difficult problems in acute gastroenterology. Once the site is identified, surgical resection is indicated. If the site cannot be found, treatment depends on the pattern of bleeding.

Continuous bleeding
Referral to a specialist unit is advisable if bleeding persists after replacement of 6 units of blood and the source cannot be found. Surgery is an alternative and depends on local expertise. The options are:
- Laparotomy with peroperative colonoscopy after lavage through an appendicostomy. The physician is well advised to attend the laparotomy, but the difficulty of performing colonoscopy in these circumstances should not be underestimated

- Segmental resection if the site can be identified
- 'Blind' hemicolectomy can rarely be justified. If the site cannot be found and surgery is essential to stop bleeding, a subtotal colectomy should be performed

Intermittent bleeding
Referral to a specialist gastroenterology unit is advisable if the site of bleeding cannot be identified after three episodes of bleeding.

Rectal bleeding in children
The differential diagnosis is:
- Intussusception—commonest at 6–12 months
- Meckel's diverticulum
- Ulcerative colitis
- Foreign body
- Juvenile polyps—usually in the descending colon
- Intestinal haemangiomas
- Child (sexual) abuse

1.6 Acute abdominal pain

Clinical diagnostic accuracy is about 50%. Metabolic and extraintestinal causes (Table 1.3) should be considered if the diagnosis is in doubt.

Causes
The type of pain, relieving factors and progress are so variable that they rarely discriminate between diseases causing acute pain (Table 1.3; Table 1.4).

Table 1.3 Causes of acute abdominal pain

Common	Less common	Rare
Appendicitis	Cholangitis	Necrosis
Biliary colic	Mesenteric infarction	hepatoma
Cholecystitis	Pyelonephritis	fibroid
Diverticulitis	Torsion	Splenic infarction
Intestinal obstruction	ovarian cyst	Pneumonia
Perforated viscus	testicle	Myocardial infarction
Pancreatitis	omentum	Diabetic ketoacidosis
Peritonitis	Rupture	Porphyria
Salpingitis	ovarian cyst	Addisonian crisis
Mesenteric adenitis	ectopic pregnancy	Lead poisoning
Renal colic	aortic aneurysm	Tabes dorsalis
'Non-specific'	Prolapsed disc	Inflammatory aneurysm
	Abscesses	Volvulus
	Exacerbation of peptic ulcer	sigmoid
	Ileitis	caecum
	Crohn's	gastric
	Yersinia spp.	Herpes zoster

Table 1.4 Patterns of acute abdominal pain

	Appendicitis	Cholecystitis	Perforated viscus	Renal colic	Pancreatitis	Diverticulitis	Salpingitis	Intestinal obstruction
Site	C/RLQ	RUQ	UQs	R/L loins	UQs	LQs	LQs	Symmetrical
Duration	12–48 h	Days	< 12 h	< 12 h	< 48 h	Days	> 24 h	< 48 h
Severity	Moderate	Severe	Severe	Severe	Severe	Moderate	Moderate	Severe
Radiation	Nil	Shoulder, back	Nil	Groin	Nil	Nil	Groin, thigh	Nil
Aggravating factors	Movement cough	Inspiration	Movement cough	Nil	Movement	Movement cough	Nil	Eating

C/RLQ, central or right lower quadrant.
RUQ, right upper quadrant.
UQs, upper quadrants.
R/L, right or left.
LQs, lower quadrants.

Discriminating questions
- Site
- Duration
- Severity
- Radiation
- Aggravating factors

Also ask about
- Vomiting (if it precedes pain, a surgical cause is less likely)
- Time last ate or drank
- Bowel disturbance
- Urinary frequency
- Date of last menstrual period
- Previous abdominal surgery

Specifically examine for
- Distension
- Visible peristalsis
- Rebound tenderness, guarding or rigidity
- Pulsatile mass and peripheral pulses
- Hernial orifices
- Rectal *and pelvic* tenderness or masses
- Bowel sounds
- Epigastric bruit (normally audible in about 10% of thin patients)
- Fever (> 39°C with rigors suggests pyelonephritis, cholangitis or pneumonia)

Investigations
Every patient with acute abdominal pain should have on admission:
- Full blood count—leucocytosis may be absent in the elderly
- Electrolytes and creatinine
- Amylase—but many causes of slight elevation other than acute pancreatitis (p. 28)
- Group and save serum
- Urine examination—including *pregnancy* test if doubtful
- Erect chest X-ray—look for basal atelectasis and gas under diaphragm
- Supine abdominal X-ray—look for biliary and renal calculi, dilated bowel (> 2.5 cm small intestine, ≥ 6.0 cm colon), air in the biliary tree (p. 422)
- ECG
- Blood cultures—if febrile
- Abdominal ultrasound—the most discriminating investigation to identify appendicitis, cholecystitis, renal, or pelvic inflammatory disease
- Abdominal CT scan is indicated when ultrasound is technically difficult (often due to bowel gas or obesity) or does not identify a specific cause for acute abdominal pain. It is the initial imaging procedure of choice for suspected pancreatitis

Management—general principles
- Analgesia—do not withhold opiates for severe pain 'pending a surgical opinion', if the diagnosis is clear

- Perforation, peritonitis, or obstruction needs emergency surgery
- Observation overnight often clarifies a difficult diagnosis
- Nil by mouth until a decision about surgery has been made
- Specific management of common causes of abdominal pain are discussed below

Appendicitis
See Section 7.4 (p. 236).

Biliary colic

Distinguishing features
- Biliary colic typically causes a few minutes of right upper quadrant pain, with intervals of 1 h, and subsides after several hours. The pain may be exclusively high epigastric in location. Recurrent colic is a feature of chronic cholecystitis
- Fever, leucocytosis or pain lasting more than 12 h is likely to be due to acute cholecystitis
- Murphy's sign (tenderness in the right upper quadrant on inspiration) is positive in acute cholecystitis
- Flatulence, distension, fat intolerance and nausea are frequent but non-specific, and occur in other common conditions, especially irritable bowel syndrome (IBS) or non-ulcer dyspepsia
- Daily pain is unlikely to be due to biliary colic, even if gallstones are present

Management
- Ultrasonography will detect gallstones, although difficult in the obese and those with a fibrosed gall bladder. Repeat ultrasound after a fatty meal is a test of gall bladder function, and is abnormal (no contraction) in acute or chronic cholecystitis
- Other laboratory investigations are usually unhelpful, but a transient (<48 h) elevation in aspartate transaminase (AST) may occur in uncomplicated biliary colic
- Cholecystectomy is appropriate if symptoms are typical (Table 1.4, p. 22). Non-surgical options are discussed on p. 193

Acute cholecystitis

Distinguishing features
- Fever and persistent pain distinguish acute cholecystitis from biliary colic or chronic cholecystitis
- Impaction of a gallstone in the cystic duct causes > 90%
- Typical pain (Table 1.4, p. 22) occurs in < 50%
- Pain may be provoked by a fatty meal and builds up to a peak over 60 min, unlike the short spasms of biliary colic
- Fever develops after 12 h due to bacterial invasion and pain then becomes continuous
- Murphy's sign is sensitive, but not specific
- Calcified calculi (15%) and very rarely gas within biliary tree due to gas-forming organisms or a spontaneous choledochoduodenal fistula may be visible on plain abdominal X-ray

Complications
See Chapter 6 (p. 189).

- Recurrence (50%)
- Cholangitis due to associated common duct stones (10%)
- Mucocoele, empyema or gangrene of the gall bladder (1%)
- Biliary peritonitis (0.5%, with a mortality of 50%)
- Mirizzi's syndrome (obstructive jaundice due to external pressure on the common bile duct from inflammation around a stone impacted in the cystic duct)

Conservative management
- Confirm the diagnosis by ultrasound. Tenderness under the ultrasound probe in the presence of gallstones and a thickened gall bladder wall is effectively diagnostic. Isotope—hepatobiliary iminodiacetic acid (HIDA)—scans are also accurate, but not universally available
- Analgesia (intramuscular pethidine/meperidine 100 mg and hyoscine 20 mg, but not morphine, which can increase the pain)
- Intravenous fluids
- Nasogastric suction may be helpful, to alleviate vomiting if present
- Antibiotics (intravenous amoxycillin 500 mg three times daily and gentamicin 5 mg/kg once daily)
- Cholecystectomy at the earliest opportunity (see below)

Surgical management
- Optimum treatment is surgery on the same admission, on the next available list. Morbidity, total hospital stay, costs and mortality from complications of acute cholecystitis are lower compared to delayed cholecystectomy. Early surgery is especially appropriate in elderly patients or diabetics, because septic complications are more common
- Laparoscopic cholecystectomy is safe during acute cholecystitis in experienced hands. Cholecystostomy or percutaneous drainage of an empyema may be more appropriate in very sick elderly patients, but is rarely necessary
- The longer the interval between cholecystitis and surgery, the greater the risk of a recurrent attack: concern about an increased surgical complication rate 7–14 days after an acute attack is probably unfounded
- Other indications for surgery include signs of peritonitis and uncertainty about the diagnosis (when perforation or retrocaecal appendicitis cannot be excluded)

Cholangitis
See Section 6.4 (p. 200).

Diverticulitis
See Section 9.4 (p. 312).

Perforated viscus
The commonest cause is a perforated duodenal ulcer, followed by appendicitis, sigmoid diverticulum or carcinoma, Crohn's disease and gastric ulcers. Beware of a perforated peptic ulcer in patients already or recently in hospital for another reason.

Distinguishing features
- Sudden onset of severe, unremitting pain

- Temporary improvement 3–6 h later can trap the unwary
- Pain and peritonism may be absent in the elderly or those on steroids
- Abdomen fails to move with respiration
- Bowel sounds are usually absent
- Gas under the diaphragm on an erect chest X-ray is usual (70%), but not universal
- Lateral decubitus films for the very sick will also show free gas, but can be difficult to interpret
- Spontaneous sealing of the perforation occurs rarely

Surgical management
- Emergency surgery after vigorous intravenous resuscitation is almost invariably indicated
- Oversewing, omental patch and peritoneal lavage are customary for gastroduodenal perforation
- Hemicolectomy is indicated for right-sided colonic perforation, but distal perforation is probably best managed by resection, colostomy and rectal closure (Hartmann's procedure)
- Late complication of subphrenic abscess is best detected by ultrasound or CT scan, but an abscess may cause an immobile diaphragm, which can be readily detected by X-ray screening

Conservative management
- Indicated for the few patients in whom the risks are too high, or who refuse surgery
- Give intravenous fluids, antibiotics and nasogastric suction

Some surgeons advocate starting intravenous fluids, antibiotics and suction for 4–6 h and operating on those who do not improve, since this may have a lower mortality than emergency surgery for all patients. Whilst preoperative resuscitation is always advisable, this conservative surgical approach is not widespread.

Peritonitis

Fever, guarding, rebound tenderness and rigidity may be minimal in the elderly, the very young, patients on steroids and the immunocompromised. Bowel sounds are absent.

Causes
- Perforated viscus
- Local:
  - appendicitis
  - cholecystitis
  - diverticulitis
  - pancreatitis
  - salpingitis
- Spontaneous bacterial peritonitis (Section 5.2, p. 145)
- Continuous ambulatory peritoneal dialysis (CAPD)
- Rare:
  - tuberculous
  - sclerosing
  - granulomatous
  - periodic (familial Mediterranean fever)

Management

- Intravenous resuscitation
- Intravenous antibiotics (cefuroxime 750 mg and metronidazole 500 mg three times daily), after blood cultures
- Laparotomy
- Spontaneous bacterial peritonitis is usually due to *Escherichia coli* or *Streptococcus pneumoniae* in cirrhotic patients with ascites (p. 146). It does not display clinical features of pain, rebound and absent bowel sounds, but presents with encephalopathy or decompensation of stable chronic liver disease. Ascitic fluid should be sent for immediate Gram stain and absolute neutrophil count. Oral or intravenous ciprofloxacin 500 mg twice daily (400 mg twice daily for the intravenous form) should be started if the neutrophil count is > 250/mL, pending the result of culture. Long-term prophylaxis with ciprofloxacin is then appropriate
- CAPD peritonitis is usually caused by Gram-positive skin flora. Cloudy effluent, abdominal pain and tenderness are usual. Patients are often afebrile. Send fluid for Gram stain and absolute neutrophil count: a neutrophil count > 100/mL or the presence of organisms is diagnostic. Renal unit antibiotic policies differ, but intraperitoneal vancomycin 15 mg/L dialysate and gentamicin 4 mg/L are appropriate. Always consider silent intestinal perforation if bacteria other than skin flora are isolated. Laparotomy without further delay by an experienced surgeon is then indicated
- Tuberculous peritonitis is usually diagnosed at laparotomy, but can be suspected by a high ascitic adenosine deaminase level, although this is not widely available. Standard antituberculous chemotherapy for 9 months is advised (p. 357)

Acute pancreatitis

Acute pancreatitis affects around 200 000 people annually in the US, either as isolated or recurrent attacks. Recurrent attacks are distinguished from chronic pancreatitis by the absence of permanent impairment of exocrine or endocrine function. Initial symptoms are a poor indicator of prognosis. Complications (affecting 30%, p. 115) should be sought because early recognition improves prognosis and recovery is potentially complete. 10–15% of patients develop systemic inflammatory response syndrome (SIRS), leading to a fulminant course with pancreatic necrosis and multi-organ failure. Isolated and recurrent attacks are distinguished from chronic pancreatitis by the absence of permanent impairment of exocrine or endocrine function, but there is a spectrum of disease. Overall mortality ranges from 2–10% but this rate rises to 25% in the presence of infected pancreatic necrosis.

Distinguishing features

Abdominal pain with a serum amylase > fourfold the upper limit of normal is usually diagnostic, but late presentation (> 12 h) of a perforated duodenal ulcer, or ectopic pregnancy, may cause a similar rise in amylase

- The severity, rather than the nature, of the symptoms (pain and vomiting) characterises pancreatitis
- Diabetic coma is occasionally caused by acute pancreatitis

Predisposing factors

- Small gall stones—30–50%, more common in women, causing transient impaction at the ampulla

- No predisposing cause is found in about 15%. Many may be due to undetected microlithiasis
- Alcohol—10–40%, more common in men and in recurrent or chronic pancreatitis
- Trauma—about 5%, postoperative, post-ERCP or after blunt trauma
- Other causes of acute pancreatitis are rare:
  - drugs (azathioprine, mercaptopurine, sulphonamides, sodium valproate, antiretroviral agents)
  - pancreatic duct obstruction by benign stenosis, dyskinesia, pancreatic or ampullary carcinoma
  - pancreas divisum (congenital absence of pancreatic fusion)
  - end-stage renal failure
  - organ transplantation (drug-, viral- or lipid-related)
  - hypercalcaemia (acute or chronic pancreatitis)
  - hypertriglyceridaemia (> 10 mmol/L)
  - hypothermia
  - viral (mumps, coxsackie B4), pregnancy, hypothermia and arteritis cause isolated cases

Other abdominal causes of a moderately (< fourfold) raised serum amylase are:
- Acute-on-chronic pancreatitis in an alcoholic
- Perforated peptic ulcer (posterior perforation provokes pancreatitis)
- Ectopic pregnancy (amylase-secreting cells in the fallopian tube)
- Intestinal ischaemia, or infarction
- Aortic dissection
- Renal failure
- After any ERCP
- Consistent clinical features, a predisposing cause and an associated abnormality (such as hypocalcaemia or hypoxia) help discriminate acute pancreatitis from other causes of a moderately raised serum amylase

Complications of acute pancreatitis
- Local:
  - inflammatory mass (phlegmon)
  - pseudocyst (fluid collection; persistently raised amylase, p. 115)
  - pancreatic duct disruption (causing pseudocyst or ascites)
  - abscess (swinging pyrexia 1 week after attack)
  - jaundice (pancreatic oedema, or stones, can occlude the common bile duct)
- Paralytic ileus—exacerbates fluid and electrolyte imbalance
- Hypovolaemic shock—due to vomiting, hypoalbuminaemia, ascites or retroperitoneal haemorrhage
- Grey Turner's (flank) and Cullen's (periumbilical) signs are caused by tracking of blood-stained fluid
- Hypoxia—(PaO_2 < 8 kPa, or 60 mmHg) a prognostic factor and clinically underdiagnosed
- Hypocalcaemia—(< 2.0 mmol/L, corrected by adding 0.02 mmol/L for every g/L that the serum albumin < 40 g/L). Tetany is rare
- Acute renal failure—due to hypovolaemia, or disseminated intravascular coagulation (rare)
- Effusions—ascitic and pleural exudates with a high amylase

- Death—6–28%, depending on severity
- Recurrent attacks occur in one-third, especially in alcoholics, or if cholecystectomy for associated gallstones is delayed

Management

Establish the diagnosis
- Serum amylase is characteristically elevated > fourfold, but may be normal in up to 10%. Urinary amylase (spot sample) remains elevated for longer than serum amylase, but is not widely used
- Serum lipase elevated > threefold may be useful in patients presenting late, as it rises within 4–8 h, peaks at 24 h and returns to normal after 8–14 days. It is also more sensitive in alcohol-induced pancreatitis
- In patients with acute pancreatitis, a threefold or greater elevation in ALT suggests a gallstone aetiology with a positive predictive value of 95%
- Ultrasound may reveal pancreatic oedema and may also demonstrate gallstones if present. The sensitivity for gallstone detection is reduced to 60–80% during an acute attack of pancreatitis. Endoscopic ultrasound (EUS) is more sensitive for the detection of common bile duct calculi, but is invasive. A well-visualised normal pancreas makes pancreatitis most unlikely
- CT scan is indicated if the pancreas cannot be visualised by ultrasound or the attack is severe

Assess the severity (Table 1.5)
- Three or more factors present out of eight possible characteristics indicate severe disease (Ranson/Glasgow prognostic score, applied after 48 h). Unfortunately none may be abnormal in the early stages, and there is a move towards using the APACHE II scoring system for evaluating multisystem failure. This is widely used in intensive care units and, whilst not specific for acute pancreatitis, it does identify sick patients (score ≥ 8) at an early stage. The most important predictor of mortality is a Marshall organ failure score ≥ 2
- C-reactive protein concentration > 210 mg/L on day 2–4, or > 120 mg/L at the end of the first week, also discriminates between mild and severe pancreatitis, and is easier to apply than a multiple scoring system
- Peritoneal aspiration of more than 20 mL clear fluid, or any volume of dark fluid, also indicates severe acute pancreatitis, if Gram stain is negative and there is no odour

Table 1.5 Markers of severe pancreatitis*

White cell count > 15 × 10⁹/L
Urea > 16 mmol/L (no improvement with intravenous fluids)
Calcium < 2.0 mmol/L
Albumin < 32 g/L
Glucose > 10 mmol/L (no history of diabetes)
PO_2 < 8 kPa (60 mmHg)
AST > 200 iu/L
LDH > 600 iu/L
C-reactive protein > 150 mg/L

* Most reliable when used 48 h after onset of attack, which limits clinical applicability.

- Contrast-enhanced CT scan within the first 72 h of presentation assists in assessing the severity of pancreatitis. Necrosis predicts a high likelihood of complications such as an abscess and helps identify those who need early surgery
- Patients with severe disease have 30–40% major morbidity or mortality and greater need of intensive care management. Age (> 55 years), multiple organ failure and aetiology (post-ERCP, unknown) are associated with a higher mortality. Most patients (about 75%) have mild acute pancreatitis (mortality < 3%), but initial clinical appearances can be deceptive

Resuscitation and initial management
- Nil by mouth and nasogastric aspiration are designed to reduce pancreatic secretions
- Stop all drugs if possible
- Insert a central venous line if there is any doubt about cardiovascular stability or fluid replacement
- Intravenous crystalloid (0.9% saline) is usually sufficient for mild attacks, but some colloid (4.5% human albumin solution, or FFP) should be given for severe attacks
- Amount depends on urine output or central venous pressure, but 1500 mL colloid with 2000–3000 mL crystalloid daily are commonly needed in severe attacks
- Blood transfusion is indicated if the haematocrit is less than 0.30 (Hb < 10 g/dL)
- Early enteral feeding helps maintain mucosal function, limits absorption of endotoxins or cytokines from the gut and may reduce bacterial translocation. Nasojejunal and jejunostomy feeding avoid pancreatic stimulation and are recommended for severe pancreatitis even in the presence of ileus. Parenteral nutrition is the alternative, but causes more complications and does not provide mucosal protection
- Antibiotics for acute pancreatitis remain contentious. Currently, prophylactic broad-spectrum antibiotics (e.g. imipenem) should be reserved for patients with pancreatic necrosis

Specific treatment (See Fig. 1.4)
- Urgent ERCP (within 72 h) and sphincterotomy are indicated when there is a severe attack of gallstone pancreatitis or whenever jaundice is present
- No drugs are of proven value (including aprotinin, somatostatin, calcitonin, lexipafant), nor is peritoneal lavage helpful, even in severe attacks with haemorrhagic ascites. Surgery in the acute phase is only indicated for complications (p. 115)
- CT scan is better than ultrasound for determining prognosis: look for pancreatic necrosis, visible on a contrast-enhanced image, which is a poor sign (Fig. 4.1, p. 114). If necrosis is identified and there has been no clinical improvement within 48 h, repeat the scan to assist surgical decision-making
- CT scan should be repeated if there is persistent pain or pyrexia, or if the amylase has not returned to normal after 5 days, to detect a pseudocyst or abscess. Management of complications is discussed on p. 115

Indications for surgery
See Section 4.1 (p. 113).

Treat predisposing causes
- Urgent ERCP and sphincterotomy are indicated when there is a severe attack of gallstone pancreatitis or whenever jaundice is present

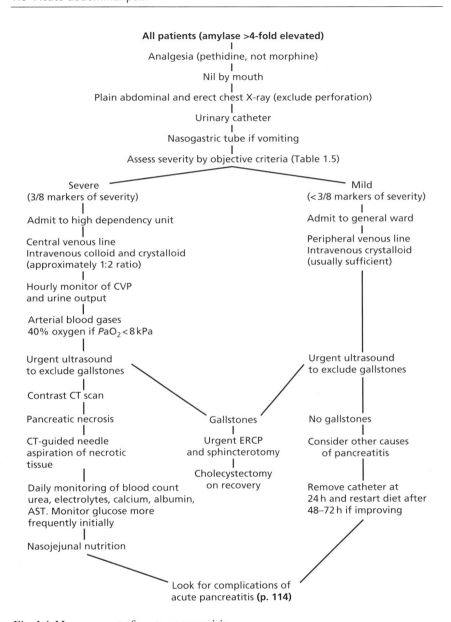

All patients (amylase >4-fold elevated)
|
Analgesia (pethidine, not morphine)
|
Nil by mouth
|
Plain abdominal and erect chest X-ray (exclude perforation)
|
Urinary catheter
|
Nasogastric tube if vomiting
|
Assess severity by objective criteria (Table 1.5)

Severe
(3/8 markers of severity)
|
Admit to high dependency unit
|
Central venous line
Intravenous colloid and crystalloid
(approximately 1:2 ratio)
|
Hourly monitor of CVP
and urine output
|
Arterial blood gases
40% oxygen if $PaO_2 < 8\,kPa$
|
Urgent ultrasound
to exclude gallstones
|
Contrast CT scan
|
Pancreatic necrosis
|
CT-guided needle
aspiration of necrotic
tissue
|
Daily monitoring of blood count
urea, electrolytes, calcium, albumin,
AST. Monitor glucose more
frequently initially
|
Nasojejunal nutrition

Mild
(<3/8 markers of severity)
|
Admit to general ward
|
Peripheral venous line
Intravenous crystalloid
(usually sufficient)
|
Urgent ultrasound
to exclude gallstones

Gallstones
Urgent ERCP
and sphincterotomy
Cholecystectomy
on recovery

No gallstones
|
Consider other causes
of pancreatitis
|
Remove catheter at
24 h and restart diet after
48–72 h if improving

Look for complications of
acute pancreatitis **(p. 114)**

Fig. 1.4 **Management of acute pancreatitis.**

- Cholecystectomy immediately after recovery from gallstone-associated pancreatitis (and always on same admission if possible), even if sphincterotomy has been performed (p. 115)
- Complete abstinence from alcohol
- Stop any implicated drugs

- Early elective ERCP for recurrent pancreatitis and sphincterotomy for ampullary dyskinesia or tumour
- Consider distal pancreatic diversion by an experienced surgeon for recurrent pancreatitis associated with ductal stenosis or pancreas divisum

Post-ERCP pancreatitis
- 3–40% of patients develop pancreatitis following ERCP
- Risk varies according to a number of factors (Table 1.6). Paradoxically, patients who need ERCP the least are the most likely to suffer a complication. Alternative approaches, such as magnetic resonance cholangiopancreatography (MRCP, p. 426), should be considered in such high-risk patients
- Somatostatin, an antisecretory agent, and gabexate, a protease inhibitor, are effective in preventing post-ERCP pancreatitis. However, these agents are not currently recommended, as they must be administered before ERCP and continued for a 12 h infusion afterward to be effective. Furthermore 13–27 patients must be treated to prevent a single case of pancreatitis
- Transsphincteric pancreatic stent placement reduces the risk of severe post-ERCP pancreatitis and is now being used in specialist centres for high-risk patients

Table 1.6 Risk factors for post-ERCP pancreatitis in prospective multivariate analyses

Definite[a]	Possible[b]	Unrelated[c]
Suspected SOD*	Female gender	Small CBD diameter[†]
Younger age	Acinar filling by contrast	SO manometry[‡]
Normal bilirubin	Absent CBD stone	Biliary sphincterotomy
Previous post-ERCP pancreatitis	Lower ERCP volume	
Difficult cannulation		
Pancreatic duct injection		
Pancreatic sphincterotomy		
Precut sphincterotomy (by endoscopists of mixed experience)		
Balloon dilation of biliary sphincter		

[a] Significant by multivariate analysis in most studies.
[b] Significant by univariate analysis in most studies.
[c] Not significant by multivariate analysis in any study.
* SOD, sphincter of Oddi dysfunction; [†] CBD, common bile duct; [‡] SO, sphincter of Oddi.

Acute intestinal ischaemia
The superior mesenteric artery supplies the jejunum and intestine to midtransverse colon (Fig. 9.5, p. 314). Acute intestinal ischaemia usually refers to mesenteric infarction and is uncommon. It is difficult to diagnose early, when surgery is most likely to be effective. The other patterns of intestinal ischaemia (mesenteric angina, focal ischaemia and ischaemic colitis) are covered in Section 9.6 (p. 319). Causes of intestinal ischaemia are shown in Table 9.6 (p. 320).

Distinguishing features
- Severe abdominal pain in an elderly patient with arterial disease
- Paucity of abdominal signs, compared with the severity of pain
- Atrial fibrillation, or vasculitis with abdominal pain

- An epigastric bruit suggests the diagnosis if present, but is frequently absent
- Rectal bleeding after the onset of pain is a late sign
- Peritonism is a late sign, when the patient is usually beyond recovery
- Marked leucocytosis $(20–30 \times 10^9/L)$ is common, but not invariable
- Haematocrit > 0.50 indicates dehydration

Management
- Mesenteric infarction without resection is invariably fatal. Early liaison with an experienced surgeon is essential because the situation is usually irretrievable by the time there is no clinical doubt about the diagnosis
- Suspect the diagnosis in a sick, elderly patient with severe abdominal pain and few signs
- Plain abdominal X-ray—often unremarkable. Paucity of gas, fluid levels or mucosal oedema (thickened small intestinal wall, or 'thumb printing' in the colon, p. 272; Fig. 9.5, p. 318) are usually late features
- Angiography does not help management in acute ischaemia, because non-obstructive infarction can occur and laparotomy is merely delayed
- Give analgesia—intravenous morphine 10 mg, then 2.5 mg aliquots every 3–4 h to control pain
- Vigorous intravenous rehydration—monitor haematocrit, central venous pressure and urine output
- Check arterial gases—metabolic acidosis responds to rehydration
- Antibiotics—intravenous cefuroxime 750 mg and metronidazole 500 mg three times daily, after blood cultures, if hypotensive
- Early exploratory laparotomy—especially for elderly patients, for diagnosis and to remove infarcted gut. A 'second look' to remove further non-viable tissue after 24 h is often advisable
- Start parenteral nutrition soon after laparotomy if there has been major (> 1 m) small bowel resection
- Mortality has been above 80% and morbidity after extensive resection is substantial (short bowel syndrome, p. 231), but a nihilistic approach (open and close laparotomy) is often unjustified. Extensive resection and early referral to an intestinal failure unit is appropriate

Abdominal pain in pregnancy (See also Section 13.1, p. 398.)
Pregnancy displaces abdominal organs, alters the pattern and signs of pathology and interferes with the mechanisms that localise abdominal sepsis. Miscarriage after surgery occurs in a quarter of patients, but this is related to the stage of disease rather than laparotomy. The risks of overlooking peritonitis are substantial and negative laparotomy is well tolerated by mother and fetus.
- Appendicitis is the most common indication for laparotomy
- Ovarian cyst torsion, haemorrhage and rupture are the next most common causes
- Biliary colic during the first or second trimester is best treated surgically to avoid the risk of acute cholecystitis
- Pancreatitis is more common and usually gallstone-related
- For all conditions, joint assessment by an experienced surgeon and obstetrician is appropriate, with ultrasound by an experienced radiologist rather than an obstetric ultrasonographer

Abdominal pain in the elderly (See also Section 13.2, p. 400.)

Elderly patients often present late and tolerate delayed diagnosis or management poorly. The intensity of pain, fever, tachycardia and leucocytosis from intra-abdominal sepsis may be minimal.

- Biliary tract disease including cholangitis accounts for 25%. Early ultrasound and, if necessary, ERCP are indicated. A low threshold for diagnosing ascending cholangitis in the elderly is mandatory: it may present solely with confusion, a high ESR and minimally elevated alkaline phosphatase (ALP)
- Intestinal obstruction and incarcerated hernias are the next most common conditions
- Appendicitis is the cause of an acute abdomen in about 10%
- Intestinal ischaemia should be considered if the severity of the pain is disproportionate to the signs

Abdominal pain in the immunocompromised

Abdominal pain in patients receiving chemotherapy for malignancy, after organ transplant or during renal replacement therapy, or in those receiving immunosuppression for other diseases, is more common than abdominal pain related to AIDS in most regions. The elderly and diabetics are relatively immunocompromised.

- Signs of perforation or abdominal sepsis may be minimal
- Neutropenic patients are prone to overwhelming sepsis. Laparotomy should not be delayed if appendicitis, diverticulitis or cholecystitis is suspected
- Neutropenic enterocolitis ('typhlitis') causes fever, diarrhoea and abdominal tenderness. The pathogenesis is unknown, but *Clostridium difficile* accounts for some and poor nutrition may contribute. Intravenous fluids, antibiotics and early surgery if perforation is suspected are appropriate

Metabolic causes

Metabolic derangements can masquerade as acute abdominal emergencies.

- Diabetic ketoacidosis—severe pain occurs in 10%, but acute pancreatitis must be excluded
- Hypercalcaemia—constipation and vomiting can occur without acute pancreatitis (Ca > 3.5 mmol/L)
- Acute adrenal insufficiency—with hyponatraemia, hyperkalaemia, elevated urea and hypotension
- Acute intermittent porphyria—neurological signs and abdominal pain, but no rash. Urine turns red on standing; porphobilinogen is detected by adding 2 mL Ehrlich's aldehyde to 2 mL urine. The pink colour is insoluble in chloroform
- Lead poisoning—ask about constipation, water supply and look at the gums for a fine blue line. Basophilic stippling and red cell lead are diagnostic
- Tabetic crisis—'lightning' pain; look for Argyll Robertson pupils and at posterior column function. It is extremely rare

Extraintestinal causes

Referred pain is more common in children and young adults.

- Lobar pneumonia—especially basal. Pneumothorax or pulmonary embolism may also cause abdominal pain

- Testicular torsion—do not forget to look, especially in teenagers
- Inferior myocardial infarction. Cardiac failure may cause severe epigastric pain due to hepatic venous congestion
- Herpes zoster—before the rash appears
- Spinal arthritis
- Root compression—classically with a thoracic meningioma; pain radiates from back to front

Munchausen's syndrome

Psychiatrically disturbed patients, who manipulate recurrent admission to hospital by simulating an acute medical condition, often describe acute abdominal pain in a convincing manner. Features that should raise suspicion are:

- 'Textbook' story of an acute abdominal condition (renal colic, peptic ulcer, biliary colic), with normal investigations
- History of surgery, or admission to hospitals in other parts of the country or abroad. Recent admissions are frequently concealed (look for signs of venesection)
- Psychiatric history, or inappropriate affect
- Neuropsychiatric disorders and acute abdominal pain can occur in acute porphyria, lead poisoning or syphilis (tabetic crisis, see above)
- Previous hospital admissions should be pursued. The patient is often well known to hospitals in one area. Once the diagnosis is documented, a description should be circulated to local hospitals, but self-discharge is usual before a photograph can be taken

Undiagnosed abdominal pain

No specific diagnosis is made in one-third of patients with acute abdominal pain. Take a careful history to identify any pattern of recurrent or acute-on-chronic abdominal pain. Complete resolution between episodes of recurrent pain makes organic disease more likely. If the pain is localised to a specific site, consider non-visceral pain in the abdominal wall. Pain from a rectus sheath haematoma or Spigelian hernia (lateral to the rectus sheath) may be very severe, but neuromuscular abdominal wall pain is more common. Otherwise the term 'non-specific abdominal pain' is best used, or 'irritable bowel' if the pain is acute-on-chronic and associated with bowel symptoms (p. 367).

Distinguishing features

- Type, site and relief of pain fail to fit a common pattern
- Abdominal bloating is common
- Vomiting occurs in 50%, often preceding pain
- Constipation should not be overlooked and can be diagnosed on plain abdominal X-ray
- Non-visceral abdominal pain is exacerbated by a finger placed on the site of pain whilst tensing the muscles of the abdominal wall, but makes little difference to pain from an irritable bowel (Carnet's sign)

Management

- Observation with oral fluids and analgesics for 24 h will usually discriminate the non-specific from the pathological cases
- Confirm that the temperature, blood count, C-reactive protein and urine examination are all normal

- Any abnormalities should be pursued, by ultrasound, small bowel radiology or a gastroenterological opinion as appropriate
- A confident diagnosis of IBS helps management (p. 340)
- Non-visceral abdominal pain can often be relieved by injection of local anaesthetic after consultation with anaesthetists or the pain team

1.7 Intestinal obstruction

Mechanical intestinal obstruction or failure of peristalsis (ileus) is life-threatening. Figure 1.5 outlines the approach to management.

Clinical features

The cardinal features are:
- Pain
- Distension
- Vomiting
- Constipation

The pain is colicky, but once strangulation occurs the pain becomes continuous and rebound tenderness is present. Vomiting can be the only feature of high jejunal obstruction.

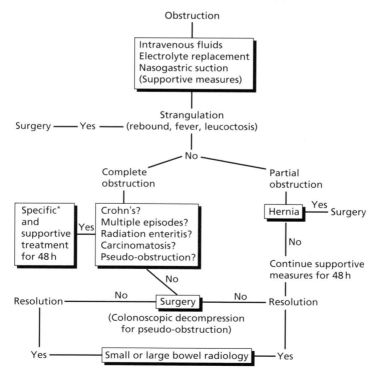

Fig. 1.5 Management of patients with intestinal obstruction.
*Specific treatment: e.g. intravenous steroids, antibiotics or neostigmine.

Subacute obstruction means incomplete occlusion of the lumen and an explosive episode of diarrhoea can follow the pain.

A succussion splash is often audible if the abdomen is shaken. Visible peristalsis may be seen. Hernial orifices must be examined carefully and previous abdominal surgery noted. Bowel sounds are increased in mechanical obstruction, but decreased in ileus.

Causes

Mechanical
- External herniae
- Adhesions
- Malignant colonic strictures

These three causes account for 75%

Less common mechanical causes
- Luminal:
  - ingested foreign bodies
  - fibrous food bolus
  - gallstone ileus
  - intussusception
- Mural:
  - sigmoid diverticular disease
  - Crohn's disease
  - NSAID-induced small intestinal strictures
  - radiation enteritis
  - ileocaecal tuberculosis
  - malignant small bowel strictures (carcinoid, lymphoma, carcinoma)
- Extrinsic:
  - volvulus (sigmoid, caecal, gastric)
  - internal herniation (through mesenteric foramina)

Ileus
- Following laparotomy
- Retroperitoneal lesions:
  - pancreatitis
  - haemorrhage
  - ureteric obstruction
- Drugs—anticholinergics and opiates, among others
- Metabolic:
  - diabetic ketoacidosis
  - acute renal failure
  - hypokalaemia
- Intestinal infarction
- Pseudo-obstruction

Investigations
- Plain abdominal X-ray—the upper limit of normal diameter of the small intestine is 2.5 cm and of the colon is 6.0 cm. Supine films alone are sufficient for diagnosis.

Look for mucosal oedema, the site that luminal gas disappears, displacement of bowel loops by a mass, and air in the bowel wall or biliary tree. An occasional fluid level on an erect film is normal. On an erect chest X-ray, look for air under the diaphragm. It remains the investigation of choice
- CT scan—often helpful in determining the site and likely cause of partial bowel obstruction
- Blood tests—look for hypokalaemia or high urea. Leucocytosis suggests strangulation. Crossmatch 2 units prior to surgery
- Arterial gases—metabolic alkalosis occurs with severe vomiting

Management (Fig. 1.5, p. 36)
- Nasogastric suction
- Replace fluid and electrolytes—5 L 0.9% saline and 200 mmol KCl may be needed in the first 24 h. Sequestered fluid in obstructed bowel is not measured, so adjust infusion rate according to the urine output and central venous pressure in very sick patients
- Assess concomitant medical problems—drugs may not have been absorbed
- Relieve the obstruction—the site governs the type of operation. Suspicion of strangulation demands urgent surgery. Non-operative manoeuvres are initially indicated for ileus, pseudo-obstruction, volvulus, or intussusception
- Monitor:
  - urine output
  - nasogastric aspirate
  - central venous pressure in the shocked or elderly
  - daily electrolytes

Ileus
- Nasogastric suction, maintaining serum potassium at 4.0–4.5 mmol/L, intravenous fluids and patience are usually sufficient
- Check that anticholinergic drugs are not prescribed and decrease opiate analgesia to a minimum
- Try metoclopramide 10 mg intravenously three times daily, or erythromycin 500 mg four times daily (as a motilin agonist), as prokinetic agents
- Consider parenteral nutrition if resolution is delayed for longer than 72 h
- Exclude mechanical obstruction by contrast radiology, if ileus persists after a few days

Volvulus
- Sigmoid volvulus—common in developing countries, elderly males and the mentally handicapped. Plain X-ray shows massive sigmoid distension. Colonoscopy is more effective than a deflating rectal tube and should be attempted before surgery
- Caecal volvulus—obstruction is often incomplete initially but recurs without surgery, so laparotomy is advisable
- Gastric volvulus—associated with diaphragmatic eventration, visible on plain chest and abdominal X-rays. Distinguish from 'acute gastric dilatation', which is a misnomer for gastric ileus, caused by poor attention to nasogastric suction and electrolyte balance. Surgery is needed for gastric volvulus, with repair of the diaphragm

Intussusception

- Usually idiopathic in infants; due to a Meckel's diverticulum in adolescence; or a polyp or carcinoma in adults
- Intermittent pain, rectal bleeding, small intestinal fluid levels and an absent caecal gas shadow suggest the diagnosis. Facial pallor during pain occurs in infants
- Ultrasound in experienced hands is diagnostic and the recommended initial investigation, although barium enema may be both diagnostic and therapeutic in the early stages

Pseudo-obstruction

- Clinical features of intestinal obstruction without a mechanical cause. The motility disorder commonly affects the whole gastrointestinal tract, although it is colonic distension that is often most prominent
- Consider the diagnosis in the elderly and mentally handicapped, or when obstruction is associated with other disorders (myocardial infarction, pneumonia, Parkinson's disease)
- An urgent single contrast barium enema is often necessary to distinguish pseudo-obstruction from mechanical obstruction, and occasionally has a therapeutic effect
- Stop causative drugs (opiates, phenothiazines, tricyclics, clonidine) and treat associated disease
- Do not allow the patient to remain supine, but ensure mobility or turning regularly, including into the prone or head-down position as this may help deflation
- Intravenous neostigmine 2 mg, repeated if necessary, may have a dramatic effect in relieving pseudo-obstruction. There is usually a relative contraindication (other drugs, cardiovascular, or respiratory disease), but liase with an experienced anaesthetist and monitor for bradycardia
- Erythromycin 2 g daily as a prokinetic (motilin-like activity), stimulant laxatives (e.g. senna) rarely help, and lactulose may increase intraluminal gas. Enemas should be used with care as perforation can occur
- Repeat plain abdominal X-ray after 24 h to monitor caecal diameter
- 90% resolve spontaneously, but colonoscopic decompression is warranted if pain is severe, or the caecum > 10 cm. Surgery should be avoided if at all possible, but caecostomy is appropriate if two attempts at colonoscopic decompression fail and symptoms persist
- Chronic intestinal pseudo-obstruction is a feature of systemic sclerosis, neuromuscular diseases and amyloidosis amongst others. Severe dysmotility syndrome causes severe abdominal pain and episodes of functional intestinal obstruction. It is usually associated with previous surgery for functional disease (e.g. slow transit constipation), opioid dependence and may cause intestinal failure requiring home parenteral nutrition. Referral to a specialist centre is appropriate

1.8 Toxic dilatation of the colon

Dilatation of the colon with signs of systemic upset ('toxic') is becoming less common as acute attacks of ulcerative colitis are recognised and appropriately treated (p. 308). The danger if surgery is inappropriately delayed is colonic perforation, which still carries a high mortality.

Clinical features

- Colitis—usually caused by severe ulcerative colitis, but can occur in Crohn's colitis, and rarely in ischaemic, or infective, colitis (*Yersinia enterocolitica*, *Campylobacter* spp., *Cl. difficile*, p. 283)
- Fever > 37.8°C
- Neutrophils > $10 \times 10^9/L$
- Tachycardia > 90 b.p.m.
- Radiological colonic dilatation (widest diameter ≥ 6.0 cm in transverse colon; Fig. 1.6)
- Clinical appearance can be deceptive due to steroids

Management

Patients presenting with dilatation should start intensive medical treatment (see below) and the response should be carefully assessed after 24 h. About half respond, but a decision to continue for a further 24 h or proceed to emergency colectomy must be made by a senior gastroenterologist in consultation with a colorectal surgeon. Patients who recover continue treatment as for severe colitis (p. 275). When dilatation develops during intensive medical treatment for colitis, colectomy is indicated without further delay.

Diagnosis

- Always take a plain abdominal X-ray on admission in patients with severe colitis (p. 275). Mucosal islands (polypoid mucosal swellings projecting into the colonic lumen; Fig. 1.6), in addition to dilatation indicate very severe ulceration and predict the need for colectomy. The presence of three or more distended loops of small bowel is also associated with the need for colectomy. The X-ray should be repeated daily until clinical improvement or surgery occurs
- Stool culture and faecal *Cl. difficile* toxin assay
- Blood cultures
- Flexible sigmoidoscopy and rectal mucosal biopsy to confirm colitis, but colonoscopy or barium enema are dangerous and should be avoided

Supportive therapy

- Vigorously correct fluid and electrolyte imbalance with intravenous fluids and KCl supplements (serum K 4.0–4.5 mmol/L)
- Nil by mouth
- Involve the surgeons as soon as the diagnosis is made
- 4-hourly observation of pulse, temperature and BP, as well as fluid balance and meticulous stool chart, since nursing observations are essential prognostic factors when deciding the timing of colectomy (p. 275)
- Examine the patient at least twice daily (check pulse, abdominal tenderness, temperature and stool chart)
- Monitor daily full blood count, C-reactive protein, electrolytes and maximum colonic diameter on plain abdominal X-ray

Specific therapy

- Stop antidiarrhoeal agents, opiates and anticholinergic drugs

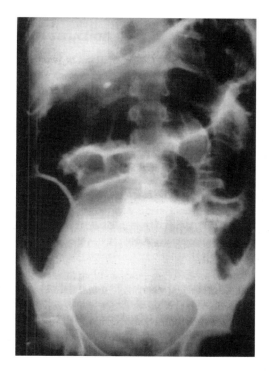

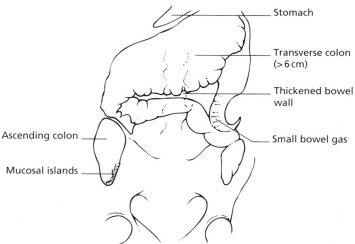

Fig. 1.6 Toxic dilatation of the colon in ulcerative colitis. Plain abdominal radiograph in toxic megacolon showing a grossly dilated transverse colon with mucosal islands in the ascending colon.

- Intravenous hydrocortisone 100 mg four times daily or methylprednisolone 20 mg three times daily, for ulcerative colitis or Crohn's disease
- Rectal hydrocortisone 100 mg in 100 mL twice daily (p. 274)
- There is no evidence that antibiotics alter outcome

Indications for emergency colectomy

The decision is usually difficult, but prolonged medical treatment increases mortality, even in young patients. If objective signs (pulse, temperature) are improving after 24 h, a further 24 h trial of medical treatment may be justified. This decision should be taken by a senior physician, jointly with the surgeons. Indications for colectomy in the presence of a dilated colon are:

- Failure to improve clinically (no change in stool frequency, tachycardia or temperature) or radiologically within 24 h
- Signs of perforation (may be minimal, due to steroids)
- Mucosal islands as well as dilatation (because such severe ulceration is very unlikely to respond to steroids)
- Severe ulcerative colitis *without* colonic dilatation is slightly different, but early decision-making on surgery is still essential. If, after 3 days' intravenous treatment, the stool frequency is > 8/day, or the frequency is 3–8/day together with a C-reactive protein > 45 mg/L, then there is 85% chance that colectomy will be needed on that admission (p. 275)

1.9 Acute hepatic failure

Acute hepatic failure occurs in a previously normal liver and is either acute or late onset (subacute). The time of onset and mortality distinguish the two types, although other features and management are similar.

The main differential diagnosis is between acute and acute-on-chronic liver failure (Table 1.8, p. 43). The potential for complete recovery distinguishes acute failure, although it has a worse prognosis.

Clinical features

Hyperacute hepatic failure
- Encephalopathy within 7 days of the onset of jaundice (after paracetamol/acetaminophen)
- Encephalopathy includes all stages from personality change to coma. The grade may change rapidly (Table 1.7)
- Paradoxically, this group has the highest likelihood of recovery with medical management

Acute liver failure
- Encephalopathy develops 8–28 days after the onset of jaundice (viral or drug-induced)
- This group has a high mortality and marked prolongation of prothrombin time

Subacute liver failure
- Encephalopathy after an interval of 4–12 weeks after the onset of jaundice (any cause)
- Less marked prolongation of prothrombin time, but mortality remains high

Table 1.7 Grade of hepatic encephalopathy

Grade	Features
1	Altered mood or behaviour
2	Drowsy
3	Stupor
4	Coma
5	Coma with no response to painful stimuli

Associated features
- Fetor hepaticus—characteristic smell of 'pear-drops' (acetone) in breath
- Jaundice—may be minimal in the early stages
- Liver size—usually small, due to hepatic necrosis. If enlarged, acute-on-chronic liver failure (Table 1.8) or Budd–Chiari syndrome is more likely
- Spleen—usually not palpable
- No single feature entirely discriminates between acute and acute-on-chronic hepatic failure. The history is the best guide

Causes
- Acetaminophen/paracetamol overdose and cryptogenic are the commonest
- Acetaminophen/paracetamol—presentation a few days after apparent recovery from poisoning is typical
- Cryptogenic (or non-A–non-B–non-C viral hepatitis, NANBNC)—the commonest cause after acetaminophen/paracetamol
- Viral—hepatitis B or D (δ agent). Rare after hepatitis A, C or E (community-acquired non-A, non-B), yellow fever or leptospirosis
- Drugs—acetaminophen/paracetamol (especially associated with alcohol), halothane, isoniazid
- Alcohol—occasionally without underlying liver disease, but usually acute-on-chronic
- Wilson's disease—haemolysis is a feature
- Budd–Chiari syndrome—ascites and abdominal pain are often prominent
- Fatty liver of pregnancy—third trimester (p. 398)
- HELLP syndrome (haemolysis, elevated liver enzymes and low platelet count)—a severe complication of pre-eclampsia in pregnancy (p. 398)

Table 1.8 Clinical features of acute versus acute-on-chronic hepatic failure

	Acute	Acute on chronic
History	Short	Long
Nutrition	Good	Poor
Liver	Small/Normal	Usually enlarged
Spleen	Impalpable	Enlarged
Spiders	Absent	Many
Encephalopathy	Early	Late
Jaundice	Late	Early
Ascites	Late	Early

Investigations

Blood tests
- Coagulation studies, glucose and potassium immediately and creatinine as soon as possible
- Full blood count, group and save, bilirubin, albumin, AST, amylase
- Hepatitis serology (including hepatitis B core IgM), acetaminophen/paracetamol levels, serum copper and caeruloplasmin (24 h urinary copper if Wilson's suspected Acetaminophen/paracetamol is often undetectable by the time acute liver failure presents

Other
- Chest X-ray
- Ultrasound of liver and pancreas. Hepatic vein Doppler studies if Budd–Chiari syndrome is suspected
- Blood cultures—even if afebrile
- EEG—may be diagnostic when there is doubt, but is seldom necessary

Management

General
- Intensive care nursing
- Insert a central venous line early to ensure good hydration. Aggressive early rehydration appears to improve outcome. Patients drink little because of nausea or encephalopathy. Hypovolaemia impairs hepatic and renal perfusion
- Monitor urine output, blood glucose and vital signs, every hour
- Check serum potassium and coagulation studies twice daily for the first 48 h, then daily with full blood count, creatinine and albumin
- Avoid giving FFP as prothrombin time/INR are the best guide to liver function, severity and outcome
- Reassess the grade of encephalopathy (Table 1.7), ascites and fluid balance once or twice daily

Specific therapy
- Commence N-acetyl cysteine infusion for significant acetaminophen/paracetamol poisoning and continue infusion until coagulation returns to normal
- Inotropic support if hypotensive

Encephalopathy
- Avoid sedation if possible, but chlordiazepoxide is appropriate for alcohol withdrawal (Fig. 5.8, p. 177)
- Protect the airway as encephalopathy progresses beyond grade 2 (Table 1.7, p. 43)
- Intracranial pressure monitoring is appropriate in grade 4 encephalopathy (usually when the patient has been transferred to a liver unit). Mannitol 0.3–1.0 g/kg is given when intracranial pressure is increased provided not anuric. Oxygen and inotropic support are also necessary. Phenytoin decreases subclinical seizure activity and cerebral oedema

Hypoglycaemia and hypokalaemia

- 10% dextrose 100 mL/h with KCl 40 mmol/L, but 20–50% dextrose may be needed if hypoglycaemia is severe
- Empirical antibiotics (see below)

Bleeding

- Avoid arterial punctures
- FFP if clinically significant bleeding occurs
- Acid suppression (omeprazole 20 mg orally, or sucralfate 2 g three times daily) is often given to reduce stress-induced gastric erosions, but the evidence of benefit is debated

Renal failure

- Over 50% develop renal impairment. Good hydration is the key to preventing renal failure, but hepatotoxic drugs may be directly nephrotoxic. Hepatorenal syndrome (Section 5.3, p. 149) may be defined as doubling of serum creatinine to > 200 µmol/L in < 2 weeks, together with a low urinary sodium (< 5 mmol/L), in the absence of hypovolaemia. Although two types (early and late) are described, the differences are largely semantic
- Serum urea is falsely low in severe liver disease, so creatinine should be measured, but a bilirubin > 200 µmol/L interferes with creatinine assay
- Hepatorenal syndrome has a dreadful prognosis, although terlipressin, where available, has an increasing therapeutic role. The optimum dose, duration and amount of additional albumin are still being assessed. Terlipressin 0.5 mg twice daily (less than for variceal bleeding), with 20% albumin 1 g/kg (i.e. 60 kg man = 300 mL 20% albumin) is appropriate. Increase terlipressin to 1 mg four times daily if no fall in creatinine after 48 h
- Haemofiltration or dialysis is rarely indicated because the prognosis of established renal and liver failure is so poor. Discussion between consultant hepatologist and renal physician is appropriate

Infection

- Meticulous care of intravenous and urinary catheters
- Blood, urine and catheter cultures are essential and must be performed before starting antibiotics
- Antibiotics are recommended, because patients are critically ill and signs of sepsis are commonly absent. Intravenous cefuroxime 750 mg three times daily is appropriate, until culture results are available

Indications for transplant

Deciding when the chance of spontaneous recovery is less than the risks of a liver transplant is difficult. Discuss the situation with the nearest transplant centre at an early stage.

Transfer is generally recommended in the following circumstances

(Tables 1.9 and 1.10)

- The prothrombin time (measured in seconds) at the time of referral is greater than the interval (hours) between poisoning and referral
- Prothrombin time exceeds 50 s

Table 1.9 Guidelines for referral to a liver unit following acetaminophen/paracetamol overdose

Day 2	Day 3	Day 4
Arterial pH < 7.30	Arterial pH < 7.30	INR > 6.0 or PT > 75 s
INR > 3.0 or PT > 50 s	INR > 4.5 or PT > 60 s	Progressive rise in PT
Oliguria	Oliguria	Oliguria
Creatinine > 200 µmol/L	Creatinine > 200 µmol/L	Creatinine > 300 µmol/L
Hypoglycaemia	Encephalopathy	Encephalopathy

PT, prothrombin time.

Table 1.10 Guidelines for referral to a liver unit for non-acetaminophen/paracetamol-induced liver failure

Hyperacute	Acute	Subacute
Encephalopathy	Encephalopathy	Encephalopathy
PT > 30 s	PT > 30 s	PT > 20 s
Renal failure	Renal failure	Renal failure
		Serum sodium < 130 mmol/L
		Shrinking liver volume

PT, prothrombin time.

- Metabolic acidosis at presentation
- All patients with established encephalopathy. Table 1.11 shows the criteria used for transplantation in fulminant hepatic failure at King's College Hospital, London, but it is too late to transfer a patient at this stage. Alcohol abuse is a relative, but not absolute, contraindication to transplantation
- In one study 17/92 patients admitted to a liver unit with paracetamol poisoning were listed for transplantation. 70% of those transplanted survived compared to 14% who were listed but not transplanted. The overall mortality was 32%

Take into account
- Age (< 60 years)
- Previous liver function (should have been normal)
- Ability to cope with post-transplant regimen (Box 5.2, p. 183)

Before and during transfer
- Insert a central venous line if the prothrombin time exceeds 30 s (INR 2.0) or if there is renal dysfunction. Good hydration and circulation improve outcome
- Give 10% glucose 100 mL/h with 40 mmol/L KCl to prevent hypoglycaemia or hypokalaemia
- Give 20% mannitol 20 mL/h if encephalopathic before transfer
- Intubate and ventilate patients with advanced encephalopathy before transfer, because cerebral oedema is exacerbated by movement

Prognosis

Factors
- Grade of encephalopathy—15% survival without transplant, when grade 3–4

Table 1.11 Criteria for liver transplant in fulminant failure

Acetaminophen/ paracetamol cases	Non-acetaminophen/ paracetamol cases

Arterial pH < 7.30
or all of the following
   PT > 100 s
   Creatinine > 300 µmol/L
   Grade 3–4 encephalopathy
	INR > 6.7 or PT > 100 s
	or any three of the following
	   Aetiology non-A, non-B or drug reaction
	   Age < 10 or > 40 years
	   Jaundice > 7 days before encephalopathy
	   INR > 4.0 or PT > 50 s
	   Bilirubin > 300 µmol/L

PT, prothrombin time.

- Age:
  - > 40 years 15% survival
  - < 30 years 40% survival
- Albumin:
  - > 35 g/L 80% survival
  - < 30 g/L 20% survival
- Cause—drug reactions and non-A–non-B (hepatitis C) induced failure have a worse prognosis than other causes
- Onset—late onset has a worse prognosis than fulminant failure

Transplant in acute liver failure
- 65% survive, but this is improving
- Auxiliary liver transplantation until the original liver recovers has proved disappointing
- The role of Molecular Adsorbant Recirculating System (MARS) in hepatorenal syndrome and as a bridge to transplantation is being evaluated

2 Oesophagus

2.1 Dysphagia

Causes

Acute or progressive dysphagia demands urgent investigation. Oropharyngeal and oesophageal causes are recognised (Table 2.1). Bolus obstruction is covered in Section 1.2, p. 4.

Clinical features

A careful history usually distinguishes between oropharyngeal and oesophageal causes (Fig. 2.1). Four questions about the dysphagia are essential: interval, type of food, pattern and associated features.

Interval

• Difficulty in initiating swallowing, repeated attempts at swallowing or dysphagia within a second of starting to swallow characterise oropharyngeal dysphagia

Table 2.1 Causes of dysphagia

	Oropharyngeal	Oesophageal
Common	Aphthous ulcers	Oesophagitis
	Candidiasis	Oesophageal dysmotility
	Stroke	Peptic stricture
		Carcinoma
		oesophagus
		cardia
Unusual	Parkinson's disease	Motor disorders
	Globus hystericus	achalasia
	Pseudobulbar palsy	diffuse spasm
	Motor neurone disease	systemic sclerosis
	Pharyngeal pouch	polymyositis
	Xerostomia	Oesophageal infection
		External pressure
		bronchial carcinoma
		mediastinal nodes
		aortic aneurysm
		Postcricoid web
		Schatzki's ring
		Radiation stricture
Rare	Oral tumours	Corrosive/pill stricture
	Syringobulbia	Aberrant vessels
	Bulbar poliomyelitis	Left atrial enlargement
	Muscular dystrophy	Retrosternal goitre
	Botulism	Chagas' disease

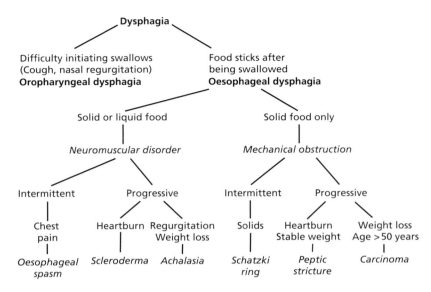

Fig. 2.1 Diagnosis of dysphagia.

- Dysphagia a few seconds after starting to swallow indicates an oesophageal cause
- Where the patient points to is no help in locating the site of the lesion

Type of food
- Ask if dysphagia is for liquids (usually pharyngeal), solids (mechanical oesophageal cause likely) or both (oesophageal dysmotility more likely)
- Exacerbation by hot or cold liquids is common in oesophagitis

Pattern
- Progressive dysphagia indicates an organic cause, such as carcinoma, benign stricture or achalasia
- Intermittent symptoms are common in oesophageal dysmotility, diverticula, web or ring
- Short (< 3 months), progressive history indicates malignancy
- A 'lump in the throat' as the only symptom is unlikely to have a mechanical cause

Associated features
- Weight loss confirms that an organic cause is probable, but lack of weight loss is of no diagnostic value
- A history of heartburn suggests a peptic stricture, although when a patient presents with dysphagia, heartburn may no longer be present
- Cough indicates spillover into the bronchial tree, commonly due to oropharyngeal dysphagia, or achalasia when at night. Very rarely it is due to an oesophagobronchial fistula
- Odynophagia (pain during swallowing) often accompanies dysphagia in oesophagitis, achalasia, or diffuse oesophageal spasm

- Examine the mouth and teeth or dentures, and feel for supraclavicular nodes (from carcinoma of the cardia)
- Look for signs of systemic disease (anaemia, systemic sclerosis, or neurological disorders)

Urgent investigations

- Indicated when dysphagia is for solids alone, when symptoms are progressive or when there is associated weight loss
- Consult the radiologist or gastroenterologist to arrange urgent investigation
- Chest X-ray—look for a hilar tumour, mediastinal fluid level, absent gastric bubble or right lower lobe consolidation (aspiration)
- Barium swallow—within 48 h. A smooth, tapering stricture is often benign. Irregularity or asymmetry suggests malignancy (Fig. 2.3, p. 60 and Fig. 2.4, p. 63)
- Endoscopy—*after* a barium swallow. Allow 12 h for barium to clear: it can block the endoscope
- Blood tests—anaemia may be due to malignancy, poor nutrition, bleeding, or Plummer–Vinson syndrome (p. 61). A high urea usually reflects dehydration

Elective investigations

- Barium swallow, chest X-ray and endoscopy can be performed electively in patients with intermittent dysphagia without weight loss, or when symptoms suggest oesophageal motility disorders
- Cine or bread/marshmallow barium swallow, or oesophageal manometry is usually appropriate if the barium swallow is normal (p. 74)
- ENT assessment is indicated for most pharyngeal causes of dysphagia
- Pulmonary function tests (spirometry and oxygen-diffusing capacity) establish a baseline in patients with systemic sclerosis

2.2 Gastro-oesophageal reflux disease

Gastro–oesophageal reflux symptoms occur monthly in almost 50% and weekly in 20% of US males, but may be asymptomatic. Abnormal reflux is predominantly caused by dysfunction of the lower oesphageal sphincter (frequent transient relaxations) and not necessarily by a hiatus hernia. Delayed clearance of refluxate prolongs mucosal exposure to a low pH (< 4), which damages the oesophageal mucosal barrier and initiates oesophagitis. In addition to acid, bile acids and pepsin also disrupt mucosal integrity or provoke oesophageal dysmotility. Peptic stricture of the oesophagus is an unusual complication, in view of the high prevalence of gastro-oesophageal reflux. Prolonged, symptomatic gastro-oesophageal reflux increases the risk of oesophageal adenocarcinoma by about eightfold. It is not yet clear whether potent acid suppression reduces this risk.

Clinical features

- Heartburn—retrosternal pain related to meals, lying down, stooping, straining and occasionally to exercise

- Regurgitation of acid or bile. Patients often have difficulty in describing the taste, usually bitter or sour
- Dysphagia may be due to peristaltic dysfunction. Pain during swallowing (odynophagia) is unusual unless there is severe oesophagitis or a stricture (when dysphagia for solids is also present)
- Excess salivation (water brash), usually during pain
- Relief by antacids
- Chest pain, related to posture or exercise (both of which increase intra-abdominal pressure), can be difficult to distinguish from angina (p. 74)
- Nocturnal asthma (cough or wheeze) may be the only symptom, and can be relieved by treatment of reflux
- Oesophagitis can be asymptomatic. There is no clear relation between symptom severity and endoscopic severity of oesophagitis, although the severity of symptoms correlates with increasing risk of adenocarcinoma

Hiatus hernia

The common sliding hiatus hernia is compatible with normal lower oesophageal sphincter function. It is not necessarily pathological and no symptoms can be attributed to the hernia itself. Symptoms are due to oesophagitis or oesophageal dysmotility provoked by reflux.

- More than 30% of patients over 50 years have a hiatus hernia and less than half have symptomatic gastro-oesophageal reflux
- A report of a sliding hiatus hernia on barium radiology is not a diagnosis. If a patient's symptoms warrant investigation, endoscopy to identify oesophagitis is appropriate, with further investigation if this is normal
- Never accept a hiatus hernia as a cause of iron-deficiency anaemia—there is usually another cause, such as a silent caecal carcinoma
- Rolling (paraoesophageal) or incarcerated hiatal herniae are diagnosed radiologically. A chest X-ray may show a fluid level behind the heart. Episodic pain and vomiting are indications for a barium meal, as partial or complete gastric volvulus may occur, for which surgery is needed

Investigations

- Typical symptoms of gastro-oesophageal reflux do not require investigation unless they are frequent, severe or progressive
- Endoscopy should be considered if symptoms are atypical (partial relief by PPI, associated epigastric pain or associated symptoms) to evaluate the severity of oesophagitis or to identify Barrett's oesophagus
- It is common to get symptomatic reflux with no signs of oesophagitis at endoscopy
- Macroscopic oesophagitis indicates reflux, but the severity does not correlate with symptoms.
- If Barrett's oesophagus (see below) is found, multiple biopsies should be taken
- Iron-deficiency anaemia should not be attributed to oesophagitis but can rarely occur in patients with severe ulcerative oesophagitis
- *H. pylori* is unrelated to (or negatively associated with) reflux oesophagitis

- A therapeutic trial of a PPI is a reliable method of confirming the diagnosis. Debate continues about whether an endoscopy is necessary if symptoms are relieved
- 24 h oesophageal pH monitoring is indicated when it is difficult to distinguish symptomatic reflux from other causes of chest pain (p. 74), but is not part of routine management

General measures

General measures to reduce reflux are more important than drugs in most patients.
- Reduce fat intake (fat promotes reflux by delaying gastric emptying)
- Weight reduction (height and weight charts: Appendix 3, p. 451; reducing diet: p. 386)
- Stop smoking
- Raise the head of the bed by about 10 cm, using blocks or bricks (especially if symptoms are nocturnal)
- Small, regular meals
- Allow 3 h between last meal and retiring at night
- Avoid hot drinks or alcohol before bed
- Avoid drugs that adversely affect oesophageal motility (nitrates, anticholinergic agents, antidepressants, theophylline compounds), or that damage the oesophageal mucosa (NSAIDs, slow-release potassium)
- Use antacids or alginates (e.g. Gaviscon, Maalox, Mylanta) for initial symptomatic relief. There is no evidence that one is better than another, but none will heal oesophagitis

Management

If general measures alone are insufficient, drug treatment is indicated. Controversy persists about the best approach, but PPIs are unequivocally the most effective treatment and are best given in the morning. At first presentation, liquid antacids or alginates are more cost-effective than H$_2$-receptor antagonists, since 50% respond equally well to either. After antacids or alginates, an incremental approach is recommended, using the minimum effective treatment to relieve symptoms. Only a minority of patients with reflux have severe oesophagitis (Fig. 2.2).
- There is probably little difference between the PPIs (esomeprazole, lansoprazole, omeprazole, pantoprazole, rabeprazole) in terms of efficacy or side-effect profile in most patients, although costs may vary. Many hospitals and practices have their own prescribing policy. For rare patients, incremental doses above 40 mg of omeprazole, esomeprazole, or rabeprazole may enhance acid suppression, in contrast to a dose ceiling with lansoprazole 30 mg or pantoprazole 40 mg
- Intermittent treatment of recurrent symptoms is often necessary. This is safe and effective in the long term (see national guidelines, such as www.nice.org.uk/CG017)
- Symptomatic erosive oesophagitis relapses within 6 months in 80% on no maintenance treatment, 40% on ranitidine 300 mg or omeprazole 10 mg daily and 15% on omeprazole 20 mg daily, but these represent a small proportion of all patients with reflux
- Maintenance treatment with lansoprazole 15–30 mg daily, omeprazole 20–40 mg or rabeprazole 10–20 mg daily is indicated for patients with refractory symptoms or confluent oesophagitis, Barrett's oesophagus or a peptic stricture

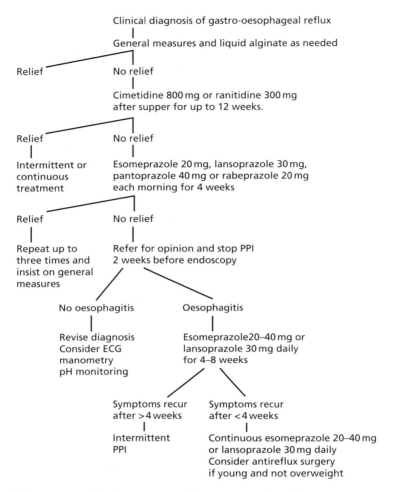

Fig. 2.2 **Management plan for symptomatic gastro-oesophageal reflux.**

- Concerns about long-term sequelae of PPIs appear unfounded, but postmarketing surveillance continues. Interference with vitamin B_{12} absorption, intestinal bacterial overgrowth, pronounced hypergastrinaemia with G-cell hyperplasia and accelerated atrophic gastritis in those with *H. pylori* are areas of interest in long-term treatment
- The current consensus is to eradicate *H. pylori* in patients who need PPIs long term
- Overweight, smoking boozers characteristically continue to have symptoms

Refractory symptoms

Symptoms that persist despite treatment with a PPI (such as omeprazole up to 40 mg, lansoprazole 30 mg, rabeprazole 20 mg daily) are usually due to coexistent oesophageal dysmotility, or a non-oesophageal cause.

- Retake the history. Abdominal bloating is common in oesophageal dysmotility. Exercise-related pain may be angina. Confirm compliance with therapy
- Consider endoscopy. Stop PPIs prior to endoscopy if oesophagitis has not previously been identified. Otherwise continue treatment, since up to 15% fail to respond
- If the endoscopy is normal, arrange oesophageal manometry or a bread/marshmallow barium swallow to exclude achalasia or oesophageal dysmotility. 24 h manometry may be needed to identify oesphageal spasm
- Arrange 24 h pH monitoring (p. 430) if radiology or manometry is normal, or investigate for non-oesophageal causes by abdominal ultrasound or exercise test as appropriate

Indications for antireflux surgery

Surgery is rarely indicated. Laparoscopic antireflux surgery currently has similar risks (lack of efficacy, postoperative stricture, vagal denervation, inability to belch, splenic or oesophageal damage) to open procedures. Mortality is 1%, but results can be good in well-selected patients in experienced hands.

Consider surgery by an experienced surgeon if all the following criteria are met:
- Severe symptoms persist despite all medical treatments vigorously applied. Symptoms of volume reflux (water brash or fluid regurgitation into the mouth) have traditionally favoured surgery, but the concept of volume reflux is now questioned
- pH monitoring confirms objective evidence of gross reflux
- Oesophageal manometry has excluded a specific dysmotility syndrome (e.g. achalasia, scleroderma, diffuse oesophageal spasm)
- Age < 65 years (surgery may still be considered in older, medically fit individuals)
- Some individuals (particularly younger patients) may opt for fundoplication because of concerns regarding the safety and/or cost of long-term PPI therapy even when symptoms are well controlled on PPIs. They should know that the mortality of laparoscopic or open fundoplication is about 1%, serious morbidity is around 10% and that no patient is known directly to have died from PPIs

Endoscopic antireflux procedures

- Endoscopic stapling or suturing devices to reduce reflux are being developed, but at present the same selection procedures as for antireflux procedures should apply
- Complications from mechanical antireflux procedures can be intractable and this hazard should be compared with the tolerability and safety of medication

Barrett's oesophagus

Fifty years after the description associating Barrett's oesophagus with oesophageal carcinoma, diagnostic criteria remain debated. Division into long segment (> 5 cm), short segment (< 5 cm) and ultrashort segment (biopsy evidence only) are of potential clinical importance, since the risk of carcinoma relates to the length of metaplasia. However, > 15% of the population have intestinal metaplasia proximal to the gastro-oesophageal junction, and the implications are unclear.

Features

- Endoscopic evidence, confirmed by biopsy, of columnar-lined oesophagus more than 3 cm proximal to the gastro-oesophageal junction (UK), or intestinal metaplasia proximal to the gastro-oesophageal junction (USA)
- Oesophageal carcinoma develops in 1–5% and dysplasia in 10% over 5 years if Barrett's is > 3 cm in extent, although controversy about the estimated risk persists
- The risk of carcinoma appears to be related to the length of Barrett's oesophagus

Management

- Multiple biopsies every 2 cm are needed to exclude dysplasia at diagnosis
- Prescribe full dose PPI (equivalent to omperazole 40 mg, lansoprazole 30 mg, rabeprazole 20 mg daily). Long-term treatment is indicated, because Barrett's oesophagus is assumed to be a consequence of severe gastro-oesophageal reflux
- Discuss the diagnosis in the context of the individual patient. The risk of cancer is usually small (since most patients are older, or have a short segment of Barrett's) and needless anxiety can be created by generalisations about premalignant conditions
- Annual surveillance endoscopy has not been shown to reduce mortality, but cancers detected by surveillance have a better survival than those presenting in the normal course of events. The issues should be discussed with individual patients and a joint decision made. There is no point in surveillance if oesophagectomy is not an option (due to age, comorbidity) if cancer is detected
- Low-grade dysplasia does not necessarily progress. It is reasonable to continue vigorous antisecretory therapy and repeat endoscopy every 6–12 months for as long as patients remain surgical candidates
- High-grade dysplasia also does not always progress to carcinoma, but if confirmed on repeat endoscopy (within 3 months) or multiple foci are detected in young patients, oesophagectomy should be considered
- Photodynamic therapy and ablation of Barrett's epithelium by endoscopic argon beamer remain experimental techniques

Oesophageal ulcers

Features

- Associated with severe oesophagitis or Barrett's oesophagus
- Endoscopy, biopsy and brush cytology are needed to exclude malignancy

Management

- Check that biopsies and brushings for cytology have been taken at endoscopy
- Prescribe full dose PPI (lansoprazole 30 mg or omeprazole 40 mg daily) for 8 weeks
- Repeat the endoscopy, biopsy and brushings after 8 weeks to confirm healing. Do not stop the PPI
- Long-term treatment with a PPI is appropriate for peptic oesophageal ulcers, because these indicate severe reflux with a high recurrence rate

- Refer for surgery if high-grade dysplasia is detected in ulcers that persist despite treatment

Alkaline reflux

Bile, pancreatic enzymes and bicarbonate due to duodenogastric reflux, as well as acid and pepsin, can cause oesophagitis. This occurs particularly after partial gastrectomy. Biliary reflux at endoscopy is normal if the patient is retching.

- Oesophagitis with a pH > 4 at all times during ambulatory monitoring is necessary for diagnosis
- General measures and antacids should be tried. Sucralfate binds bile and may help, but needs to be given four times daily to heal oesophagitis. Dilute hydrochloric acid BP (0.1 mL in 10 mL water) would be logical and is said to be better than placebo for heartburn in pregnancy, but is not in general use
- Surgical (Roux-en-Y) revision is reserved for severe, intolerable symptoms

2.3 Benign strictures

Causes

- Peptic—95%
- Anastomotic—following a surgical procedure
- Radiotherapy—for carcinoma of the breast or bronchus. Stenosis after radiotherapy for oesophageal carcinoma is almost always malignant
- Corrosives—bleach (p. 7) or drugs such as slow-release potassium tablets. Patients taking NSAIDs have a higher incidence of strictures. Pills (tetracycline tablets, slow-release potassium) may cause strictures. Advise elderly patients with poor oesophageal motility to take such drugs when standing, with plenty of fluid
- Mucocutaneous disorders—epidermolysis bullosa and oesophageal lichen planus are very rare

Clinical features

Dysphagia is the main symptom (p. 51; Fig. 2.1, p. 52) and reflux is usually present. The main differential diagnosis is carcinoma. Dysphagia for < 3 months or rapid weight loss favour carcinoma.

Investigations and management

Initial investigations
- As for dysphagia (p. 53 and Fig. 2.3, p. 60)
- Check the results of biopsies *and* brushings

Dilatation
- Endoscopic dilatation as an outpatient procedure is safe in experienced hands. The technique is beyond the scope of this book (Appendix 2, p. 442)

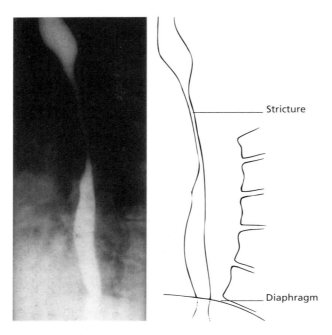

Fig. 2.3 Radiological appearances of benign oesophageal stricture. Barium swallow showing a smooth stricture in the mid-oesophagus. Negative biopsies and cytology from the stricture confirmed its benign nature.

- A subsequent chest X-ray is not necessary unless pain occurs or perforation is suspected
- Repeat dilatations may be needed. Encourage the patient to make appointments directly with the endoscopy unit if dysphagia recurs, to save time
- Recurrent symptoms < 4 weeks after dilatation suggests carcinoma

Other advice
- Ensure that the patient remains on full dose PPI (e.g. lansoprazole 30 mg, omeprazole 40 mg, rabeprazole 20 mg daily) long term, because this substantially reduces the risk of recurrent strictures
- Prevention of oesophageal obstruction (p. 5)

2.4 Oesophageal carcinoma

Oesophageal carcinoma accounts for 2% of all cancers. The incidence is increasing rapidly for unknown reasons, but may be due to the increasing prevalence of reflux. Whilst only 30% are resectable and 5-year survival is 10% in European studies, palliation is vital because inability to swallow saliva after oesophageal obstruction is a miserable way to die. Carcinoma of the cardia may mimic carcinoma of the lower third oesophagus, or achalasia (p. 65).

Causes

The cause is usually unknown. The importance of different factors varies in different parts of the world. Associations are:

- Gastro-oesophageal reflux (eightfold increase for adenocarcinoma, not for squamous carcinoma)
- Alcohol
- Tobacco
- Barrett's oesophagus (p. 57)—the degree of risk is debated. Carcinoma in Barrett's oesophagus occurs before the diagnosis of Barrett's is known in 98%
- Following corrosive injury (p. 7)
- Achalasia (p. 65)—the risk (< 1%) is less than previously considered
- Iron-deficiency anaemia and postcricoid web, with high oesophageal carcinoma (Patterson–Brown–Kelly or Plummer–Vinson syndrome)—10 times commoner in women, often aged 40–50 years
- Geographical: Caspian littoral (northern Iran: commonest malignancy, although alcohol not consumed); northern China (20 times more common than in Britain); Transkei (South Africa). Selenium or molybdenum deficiency, aflatoxin contamination of cereals and nitrosamines are postulated reasons for this variation
- Familial tylosis (palmar hyperkeratosis) is exceedingly rare

Clinical features

Progressive dysphagia and weight loss are typical, but pain and hoarseness of the voice may occur due to local spread. Patients are usually aged 60–80 years. Rapidly recurrent dysphagia after dilatation should be considered malignant until proven otherwise.

Pathology

- Cervical or midthoracic carcinomas are usually squamous
- Dysplasia may precede carcinoma
- Distal oesophageal tumours are often adenocarcinomas due to spread from the gastric fundus, or malignant change in Barrett's oesophagus. The incidence is increasing by 3–7% per year
- Pathology influences adjuvant therapy (see below)

Spread

- Local invasion along submucosal lymphatics, or directly into mediastinal nodes is the rule
- Hiccups or a persistent midthoracic ache are ominous, indicating diaphragmatic or mediastinal invasion
- Oesophagobronchial fistula, recurrent laryngeal nerve palsy and atrial fibrillation may occur
- Death usually precedes distant metastases

Investigations

Diagnostic
- Barium swallow (Fig. 2.4, p. 63) remains the most useful initial investigation
- Endoscopy, biopsy and brushings (98% detection rate), for a tissue diagnosis
- Endoscopists should define the upper and lower limits of macroscopic tumour

Look for complications
- Chest X-ray—mediastinal lymphadenopathy, evidence of aspiration
- EUS—better than CT scan or MRI for staging mural invasion, nodal involvement and assessing operability (Fig. 2.4)
- Other head and neck tumours are common (about 10%) in squamous oesophageal carcinoma

Surgical assessment
- Thoracoabdominal CT scan, with a specific request to look for nodal involvement. It may underestimate mural and lymph node invasion and should be compared with EUS (Fig. 2.4)
- Take into account age, cardiorespiratory disease and nutrition
- 'Operability' (patients considered able to survive an operation and live for more than 4 weeks) does not imply resectability
- Pulmonary function tests (including arterial gases), to estimate respiratory reserve
- The presence of lymph nodes is an indication for adjuvant therapy prior to surgery

Management
The objectives are to relieve dysphagia, prolong survival and to cure a minority. There is no ideal treatment; the site and type of the carcinoma and the general health of the patient determine the approach. Operability is the first decision.

Surgery
- Indicated for fit patients under 70 years without evidence of local invasion, when satisfactory resection can be achieved. This is less than one-third of patients with oesophageal cancer
- An experienced oesophageal surgeon, perioperative nutritional support and good physiotherapy are important
- Subtotal oesophagectomy and formation of a gastric tube is usually appropriate, usually requiring separate thoracic and abdominal incisions
- Operative mortality is < 10% in experienced hands
- Surgery alone can only be expected to cure disease confined to the oesophageal wall
- The advent of endoscopically placed self-expanding metal stents has made it difficult to justify surgery for palliation alone

Radical radiotherapy
- Squamous carcinomas that are postcricoid or in the upper third may be radiosensitive

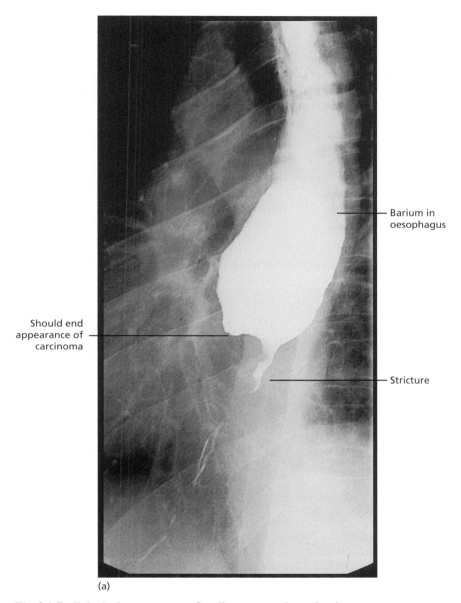

Barium in
oesophagus

Should end
appearance of
carcinoma

Stricture

(a)

Fig. 2.4 Radiological appearances of malignant oesophageal stricture.
(a) Barium swallow showing irregular stricturing in the lower oesophagus due to a carcinoma.
The oesophageal wall is thickened by the tumour. *(Continued)*

- Commonly converted into palliative therapy because of side-effects. Radiotherapy
  alone relieves dysphagia in < 50%, so continued endoscopic dilatation is necessary

Palliation
- For most (70%) patients

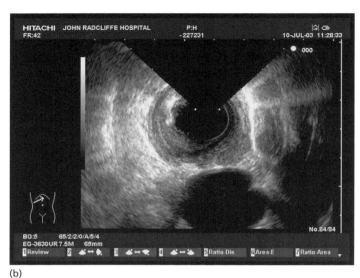

(b)

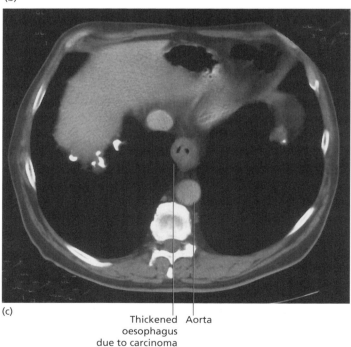

(c)

Thickened Aorta
oesophagus
due to carcinoma

Fig. 2.4 *(continued)* (b) Endoscopic ultrasound of the same tumour. EUS defines the layers, depth of tumour infiltration and nodal involvement (T3 N1 M0 in this case). Needle sampling of the node using a phased-array probe and scope can confirm tumour infiltration (as opposed to reactive change). (c) CT scan of the same tumour. Cross-sectional imaging defines the relationship to adjacent structures and likely respectability. All images are best reviewed together between radiologists, surgeons and oncologists in a multidisciplinary meeting.

- Endoscopic dilatation should be performed initially for unresectable tumours, to allow patients to swallow food and saliva
- Endoscopic placement of a self-expanding metal stent is usually optimal. These are safer and provide better palliation of dysphagia than traditional plastic stents. A variety (covered, uncovered, flanged) are available; covered stents are the tube of choice for perforated tumours. Complications include exacerbation of dysphagia in high (< 27 cm from incisors) tumours, perforation, tube migration and occlusion
- Obstructing tumours are most effectively relieved by endoscopic laser therapy, although this is not always available. Alcohol injection into the tumour through a sclerotherapy needle is cheaper and safe, but less effective
- Surgical palliation is effective in experienced hands, but morbidity is much higher than stenting
- Palliative radiotherapy may relieve pain, but is ineffective for long tumours or adenocarcinomas
- Neoadjuvant chemotherapy is showing encouraging results, especially with epirubicin and 5-fluorouracil. Specialist advice should be sought

Terminal care (p. 129)
Treatment should be carefully considered after assessing the patient, seeing the family and discussion with senior colleagues. Hydration, but not alimentation or antibiotics, is usually appropriate. Good mouth care, pharyngeal suction and liaison with the nursing staff are vital. Aspiration pneumonia is the usual cause of death.

Prognosis
- Mean survival is 10 months after diagnosis
- Overall 5-year survival is about 5%, which has changed little in the last 40 years
- In the minority (30%) who are selected for 'curative' surgery, 5-year survival is up to 25%. This is similar to the results of radical radiotherapy, but there are no direct comparative trials for equivalent stages of disease

2.5 Achalasia

Achalasia is a motility disorder characterised by absent peristalsis in the body of the oesophagus, increased lower oesophageal sphincter pressure (> 40 mmHg) and failure of sphincter relaxation during swallowing. It is due to degeneration of the myenteric plexus of unknown cause. Carcinoma of the cardia must be excluded.

Clinical features
- Occurs at any age
- Dysphagia—all patients. Unlike a stricture, dysphagia for liquids as well as solids occurs early (Fig. 2.1, p. 52). Slowly progressive; swallowing may be helped by a trick movement of the head, or Valsalva's manoeuvre
- Regurgitation—70%; undigested food, with aspiration

- Weight loss—quite common
- Pain—substernal cramps may be severe and precede dysphagia
- Symptoms for < 1 year and age > 50 years, with weight loss, suggest carcinoma
- Achalasia may present at an advanced stage. Megaoesophagus is a late manifestation that has been reported to cause respiratory obstruction (stridor). The risk of oesophageal carcinoma is increased in megaoesophagus
- Carcinoma of the cardia, gastric lymphoma, diffuse spasm, systemic sclerosis, Chagas' disease (South American trypanosomiasis), neurofibromas and amyloidosis can simulate achalasia

Investigations
- Chest X-ray—an oesophageal fluid level at the aortic knuckle and right lower lobe consolidation, or fibrosis, may be present. The gastric air bubble is characteristically absent
- Barium swallow—food debris in the oesophagus with a smooth, tapered distal narrowing and aperistaltic contractions when recumbent are characteristic. Oesophageal dilatation develops later. A video or bread/marshmallow barium swallow may elucidate difficult cases (Fig. 2.5)

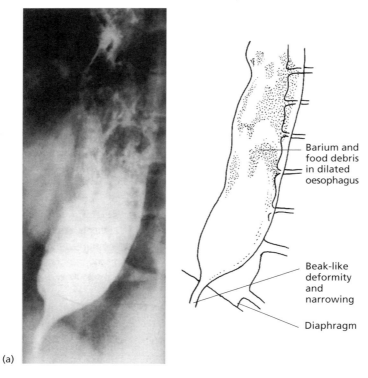

Barium and food debris in dilated oesophagus

Beak-like deformity and narrowing

Diaphragm

(a)

Fig 2.5 Achalasia. (a) Barium swallow showing achalasia with dilatation of the oesophagus. Barium is mixing with food residue in the oesophagus. The oesophagus narrows to a typical beak-like deformity at the level of the cardia. *(Continued)*

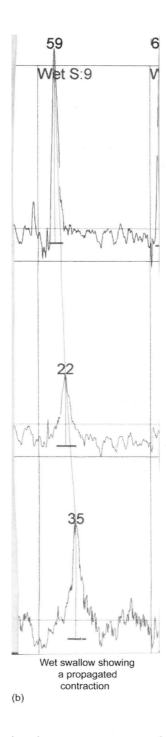

Wet swallow showing
a propagated
contraction

(b)

Fig 2.5 *(continued)* (b) Oesophageal manometry trace—normal. Note the propagation of the contractile wave (pressure against time at different probe sites) and appropriate relaxation of the gastro–oesophageal sphincter.

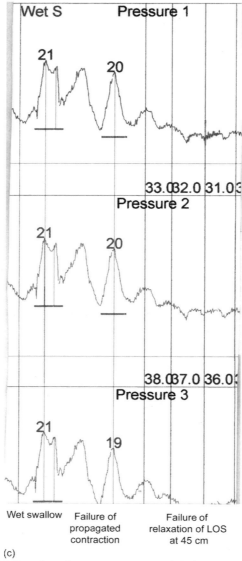

Fig 2.5 *(continued)* (c) Oesophageal manometry trace—achalasia. Note both the failure of propagation of contraction and the failure of relaxation of the gastro-oesophageal sphincter.

- Endoscopy must always be performed to exclude a stricture and to examine the cardia for carcinoma. Once food debris is negotiated the endoscope easily passes the lower oesophageal sphincter
- Manometry (p. 430) may be the only way to distinguish oesophageal spasm from achalasia and should be performed if dysphagia persists despite a normal barium swallow (Fig. 2.5 and p. 74)

Management

The choice is between endoscopic dilatation and surgery (Heller's cardiomyotomy). Dilatation is often preferred by the patient, with surgery reserved for recurrent symptoms. Drugs have no role.

Botulinum toxin

- Intrasphincteric injections of botulinum toxin (25 MU into each of four quadrants of the lower oesophageal sphincter using an endoscope and sclerotherapy needle) paralyse the hypertensive sphincter and abolish dysphagia in 60% of patients for 6–9 months
- The toxin is expensive and sphincter tone returns with time, with recurrence of dysphagia, but the risk of perforation with pneumatic dilatation is avoided
- This treatment is best performed in specialist units, but should only be considered for frail elderly patients because of the high risk of recurrence

Dilatation

- Pneumatic balloon dilatation with X-ray screening is effective in 90% at 1 year, but repeat dilatations are often required
- Dilatation should only be performed by experienced endoscopists and the patient should normally be admitted overnight
- A chest X-ray in expiration is necessary 1 h after dilatation, before the patient eats, to look for mediastinal gas or pneumothorax. Perforation occurs in 2%

Surgery

- Indicated for young patients with high sphincter pressures, when symptoms recur after three attempts at dilatation, or if the patient prefers a definitive procedure at the outset
- Cardiomyotomy is effective in 90% and gives long-term relief. Laparoscopic cardiomyotomy is safe and as effective in experienced hands and is evolving as the procedure of choice

Complications

- Megaoesophagus is now rare
- Aspiration pneumonia can be chronic, or the presenting feature
- Carcinoma may occur in untreated achalasia, but probably not after treatment. It is less common (< 5%) than previously thought
- Treatment (dilatation or surgical) may lead to reflux, stricture, failure to relieve symptoms (reassess the diagnosis), or persistent pain, even after apparent relief of obstruction

2.6 Other conditions (See Fig. 2.6)

Oesophageal dysmotility

Accounts for many patients referred with oesophageal symptoms. Chest pain or dysphagia for liquids and solids are the presenting features. Diffuse oesophageal spasm is the best-characterised motility disorder other than achalasia, but is rare in its

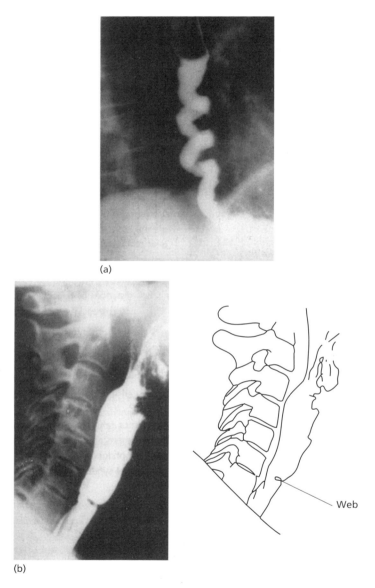

(a)

(b)

Web

Fig. 2.6 Radiological appearances of unusual causes of dysphagia.
(a) Barium swallow showing diffuse oesophageal spasm with a typical 'corkscrew' deformity.
(b) Barium swallow showing a clearly defined web arising from the anterior wall of the oesophagus and partly encircling it. A jet of barium is passing through the narrowed lumen at the level of the web. *(Continued)*

classical form. Symptoms are caused by high-amplitude, aperistaltic oesophageal contractions without a demonstrable organic lesion. When symptoms occur without typical manometric or radiological features, the term 'oesophageal dysmotility' is appropriate.

70

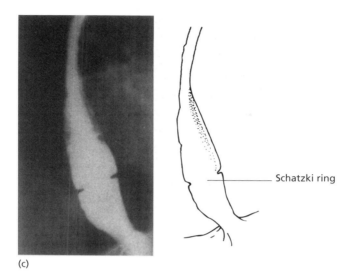

(c)

Fig. 2.6 *(continued)* (c) Barium swallow showing a narrow ring in the lower oesophagus. This is typical of the appearance of Schatzki's ring. The ring is often visible only when the oesophagus is fully distended by barium.

Symptoms
- Dysphagia—intermittent, variable intensity, for both liquids and solids (Fig. 2.1, p. 52)
- Chest pain—may mimic cardiac pain or reflux (p. 74) and be provoked by stress. A persistent ache between severe episodes usually distinguishes it from angina ('oesophagodynia'), but an identifiable oesophageal cause only accounts for 20% of non-cardiac chest pain
- Coexistent symptoms of IBS (p. 336), anxiety or depression are also common
- Weight loss is notably absent

Investigations
- Barium swallow—a corkscrew appearance is classic but unusual. Aperistaltic 'tertiary' contractions are common when recumbent, but stasis does not occur, unlike achalasia (Fig. 2.5, p. 66). Similar asymptomatic changes can occur in the elderly
- Manometry—diagnostic if positive. Repetitive contractions, high-amplitude waves and periods of normal peristalsis are typical, but occur together in a minority (< 10%). Negative results on static testing do not exclude the diagnosis; ambulatory monitoring increases the yield, but the gain is small because abnormal motility may not relate to symptom events
- Endoscopy—should be normal, but helps exclude oesophagitis or a stricture

Treatment
- Symptoms are difficult to relieve totally. Reassurance that the pain is not cardiac is essential, also explaining that the drugs prescribed are often used for angina

- A PPI (lansoprazole 30 mg or omeprazole 20–40 mg daily) should be tried first since dysmotility may be provoked by acid reflux
- Isosorbide dinitrate 5–10 mg sublingually four times daily or nifedipine 5–10 mg three times daily are adjunctive treatments, but response is unpredictable and side-effects (e.g. headache) are common and often not well tolerated
- Prokinetic agents may make symptoms worse
- Empirical treatment with amitriptyline in low dose (10–30 mg daily) can help
- Pneumatic dilatation or botulinum toxin injection should be reserved for the most severe cases with focal high pressure on oesophageal manometry, because the outcome is unpredictable

Oesophageal webs
- Not circumferential, unlike rings (Fig. 2.6, p. 70)
- Demonstrated radiologically, but difficult to see at endoscopy
- May be associated with mucocutaneous disorders such as epidermolysis bullosa
- Check for iron-deficiency anaemia, associated with a postcricoid web and high oesophageal carcinoma (Plummer–Vinson syndrome)
- Exclude carcinoma of the upper third of the oesophagus by careful radiology and endoscopy. ENT advice may be necessary

Schatzki's ring
- Circumferential contraction in the middle or lower third, usually diagnosed radiologically rather than by endoscopy (Fig. 2.6, p. 71)
- Typically causes intermittent dysphagia for solids over a long period, but often asymptomatic and of no significance
- If dysphagia is present, dilatation is justified after biopsy. Occasionally pneumatic dilatation is necessary

Diverticula
- Pharyngeal pouches (Zenker's diverticulum) present with intermittent dysphagia and regurgitation in the elderly. Regurgitation of fluid when recumbent may lead to aspiration
- An ENT opinion is advisable after diagnosis by barium swallow taking care to show the upper oesophagus
- Routine endoscopy is not indicated and may be dangerous if oesophageal intubation is not carefully performed under direct vision
- Surgical excision with cricopharyngeal myotomy is the treatment of choice for symptoms. Endoscopic excision by an experienced ENT surgeon is effective
- Mid-oesophageal and epiphrenic diverticula are an endoscopic hazard, but of no other consequence

Systemic sclerosis
- Dysphagia and heartburn with Raynaud's phenomenon are characteristic
- Recurrent strictures caused by reflux and stasis are the principal problem

- CREST syndrome (digital calcinosis, Raynaud's phenomenon, dysphagia, sclerodactyly and telangiectasia) should be distinguished clinically from systemic sclerosis, because it has a better prognosis
- PPIs at doses higher than standard recommended dosage (e.g. omeprazole 80 mg/day or more) are the best treatment, because standard antireflux treatment is ineffective
- Endoscopic dilatation is necessary for strictures
- Antireflux surgery may make the situation worse. Refractory cases should be referred to a specialist unit
- Other gastrointestinal complications (nutritional deficiency, malabsorption due to small bowel bacterial overgrowth or constipation) should be looked for and treated

Oesophageal infections

Oesophageal infections occur in the debilitated and immunocompromised (Section 11.4, p. 363). Underlying disease should be sought and treated.

Candidiasis
- Painful dysphagia (odynophagia) with oral candidiasis is typical
- Barium swallow, blind oesophageal brushings, or endoscopy with biopsy are diagnostic
- Nystatin suspension 1–2 mL four times daily for 10 days is as effective
- Oral fluconazole 100–200 mg once daily is indicated for patients with AIDS (maintenance therapy may be needed) or if nystatin is ineffective
- Fever or neutropenia make systemic invasion likely and intravenous fluconazole is indicated

Cytomegalovirus
- Serpiginous or large ulcers in the mid-oesophagus cause painful dysphagia in the immunocompromised
- Oesophageal biopsy is diagnostic (epithelial inclusion bodies)
- Ganciclovir (intravenous 5 mg/kg over 1 h, twice daily) for 14 days is only appropriate for severe infection. Recurrence is common

Herpes simplex
- Small, circumscribed ulcers in the mid-oesophagus are seen endoscopically. Ulcers may coalesce or bleed
- Electron microscopy of brushings transported in 4% glutaraldehyde is diagnostic
- Intravenous acyclovir 5 mg/kg three times daily, until tablets can be swallowed (200 mg five times daily for 5 days)

Rumination and regurgitation

Rumination is the chewing of regurgitated food that is then swallowed or spat out. Regurgitation is effortless and involuntary, although it may be a learned habit or indicate psychiatric disease such as bulimia or an anxiety state. It should be distinguished from recurrent vomiting by the lack of nausea and from gastro-oesophageal reflux in which bitter liquid reaches the mouth. Recognition of the disorder and 'unlearning' the habit through biofeedback techniques may help.

2.7 Clinical dilemmas

General advice for diagnostic dilemmas is given in Appendix 4 (p. 455).

Causes of chest pain

20–40% of patients with chest pain, normal exercise ECG and normal angiography have an oesophageal disorder. The pain may be severe, wake patients from sleep, or occur during emotional stress.

- Confirm the history—especially the duration and type of pain, provoking and relieving factors
- Oesophageal reflux and diffuse oesophageal spasm most commonly mimic angina
- An endoscopy to identify oesophagitis is indicated. Although a therapeutic trial of a PPI may be appropriate, patients must avoid acid–suppressing medication for 3 weeks prior to endoscopy
- Oesophageal manometry and 24 h pH monitoring with symptom recording should be performed after referral to a specialist centre. Provocation tests (edrophonium for spasm or acid perfusion (Bernstein test) for reflux) occasionally help (p. 430)
- A video barium swallow in the recumbent position is an alternative method of diagnosing dysmotility

Dysphagia with a 'normal' barium swallow

Globus hystericus is not the only cause. Diffuse spasm, achalasia and strictures may be overlooked.

- Confirm the history—especially whether dysphagia is for solids or liquids and the duration of symptoms
- Document the present weight and any loss
- Check the films:
  Is it the correct patient?
  Do the films show the entire oesophagus?
- Arrange a bread/marshmallow barium swallow recorded on video, after discussion with the radiologist
- Referral for manometry (p. 430) is indicated for persistent symptoms. Obscure cases of diffuse spasm or achalasia may be detected

3 Stomach and Duodenum

3.1 Dyspepsia

- Dyspepsia (indigestion) is defined as chronic or recurrent pain or discomfort centred in the upper abdomen (epigastrium)
- The annual prevalence in Western Europe and the USA is 25%, accounting for 5% of all primary care consultations
- Although frequently grouped together, dyspepsia should be distinguished, where possible, from gastro-oesophageal reflux disease (GORD, Chapter 2). The management of patients with the two symptom complexes differs substantially
- Dyspepsia due to organic disease must be detected and distinguished from 'non-ulcer dyspepsia' or 'functional dyspepsia', so that specific treatment can be given. Table 3.1 shows the differential diagnosis of epigastric pain

Clinical features

Common symptoms
- Epigastric, usually central upper abdominal, or retrosternal discomfort related to eating, specific foods, hunger or time of day
- Heaviness, unease, postprandial fullness or early satiety are common descriptive terms, often associated with flatulence or borborygmi
- Heartburn and acid brash are more likely to indicate underlying GORD than dyspepsia

Indicators of organic disease

Examination
- Epigastric tenderness is non-specific
- Palpate carefully for an upper abdominal mass
- Feel for supraclavicular nodes and hepatomegaly
- Check for ascites

Table 3.1 Differential diagnosis of postprandial epigastric pain

Common	Uncommon*	Rare
Non-ulcer dyspepsia	Biliary colic	Chronic pancreatitis
Duodenal ulcer	Gastro-oesophageal reflux	Small intestinal stricture
Gastric ulcer	Oesophagitis	Mesenteric ischaemia
Duodenitis		Myocardial ischaemia
Gastric cancer		

*Although these conditions are common, they do not usually present with epigastric pain after meals.

Investigations
- Not all patients need investigation
- Patients with predominant symptoms of GORD should first be identified and excluded
- Most low-risk patients who are *H. pylori*-negative will have non-ulcer dyspepsia, and treatment should be directed at the most troublesome symptom (see Non-ulcer dyspepsia below). The main caveat is an increasing incidence of *H. pylori*-negative ulcers. This should be carefully considered when treating patients with non-ulcer dyspepsia

Helicobacter testing
- Testing for *H. pylori* (by serology or breath testing, p. 431) *without* endoscopy has been shown to be more cost-effective for new onset dyspepsia, cause less patient distress and achieve equivalent satisfaction levels as endoscopy
- The argument is that gastric carcinoma exceptionally rarely presents without alarm symptoms (Box 3.1) at any age and that outcome is no different between those with and without alarm symptoms. Peptic ulcers are almost all *H. pylori*-positive and treated effectively with eradication therapy
- This is a radical change to previous practice, but has been instituted in some areas and is likely to gain wider acceptance
- Low-risk patients with residual symptoms following *H. pylori* eradication should be managed in the same way as patients who originally test *H. pylori*-negative (see Non-ulcer dyspepsia below)

Endoscopy
Early endoscopy should be considered for
- Patients > 55 years (the age threshold should be defined by the local epidemiology of gastric cancer)
- All patients with alarm symptoms (Box 3.1), regardless of age
- All patients with history of NSAID usage regardless of age

Specific investigations
- Blood tests—anaemia, a high platelet count or ESR and abnormal liver function tests indicate an organic cause

---

Box 3.1 Dyspepsia alarm symptoms and signs indicating a greater likelihood of serious disease

---

Unintentional weight loss
Dysphagia
Recurrent vomiting
Symptoms of gastrointestinal blood loss
Iron-deficiency anaemia (except pre-menopausal women)
Epigastric pain severe enough to hospitalise a patient
Ulcerogenic medication (e.g. NSAIDs, steroids)
Epigastric mass
Previous gastric ulcer
Concomitant disease with possible gastrointestinal involvement

- Barium meal—only indicated in preference to endoscopy if endoscopy is difficult or impossible or oesophagogastric anatomy needs defining. Anastomoses can confuse endoscopists and it is easier to evaluate pyloric stenosis by barium meal
- Ultrasound of the gall bladder and pancreas, if the endoscopy is normal

Organic dyspepsia

Dyspepsia due to lesions readily identified on routine investigation:

- Duodenal or gastric ulcer
- Duodenitis—usually part of the duodenal ulcer diathesis (Section 3.8, p. 101)
- Gastric cancer
- Reflux oesophagitis
- Gastritis—this is controversial. It is best considered a histological diagnosis
- Cholelithiasis—pain is usually severe
- Management of organic disease is discussed in the appropriate sections

Non-ulcer (functional) dyspepsia

Defined as upper abdominal discomfort related to meals, lasting for more than 4 weeks and for which no cause can be found after investigation. Attempts have been made to classify non-ulcer dyspepsia (NUD) into discrete symptom groups. Although this does not predict underlying disease, it may help predict the response to particular therapy.

Ulcer-type non-ulcer dyspepsia

- Epigastric pain:
  - may be described as epigastric burning
  - may be episodic, occasionally at night
- Relieved by antacids or food, or worse after meals
- No ulcer, past or present

Dysmotility-type non-ulcer dyspepsia

- Upper abdominal pain:
  - poorly localised
  - variable character
  - not at night
  - continuous, rather than episodic
- Abdominal distension
- Premature satiety
- Nausea—but vomiting is unusual
- Food intolerance—variable, but often several types of food

Reflux-type non-ulcer dyspepsia

- Retrosternal discomfort:
  - on stooping
  - after large meals
  - on lying flat
  - temporary relief from antacids
- Recent weight gain

- Smoker
- Cyclical severity
- No endoscopic or histological evidence of oesophagitis

It should be noted that there is often considerable symptom overlap and that many also have symptoms of IBS (p. 335).

There remain some patients who have upper abdominal pain after meals, who do not fit into one of these patterns. Features common to all patients with NUD are:
- The patient remains well
- Weight is steady or fluctuating
- Normal investigations

Treatment of non-ulcer dyspepsia
- Explanation and reassurance are essential
- Lifestyle changes (regular meals, weight loss, less alcohol, stopping smoking) often help
- Drugs should only be used when symptoms are intolerable. The following recommendations are made, but controlled trials have either not shown clear benefits from drug treatments, or have not been performed
- If not already tried, antacids should be given for NUD. Patients with reflux-type NUD are more likely to benefit. Subsequent empirical management may be influenced by the symptom pattern:
  - Dysmotility-type—prokinetic agents (e.g. domperidone 10 mg three times daily, or metoclopramide 10 mg three times daily) have been shown to be superior to placebo. Antispasmodics, e.g. hyoscine 10–20 mg, three times daily may occasionally be helpful
  - Ulcer-type—PPIs (e.g. omeprazole 20 mg, lansoprazole 30 mg or rabeprazole 20 mg daily) are more effective than H_2 antagonists and will heal *H. pylori*-negative ulcers
  - Reflux type—heartburn may become the predominant symptom after *H. pylori* eradication. A therapeutic trial of a PPI is reasonable (and difficult to avoid), but if symptoms persist, this effectively excludes an acid-related disorder and treatment should be stopped. If symptoms are controlled by empirical therapy, a trial of treatment withdrawal is appropriate, with therapy repeated if symptoms recur. Eradication therapy is appropriate for *H. pylori*-positive patients who have not previously had eradication therapy. This remains controversial, because 15 infected patients need to be treated to cure one patient with NUD, but may be equivalent to other empirical treatment. If symptoms persist, try switching treatment (e.g. from a prokinetic to a PPI). As needed therapy with a PPI is safe and may be effective
- Only if symptoms persist is referral for endoscopy appropriate
- Patients with resistant NUD may respond to an exclusion diet, or other measures to treat an irritable bowel (p. 392)

3.2 Nausea and vomiting

The timing, amount and content of the vomitus are important. Associated symptoms often indicate the cause, since isolated nausea and vomiting are rarely organic.

Causes

The list of causes is long and the likelihood depends on the clinical circumstances.

Gastrointestinal disease

Mechanical obstruction
- Pyloric stenosis
- Achalasia
- Small bowel obstruction

Functional gastrointestinal disorders
- Gastroparesis
- Intestinal pseudo-obstruction
- Non-ulcer dyspepsia
- Irritable bowel syndrome

Organic gastrointestinal disease
- Peptic ulcer (especially pyloric canal ulcers)
- Pancreatitis
- Hepatitis
- Cholecystitis
- Mesenteric ischaemia

Drugs

Chemotherapy
- Cisplatinum
- Methotrexate
- Tamoxifen

Analgesics
- NSAIDs
- Opiates

Cardiovascular drugs
- Digoxin
- Antiarrthymics
- β-blockers
- Diuretics

Hormonal drugs
- Oral contraceptive
- Oral hypoglycaemics

Antibiotics/Antivirals
- Erythromycin
- Sulphonamides
- Acyclovir

Gastrointestinal drugs
- Azathioprine
- Sulfasalazine

CNS active drugs
- Antiparkinsonian drugs
- Anticonvulsants

Alcohol
Nicotine (including patches)

Infectious
- Gastroenteritis
- Non-gastrointestinal

Endocrine
- Pregnancy (easy to forget!)
- Diabetic ketoacidosis
- Hyperthyroidism
- Addison's disease
- Hyper- and hypoparathyroidism

Metabolic
- Uraemia
- Hypercalcaemia
- Hyponatraemia
- Acute intermittent porphyria

Neurological
- Migraine
- Raised intracranial pressure
- Seizures
- Demyelination
- Labyrinthine disorders
- Motion sickness
- Labyrinthitis
- Meniere's disease
- Tumours (especially near the fourth ventricle)
- Fluorescein angiography

Psychiatric
- Anorexia nervosa
- Bulimia nervosa
- Pyschogenic vomiting
- Pain

- Depression
- Cyclic vomiting syndrome

Post-operative miscellaneous

Cardiac
- Myocardial infarction
- Congestive heart failure

Starvation

Investigations and management

Assessment
- Look for signs of dehydration
- Look for visible peristalsis and abdominal herniae. Feel for a mass and listen for a gastric succussion splash and bowel sounds
- Inspect the teeth for loss of dental enamel, which may indicate recurrent vomiting due to bulimia or severe reflux disease
- Carry out a neurological examination
- Examine the vomitus for volume, blood and bile (the latter indicates patent pylorus)
- Check the urine—osmolality, glucose and a pregnancy test
- Request serum electrolytes, urea, random glucose and calcium
- Metabolic alkalosis (pH > 7.44, $PaCO_2$ > 45 mmHg or 6.0 kPa) only occurs in severe vomiting
- Arrange an endoscopy if vomiting is persistent (p. 84)

Drug therapies
There are two broad drug groups—centrally acting antiemetics and peripherally acting prokinetics:
- Phenothiazines (e.g. prochlorperazine 25 mg suppository or 12.5 mg intramuscularly) act centrally through an antidopaminergic mechanism. Useful for vomiting due to metabolic, drug-induced, postoperative, or vestibular causes. Side-effects include sedation, orthostatic hypotension, or extrapyramidal symptoms.
- Domperidone (10–20 mg orally or 60 mg suppository, where available) or metoclopramide (10 mg three times daily) exert both antiemetic and prokinetic effects. Domperidone does not cross the blood brain barrier and is free of extrapyramidal effects, so is preferable to metoclopramide in the elderly or patients aged < 21 years.
- 5-HT_3 antagonists (e.g. ondansetron 8 mg three times daily) act centrally on the chemoreceptor trigger zone and are particular useful in drug-induced nausea.
- Antihistamines with H_1 receptor antagonistic properties (e.g. diphenhydramine 25–50 mg three times daily) are useful in vomiting of labyrinthine origin including motion sickness, vertigo and migraine.
- Dexamethasone, lorazepam, methotrimeprazine, and combination therapy are effective in special circumstances (below)

Specific clinical situations

Pregnancy
- Avoid all drugs if at all possible. Ginger may be helpful but is unproven
- Phenothiazines (promethazine 25 mg oral/injection) and antihistamines (cyclizine) may be given in the first trimester
- Thiamine 100 mg daily may also help
- Recurrent vomiting is likely to provoke oesophagitis and further vomiting. A PPI (although unlicensed in pregnancy) can break the cycle and appears to be safe
- Corticosteroids (dexamethasone), enteral or very rarely parenteral nutrition may be necessary for intractable hyperemesis gravidarum

Gastroparesis
- Meticulous glycaemic control may reverse gastroparesis in diabetics
- Erythromycin (motilin agonist) 4 g daily and other prokinetics are tried more in hope than expectation
- Percutaneous endoscopic gastrostomy with a jejunal extension (PEG-J, p. 401) secures nutrition and assists glycaemic control in insulin-dependent diabetics
- Gastric pacing remains experimental
- Subtotal gastrectomy is a last resort, but results are disappointing.

Chemotherapy and radiation-related nausea and vomiting
- A combination of a 5-HT$_3$ antagonist (e.g. oral ondansetron 8 mg three times daily, for 48 h) and dexamethasone (intravenous 8 mg immediately prior) is usually effective for prevention
- Prevention and treatment of delayed vomiting is less effective. Combining dexamethasone and domperidone (or ondansetron) is recommended
- Benzodiazepines (lorazepam 2 mg) and relaxation therapy may be helpful by reducing anticipatory symptoms

Persistent vomiting
- Review the diagnosis, especially considering cerebral, brain stem (fourth ventricle), metabolic and mechanical causes
- Arrange an endoscopy if not already performed
- Combination therapy occasionally helps when single drugs fail
- Methotrimeprazine 100 mg by continuous subcutaneous infusion daily is useful in terminal care

In patients with chronic unexplained nausea and vomiting, lorazepam or psychological assessment may help

3.3 Helicobacter pylori (See Fig. 3.1)

H. pylori is one of the commonest human infections. It is strongly associated with gastritis (which may become atrophic), gastric and duodenal ulceration, gastric cancer, Ménétrier's disease and mucosal-associated lymphoid tissue (MALT) lymphoma.

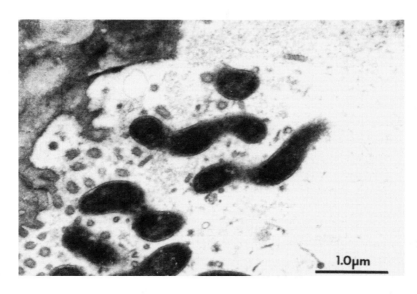

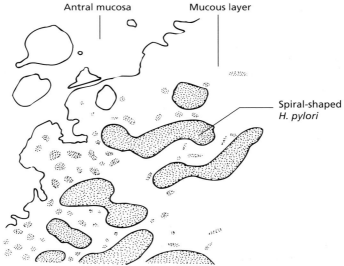

Antral mucosa   Mucous layer

Spiral-shaped
H. pylori

Fig. 3.1 Transmission electron micrograph of antral mucosa in a human patient, illustrating the spiral shape of *Helicobacter pylori*.

Associations with functional dyspepsia and NSAID-related ulcers are less certain. However, most individuals come to no harm and it may protect from GORD.

Epidemiology

• *H. pylori* is distributed worldwide. It is highly prevalent in emergent countries (80–90% colonised by the late teens), which has management implications for patients born in these countries

- In industrialised countries *H. pylori* colonisation has decreased in recent decades to 10% of teenagers, as socio-economic conditions have improved
- The infection is acquired in early childhood within families by the oro-oral, gastro-oral and faeco-oral routes
- *H. pylori* infection can be acquired through inadequately sterilised endoscopes or nasogastric tubes

Spontaneous eradication of *H. pylori* is rare, but so is reinfection

Pathophysiology

H. pylori is highly adapted to its niche in the gastric mucosa, with unique features allowing entry into mucus, attachment to epithelial cells and evasion of the host immune system. Features of clinical relevance include:

- Vac A exotoxin is secreted by the majority of *H. pylori* strains. Polymorphisms in the gene for Vac A are associated with more severe disease
- High levels of phospholipase A (PLA) enable *H. pylori* to penetrate gastric mucus. High levels of PLA are secreted by strains isolated from patients with gastric cancer
- *H. pylori* causes inflammation in the antrum (antritis) or body (corpusitis) of the stomach, although these often occur together (pangastritis, Section 3.4). Antritis is characterised by hypergastrinaemia, increased acid output and a higher risk of duodenal ulcer. Why only 2–20% with antritis develop duodenal ulcers remains unclear, but is likely to be a balance between the type of *H. pylori* and mucosal defence factors (p. 102)
- Duodenitis is caused by *H. pylori* colonisation of islands of gastric metaplasia in the duodenal bulb, which are triggered by high acid output
- *H. pylori* corpusitis is associated with gastric ulceration, gastric mucosal atrophy, decreased acid secretion and 2.5-fold increased risk of gastric cancer (p. 91)
- Reasons for predominant antritis or corpusitis remain unclear, but duration of infection or treatment with PPI are possible factors

Diagnosis of *H. pylori* infection

Non-invasive methods

Serology and breath tests have high sensitivity and specificity.

- Urea breath test
  - The most reliable method of detection and best for confirming successful eradication
  - Depends on detection of urease activity from *H. pylori* by including ^{13}C- or ^{14}C-labelled urea in a test meal. Urea is split by urease into NH_4 and CO_2 and the latter detected in expired air. ^{13}C-labelled urea has the advantage that it is non-radioactive
  - Patients must stop PPIs, antibiotics, prokinetic drugs and bismuth-containing drugs for 4 weeks and fast for 6 h before the test
  - Post-treatment tests must be delayed for 4 weeks after the end of therapy to avoid false-negative results
- Serology
  - Used for screening and epidemiological studies

- No value in confirming eradication, because Ig-G antibody titres decline very slowly
- Laboratory-based serology is reliable, but 'near-patient' or 'office' whole blood test kits are less reliable and should be validated for the local population before use
- Serology is best used for younger patients: false-negative results are more common in patients aged > 55 years, or in children. Stool antigen enzyme immunoassay
  - > 90% sensitive and specific for pretreatment diagnosis of active *H. pylori* infection
  - Particularly suitable for children
  - Patients must stop PPIs, antibiotics, prokinetic drugs and bismuth-containing drugs for 4 weeks before the test
  - Tests may be useful for follow-up of infection if carried out > 8 weeks from initial therapy, but this remains controversial

Invasive methods
All depend on endoscopic biopsies. Highly sensitive and specific, although false-negative results occur during treatment with PPIs, antibiotics or bismuth compounds. Suitable for diagnosis or assessing the result of treatment, when endoscopy is performed for other reasons. The same timings apply as for urea breath tests.
- CLO or urease test
  - Two antral biopsies are placed in a medium containing urea and a pH indicator
  - Hydrolysis of urea by *H. pylori* urease from *H. pylori* alters the pH: a pink colour develops within a few hours. Commercial kits (CLO test) are available
  - Two biopsies from the body of the stomach are needed if the patient is on PPIs, which provoke migration of *H. pylori* to the corpus
- Histology of gastric biopsies
  - Stained with Giemsa or haematoxylin and eosin
  - Two juxtapyloric biopsies are needed, as well as two biopsies from the corpus to define the histological type of gastritis (Table 3.3, p. 90)
  - Immunohistochemical stains for specific *H. pylori* antigens are available
- Culture of H. pylori
  - Gold standard, but expensive and reserved for determining antibiotic sensitivity when initial treatment has failed
  - A minority of cultures fail, so negative culture is not proof of successful treatment

Consequences of diagnosis
Once infection has been diagnosed, treatment is almost unavoidable even if it is unlikely to influence symptoms. This should be considered when testing asymptomatic individuals or those with atypical symptoms.

Indications for treatment of H. pylori
- Strongly recommended
  - Peptic ulceration (active or not, including complicated ulcers). Eradication therapy should be offered at diagnosis.
  - MALToma. 70–95% of patients with MALTomas are infected. *H. pylori* eradication therapy alone induces regression in 70–80% of cases. Lifelong surveillance is required, but such patients are best managed at tertiary referral centres (p. 100)

- Atrophic gastritis. Associated with an increased risk of progression to gastric cancer and may improve following *H. pylori* eradication
- Post-resection of gastric cancer
- First-degree relatives of gastric cancer patients
- Desire of the patient without the above (after discussion of treatment expectation and side-effects)
- Controversial
  - Prior to NSAID therapy. May reduce the incidence of peptic ulcers, but is insufficient to prevent recurrent ulcer bleeding if NSAIDs are continued. Eradication does not enhance healing of ulcers by antisecretory drugs when NSAIDs are continued
  - *H. pylori*-positive NUD
  - Patients with gastro-oesophageal reflux requiring long-term acid suppression

Treatment of *H. pylori* infection
- For first-line treatment a 1-week course of triple therapy is recommended (Table 3.2)
Testing after treatment
- Testing by urea breath test, endoscopic biopsy or stool antigen test can only be performed 4–8 weeks after treatment has been completed and drugs stopped
- It is not necessary in every patient if cost is a consideration, but should be considered essential in:
  - complicated duodenal ulcers (e.g. after haemorrhage)
  - all gastric ulcers
  - treatment of MALT lymphoma (p. 100)
- Symptomatic recurrence of an uncomplicated duodenal ulcer is a good predictor of treatment failure
- Retesting is helpful for patients who have persistent symptoms after eradication therapy. However, patients may develop reflux symptoms after eradication and this should be distinguished from ulcer recurrence or persistent infection

Treatment after eradication
- Uncomplicated duodenal ulcers—acid suppression can be stopped after *H. pylori* eradication
- Uncomplicated gastric ulcers—continue acid suppression until ulcer healing is confirmed endoscopically after 8–12 weeks
- Complicated ulcers (e.g. haemorrhage)—either continue treatment with a PPI for 4 weeks and check eradication with a breath test at 8 weeks or continue acid suppression until ulcer healing is confirmed endoscopically after 8–12 weeks
- Biopsies for *H. pylori* should be done at the subsequent endoscopy. If the patient has not stopped PPIs or H_2-receptor antagonists, biopsies must be taken from the body as well as the antrum and sent for histology
- Perforated ulcers and NSAID-associated ulcers are best treated with long-term acid suppression, since these are weakly associated with *H. pylori*. PPIs (omeprazole 10 mg, lansoprazole 15 mg daily) are best used post-perforation, but PPIs at full dose (omeprazole 20 mg, lansoprazole 30 mg daily) are probably preferable in NSAID ulcers. PPIs should be given for the duration of NSAID treatment, especially in elderly patients. PPIs are better than misoprostol for prophylaxis after an ulcer has occurred

Table 3.2 Recommended treatment options for *Helicobacter pylori*

Drug	Dose	Frequency	Duration
Recommended first-line therapy			
PPI	See below	Twice daily	
Clarithromycin	500 mg	Twice daily	1 week
Metronidazole	4-500 mg	Twice daily	
Or			
PPI	See below	Twice daily	
Amoxicillin	1000 mg	Twice daily	1 week
Metronidazole	4-500 mg	Twice daily	
Or			
PPI	See below	Twice daily	
Amoxicillin	1000 mg	Twice daily	1 week
Clarithromycin	500 mg	Twice daily	
Recommended regimens for refractory *H.pylori* infection in the absence of susceptibility data			
PPI	See below	Twice daily	
Bismuth subsalicylate (Pepto-Bismol)/tripotassium dicitratobismuthate (De-Noltab)	120 mg	Four times daily	1 week
Tetracycline	500 mg	Four times daily	
Metronidazole	4-500 mg	Three times daily	
Or			
PPI	See below	Twice daily	
Tetracycline	500 mg	Four times daily	2 weeks
Metronidazole	4-500 mg	Three times daily	
Or			
PPI	See below	Twice daily	
Amoxicillin	1000 mg	Twice daily	2 weeks
Metronidazole	4-500 mg	Three times daily	
Or			
PPI	See below	Twice daily	
Amoxicillin	1000 mg	Twice daily	10 days
Rifambutin	600 mg	Once daily	

Alternative drugs, with similar efficacy and cost
PPI = omeprazole 20 mg or lansoprazole 30 mg or pantoprazole 40 mg or rabeprazole 20 mg or esomeprazole 40 mg

Eradication failure
- 1 week triple therapy regimes eradicate > 90% infections
- If eradication fails, consider poor patient compliance. Both treatment complexity and adverse events (up to 30%) contribute. Compliance can be improved by explaining the reason for treatment, dosage schedule, post-treatment tests, and possible side-effects (most frequently diarrhoea and nausea). Discourage smoking (see below).
- Then repeat 1 week triple therapy (Table 3.2) and arrange a breath test for 4 weeks after completion of therapy
- If unsuccessful for a second time, give empirical quadruple therapy (Table 3.2) and repeat the breath test after the appropriate interval

- If the breath test remains positive, consider:
  - *Bacterial resistance.* Most commonly due to metronidazole (10–90%) caused by mutations in nitroreductase genes that interfere with intracellular activation of the genes. If likely (e.g. previous treatment with metronidazole), non-metronidazole regimens are best used. Clarithromycin is the most effective antibiotic against *H. pylori*, but resistance caused by mutations in the 23S ribosomal RNA genes is increasing. Antimicrobial sensitivity testing requires a further endoscopy to culture the organism but can identify appropriate therapy
  - *Inadequate acid suppression.* Antibiotic efficacy against *H. pylori* is pH dependent. Smoking increases gastric acidity and may explain the higher failure rate in smokers. Higher doses of a PPI (omeprazole 40 mg twice daily) may help
  - *Early reinfection.* Rare. Demonstrated by molecular tools to distinguish different isolates. Late reinfection occurs in < 1% in Europe or USA, but is higher elsewhere. Children or health care workers exposed to gastric juice are most at risk

3.4 Gastritis

Inflammation of the gastric mucosa (gastritis) is the stomach's response to infection or injury: whether gastritis is transient or related to peptic ulcer and gastric cancer depends on the site, type and cause of inflammation.

Classification

Gastritis may be immune or non-immune. The latter is by far the commonest and is usually associated with *H. pylori* colonisation of the foregut. The Sydney (1990) classification is the most acceptable, because it combines topographical and morphological details (Table 3.3).

Three types of gastritis are now recognised—acute, chronic and special forms. These are qualified by site, morphology and associated aetiology.

Site

The stomach is divided into two topographical areas—antrum and body. Gastritis in both sites is termed pangastritis.

Table 3.3 Summary of the Sydney classification of gastritis

Type	Site	Morphology	Aetiology
Acute	Antrum	Inflammation	Microbial (*H. pylori**)
Chronic	Body	Activity	Non-microbial
Special forms	Pangastritis	Atrophy	autoimmune
granulomatous		Metaplasia	alcohol
eosinophilic		*H. pylori* density	postgastrectomy
lymphocytic			NSAID
hypertrophic			chemical
reactive			Unknown

*Other microbial causes are very rare.

Morphology

The five principal features (inflammation, activity, atrophy, intestinal metaplasia and numbers of *H. pylori*) are graded as none, mild, moderate or severe.

- Inflammation reflects the number of chronic inflammatory cells in the lamina propria
- Activity means the presence of neutrophil polymorphs that characterise acute gastritis
- Atrophy evaluates the depth of gastric glands. It is positively related to gastric ulcer, or to cancer, and negatively associated with duodenal ulcer
- Intestinal metaplasia is common in chronic gastritis and in association with gastric ulcers or cancer. It may precede early gastric cancer, but is not necessarily premalignant
- Numbers of *H. pylori*, detected by Giemsa or Gram stain (culture and urease techniques only indicate presence or absence of the organism), indicate the density of infection

Other features of special forms (granulomas, eosinophils, cytomegalovirus) are not graded.

Aetiology

- Microbial—*H. pylori* (Fig. 3.1, p. 85) causes > 95% chronic gastritis. *Gastrospirillum hominis* (another spiral bacterium), cytomegalovirus, and herpes virus are very rare causes
- Non-microbial causes are listed in Table 3.3 (p. 90). Autoimmune-associated chronic gastritis is largely confined to the body of the stomach, where it causes atrophy, anacidity (achlorhydria) and vitamin B_{12} deficiency, and predisposes to cancer

Clinical features and investigations

Gastritis is a histological diagnosis and can only be adequately classified when biopsies have been taken from the body and antrum of the stomach. It does not correlate with endoscopic appearances or symptoms, and consequently does not always need treatment.

Acute gastritis

- Caused by drugs (salicylates), alcohol or trauma (stress erosions). *H. pylori*-associated acute gastritis is rarely seen, because infection is acquired in early childhood. Infection can be iatrogenic, transmitted through inadequately sterilised endoscopes or nasogastric tubes
- Often asymptomatic, but dyspepsia, retching, halitosis or haematemesis may occur
- There are no characteristic endoscopic appearances. The endoscopist is best advised to avoid the term 'gastritis' and stick to describing mucosal appearances and taking biopsies

Chronic gastritis

- Almost always caused by *H. pylori*
- Often antral, asymptomatic and stable for many years
- *H. pylori*-positive antritis predisposes to duodenal ulceration (2–20%)
- Corpusitis predisposes to gastric ulcers. A small proportion (about 3% at each stage) develop intestinal metaplasia, progress to atrophy and then to cancer
- *H. pylori* gastritis increases the risk of gastric cancer 2.5-fold (p. 86)

Autoimmune gastritis
- Autoimmune gastritis is a corpus-restricted atrophic gastritis associated with circulating antibodies to parietal cells and intrinsic factor, with or without pernicious anaemia.
- Pernicious anaemia occurs in about 10% of all patients with detectable antibodies, rising to 80% when titre > 1 : 40
- Histologically characterised by hyperplasia of G-cells (due to achlorhydria) and enterochromaffin cells. Adenocarcinoma and microcarcinoids may rarely occur
- Disease associations include autoimmune thyroiditis, adrenalitis, vitiligo and insulin-dependent diabetes mellitus

Other *H. pylori*-negative chronic gastritis
- Reactive—due to drugs, duodenogastric reflux, or after surgery
- Focal active—feature of Crohn's disease elsewhere
- Granulomas—sarcoidosis or Crohn's disease
- Eosinophilic—rare, occuring alone or with vasculitis
- Hypertrophic—(Ménétrier's disease) rare, causing weight loss and diarrhoea due to protein-losing enteropathy. Strongly associated with *H. pylori*, which should be eradicated. Rugal hypertrophy at endoscopy must be distinguished from lymphoma. Associated with adenocarcinoma
- Lymphocytic—rare, most commonly presents in the 6th decade, associated with weight loss, anorexia or epigastric pain. A varioliform pattern in the fundus may be seen at endoscopy
- 'Snake skin'—descriptive endoscopic term for portal hypertensive gastropathy (p.152)

Management
- General measures (such as avoiding alcohol, NSAIDs and smoking, although the latter not proven) are appropriate for all symptomatic patients
- *H. pylori*-positive gastritis is almost invariably treated with eradication therapy (Table 3.2, p. 89). There is little evidence of benefit, but treatment can be justified because it is not possible to predict the outcome of gastritis in any individual
- Symptomatic treatment (with antacids or drugs for non-ulcer dyspepsia, p. 80) is suitable when a specific cause cannot be identified
- Autoimmune-associated gastritis—measure serum B_{12} and if < 150 ng/L, start intramuscular hydroxycobalamin 1000 µg every 3 months for life
- Intestinal metaplasia—not an indication for treatment or repeat endoscopy, unless associated with a gastric ulcer

3.5 Gastric ulcer

Gastric ulcers are less common than duodenal ulcers before the age of 40 years, but become more common in the elderly. Ulcers on the greater curve, fundus and in the antrum are more commonly malignant. Features and treatment for gastric and duodenal ulcers are compared in Table 3.4.

Table 3.4 Practical differences between duodenal and gastric ulcers

	Duodenal	Gastric
Clinical*		
age	Mainly young	Mainly elderly
gender	Male	Either
pain	Nocturnal or before meals	Soon after eating
vomiting	Unusual	Common
appetite	Normal, increased or afraid to eat	Anorexia
weight	Stable	Loss
Endoscopy	Only for diagnosis	Repeat until healing confirmed
Biopsies	Antral for *H. pylori*	Multiple biopsies and brushings
Treatment	*H. pylori* eradication (Box 3.1)	Acid suppression if *H. pylori* negative or on NSAIDs
Relapse	Endoscopy only if clinically indicated or to *H. pylori* status	Endoscopy essential. Consider surgery
Maintenance	Failed *H. pylori* eradication complications, NSAIDs, aspirin	Failed *H. pylori* eradication NSAIDs, unacceptable operative risk
Surgery	Intractable haemorrhage, perforation, pyloric stenosis	Failure to heal, or persistent suspicion of malignancy

*None of the differences are diagnostic without endoscopy.

Causes

- More than 60% of benign, non-NSAID gastric ulcers are associated with *H. pylori*. Infection is characterised by chronic corpusitis
- Drug-related ulcers (NSAIDs, steroids) are more common in the presence of *H. pylori*. There are often few symptoms before a complication occurs. Steroids do not cause ulcers without concomitant NSAIDs
- Gastric ulcers are associated with smoking. Environmental stress may be weakly associated
- Acute ulcers or 'erosions' (small, superficial ulcers) are a separate entity and related to drugs (aspirin) or physiological stress (Cushing's or Curling's ulcers, after neurosurgery or burns, respectively)
- Contributing factors include impairment of the mucus–bicarbonate barrier, deficient gastric mucosal blood flow (possibly related to prostaglandin E_2, PGE_2) and acid-pepsin damage. Duodenogastric reflux of bile may damage the mucosa. The dictum 'no acid, no ulcer' is valid, but acid secretion in patients with gastric ulcers is frequently in the low to normal range

Clinical features

- Ulcers cannot be diagnosed reliably by history or physical examination, nor can gastric or duodenal ulcers be differentiated on clinical grounds. 'Typical' ulcer pain (epigastric, related to meals and relieved by antacids) is non-specific (Table 3.1, p. 77)
- Vomiting, weight loss or unremitting pain sometimes predominate in elderly patients with a gastric ulcer, but malignancy must be excluded by multiple-targeted biopsy and brush cytology. Some may be asymptomatic, especially NSAID-associated ulcers, perhaps because of the analgesic effect of the drug
- Complications (haematemesis or perforation, p. 17) may be the presenting feature

Investigations

Endoscopy
- Multiple-targeted rim and crater biopsies as well as brush cytology are mandatory
- When gastric ulcers are diagnosed at emergency endoscopy for bleeding, brush cytology can be taken safely, but a further endoscopy is best arranged after the bleeding has stopped, to allow biopsies to be taken
- Repeat endoscopy after 8–12 weeks of treatment should be booked at the time of diagnosis, to confirm healing. The ulcer site must be biopsied, even if the ulcer has healed. Further endoscopies, with more brushings and biopsies, are necessary for persistent ulcers until complete healing has occurred
- Symptomatic relapse after a gastric ulcer has been diagnosed is an indication for repeat endoscopy
- If a gastric ulcer is shown on a barium meal, endoscopy should be arranged for biopsies and brushings

Management

General
- *H. pylori* eradication is the first-line of treatment for uncomplicated gastric ulcers (Table 3.2, p. 89). Acid suppression is usually continued for 4 weeks or until repeat endoscopy for ulcers complicated by bleeding, but may be unnecessary
- Stop smoking—increases the healing rate and decreases relapse
- Alcohol intake—curtail if excessive (> 21 units/week for women, > 28 units/week for men), but abstinence is unnecessary

Which acid suppressant?
- All PPIs heal 90% benign gastric ulcers in 4–6 weeks. Costs vary and local policy is best followed
- H_2-receptor antagonists are now rarely used. They remain effective (up to 90% healing), but take longer to work (6–12 weeks).
- NSAID-associated gastric ulcers are best healed by full-dose PPIs, which should be continued if NSAIDs cannot be stopped

Maintenance treatment
- Indicated for patients with cardiorespiratory disease, or any disorder that would affect survival in the event of developing complications of a recurrent ulcer. Lansoprazole 15 mg or omeprazole 10 mg daily is usually sufficient
- If NSAIDs cannot be stopped (Section 3.10)

Resistant ulcers
- Ulcers that have not healed after 8 weeks of treatment must be rebiopsied and brushed for cytology, as well as taking biopsies from the antrum and corpus to check for *H. pylori* eradication

- For unhealed ulcers, prescribe second-line eradication therapy (Table 3.2, p. 89) if *H. pylori* still present, then double the dose of PPI for a further 8 weeks and arrange a repeat endoscopy
- Poor compliance is the commonest cause of failure to heal
- Persistent failure of a gastric ulcer to heal after 12–16 weeks of treatment may be due to malignancy (which can be missed, even with biopsies and brushings), and is an indication for surgery. Endoscopic ultrasound, if available, can help discriminate between benign and malignant ulceration
- Long-term PPIs are appropriate in those unfit for surgery

Indications for surgery
- Complications—bleeding (but eradicate *H. pylori* after surgery, p. 88); perforation (but continue PPIs after surgery, p. 25)
- Failure to heal after 12–16 weeks of treatment, unless the risks of operation are very high
- Relapse on maintenance therapy
- A Billroth partial gastrectomy is the standard operation, carrying < 2% operative mortality and 10–30% incidence of long-term sequelae (p. 106)

Special categories
- Giant ulcers (> 2.5 cm diameter)—carry no special risk of malignancy
- Antral ulcers—20% are malignant
- Prepyloric ulcers—behave like duodenal ulcers
- Pyloric canal ulcers—vomiting and weight loss are common; if ulceration extends through to the duodenum, consider lymphoma
- Combined gastric and duodenal ulcers—bleeding and obstruction are said to be more common

Complications
- Complications of gastric ulcers may occur without any preceding symptoms, especially in those taking NSAIDs
- 50% recur without *H. pylori* eradication therapy
- 25% bleed (Section 1.5, p. 8)
- 10% perforate (p. 25)
- Fibrosis causing deformity ('hourglass' or 'teapot' stomach) is rare. Pyloric stenosis may complicate prepyloric ulceration
- Carcinoma at the site of a 'benign' ulcer is the result of an initial misdiagnosis, rather than malignant transformation, even if the ulcer has responded to conventional treatment

3.6 Gastric carcinoma

Gastric cancer is the fourth most common cause of cancer deaths in Europe and the USA. There is widespread geographical variation in incidence and prognosis, but the incidence of cancer of the antrum and body (corpus) of the stomach is falling in the West, presumably because of falling prevalence of *H. pylori* infection. In contrast, the incidence of cancer of the cardia is rising. The reason is unknown. This cancer is three times as common in men as in women. 80% of cases are diagnosed > 65 years of age.

Aetiology

- Twin studies indicate a degree of genetic susceptibility. Genes for sporadic cancers remain undiscovered
- Blood group A is associated with a 20% increase in risk. Other genetic associations include variants in IL-1β and NAT-1 genes, which together account for 48% of the attributable risk for sporadic gastric cancer
- 3% are due to clearly inherited predisposition syndromes, including familial adenomatous polyposis (APC gene), hereditary non-polyposis colon cancer type B (mismatch repair gene), Peutz–Jeghers syndrome (unknown gene), Cowden's syndrome (unknown gene) and hereditary diffuse gastric cancer (CDH1 gene)
- Chronic *H. pylori* infection—causes gastric intestinal metaplasia in about 3% and atrophy, increasing the risk of cancer 2.5-fold. It is classified by the World Health Organization (WHO) as a class I (definite) carcinogen
- Chronic benign gastric ulcers do not predispose to cancer despite their association with *H. pylori*
- Early gastric cancer may develop at sites of intestinal metaplasia, but metaplasia is not definitely premalignant
- Gastric adenomatous polyps—unusual, but have the same malignant potential as in the colon (p. 296)
- Diet—may explain the high incidence in Japan, China and Central America, since the incidence declines in migrant populations. *N*-nitrosamines have been implicated. The prevalence of *H. pylori* is also high in these populations. Dietary protection through antioxidant effects of vitamins C, E, or beta carotene remain unproven
- Low socio-economic class—incidence five times higher in labourers than professionals, which may reflect a higher prevalence of *H. pylori* infection
- Gastric surgery—increased incidence 15 years after partial gastrectomy is probably real and may be explained by the prevalence of *H. pylori*
- Pernicious anaemia—the risk (about 1%) is increased

Clinical features

General

- Dyspepsia is usual, but non-specific, poorly related to meals and relief by simple antacids is common
- Anorexia and weight loss are common presenting features and often indicate incurable disease
- Haematemesis is unusual
- Signs are typically absent until incurable disease exists
- Metastases to the lungs (lymphangitis carcinomatosa), bone or brain may be the presenting feature. A supraclavicular node (Virchow's node, Troisier's sign), or migratory phlebothrombosis (Trousseau's sign) are uncommon

- Dermatomyositis and acanthosis nigricans are most frequently associated with gastric carcinoma, but are rare
- H_2-receptor antagonist or PPIs can temporarily relieve symptoms and heal malignant ulcers, which can be a diagnostic pitfall

Pathology
- No classification is satisfactory, but there is a spectrum from polypoid lesions through ulcers to diffuse infiltrating cancer (linitis plastica). All types are adenocarcinomas
- The degree of differentiation, local and remote spread affect the prognosis, but not histological type (mucinous, signet ring). Tumours are multiple in 10%

Early gastric cancer
- Defined as adenocarcinoma confined to the mucosa or submucosa and distinguished by an excellent prognosis (90% 5-year survival) after resection. Early gastric cancer is recognised endoscopically at a curable stage, and is probably a distinct entity rather than an early stage of the more common variety. It is often asymptomatic unless the lesion ulcerates, when dyspepsia occurs
- Endoscopy shows a superficial excavated or slightly protuberant lesion, which may look insignificant. Biopsy of any gastric lesion is therefore essential if early gastric cancer is to be diagnosed. Local venous or lymphatic metastases are sometimes present, but the prognosis can still be good

Investigations
New onset dyspepsia with alarm symptoms (Box 3.1, p. 78) demands investigation (p. 78). Once the diagnosis has been made, a search for clinically silent metastases is indicated, before a decision about treatment is made.

Diagnostic
- Endoscopy—antral ulcers, or rolled and irregular edges of an ulcer crater favour malignancy, but multiple biopsies and brushings must be taken from all gastric ulcers

Staging of disease
- Blood tests—leucoerythroblastic anaemia or abnormal liver function tests suggest incurable disease. Elevated ALP may be due to bony metastases if the γ-glutamyl-transferase is normal
- Chest X-ray—look for a pleural effusion, solitary metastasis or reticular shadowing from lymphangitis
- Spiral contrast-enhanced CT scans and EUS are the principal complementary modalities used. EUS is superior to CT for the T and N staging of gastric cancer. Spiral CT will detect 75–80% of hepatic and pulmonary metastases (Fig. 3.2)
- Laparoscopy is commonly performed, because this is the only way that peritoneal seedlings will be identified prior to full laparotomy. 40% of patients found to have peritoneal spread at an 'open and close' laparotomy die within 12 weeks

Early diagnosis
- An early diagnosis programme is one reason for the better outcome in Japan (25% overall 5-year survival) where a higher proportion of early gastric cancers are detected

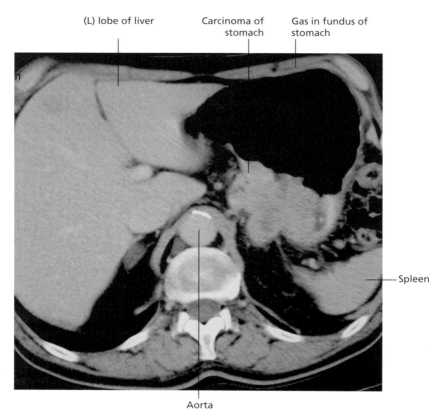

Fig. 3.2 Radiological appearances of gastric cancer. CT scan showing gastric cancer. CT scans of the stomach are easy to overinterpret if the stomach is not distended. Confirmation by endoscopy and biopsy is essential.

- Public awareness and early investigation of dyspeptic symptoms are essential to early diagnosis, but outside Japan it has not been possible to show a survival benefit in the small number of patients who present with isolated dyspepsia compared to those with alarm symptoms
- Screening asymptomatic individuals (even those with pernicious anaemia or previous gastric surgery) is not justified in Europe or the USA

Management

Surgery
- Indicated for patients aged < 75 years with no signs of metastases and otherwise in good health—less than one-third of all patients
- Radical surgery ('R2 resection') has a mortality of 10% and postgastrectomy sequelae are more common

- The operation rate, curative resection rate and survival are appreciably higher in Japan, possibly as a result of population screening, earlier detection and more aggressive surgery
- Most surgery is palliative, to relieve obstruction

Adjuvant therapy
- Post-operative chemotherapy may offer a small survival advantage. There is at present insufficient evidence for routine use and it should be used only in clinical trials under specialist oncological supervision
- First-line palliative chemotherapy with epirubicin, cisplatin and 5-fluouracil (ECF) may help patients with a good performance status and no comorbid disease
- Second-line palliative treatment with docetaxel and epirubicin may help patients who fail to respond or relapse after ECF therapy
- Chemotherapy to downstage locally advanced disease prior to surgery is under trial

Supportive therapy
- Pain may be relieved by omeprazole 20 mg daily, unless it is due to infiltration, when opiates are necessary. It is important to ensure adequate pain control
- Explanation to the family, home support and liaison with the general practitioner are vital aspects of terminal care (p. 130)

Prognosis
- Local recurrence is the main cause of failure. The prognosis will only be improved by earlier detection followed by effective surgery
- The 5-year survival for all patients is 9%
- Following curative surgery the 5-year survival in the UK is 23%
- Median survival for inoperable disease is 4 months

3.7 Other gastric tumours

Lymphoma
Gastric lymphoma includes primary gastric lymphoma (PGL) and systemic lymphoma with secondary gastric involvement (SGL).

Primary gastric lymphoma
- 5% of all gastric malignancies
- Patients are usually aged 55–70 years. Male predominance
- Relative risk increases fivefold in patients with AIDS
- By definition there is no systemic involvement until very late
- > 90% of PGL are B-cell non-Hodgkin's lymphoma. Of these, the majority are high-grade, diffuse, large-cell lymphoma. A minority are characterised as low-grade MALT lymphoma.

Clinical features
- Gastric lymphoma cannot be distinguished clinically from a benign ulcer or gastric cancer
- Weight loss, nausea and vomiting are said to occur earlier than in gastric cancer and haematemesis may be more common
- An epigastric mass is palpable in about 30%, but splenomegaly and peripheral lymphadenopathy are unusual
- Patients are usually aged 55–70 years

Diagnostic and staging investigations
- Blood tests—a microcytic anaemia and raised ESR are common
- Endoscopy—appearances are varied and may be similar to a carcinoma. Multiple ulcerated nodules, transpyloric infiltration and giant rugae favour lymphoma. Deep, multiple biopsies (best performed using jumbo forceps, saline-assisted mucosal resection or by snaring a mucosal fold) are necessary, but may still not be positive. Diagnostic laparotomy and frozen section biopsies are then indicated
- Other methods to improve the diagnostic yield from endoscopic biopsy specimens should be discussed with the pathologist and include the use of immunohistochemical techniques as well as PCR assays to detect monoclonal B-cell populations
- Endoscopic ultrasound is the procedure of choice to assess the size and depth of lesion and the presence of perigastric lesions
- Spiral CT is recommended to evaluate lymph nodes above and below the diaphragm
- Bone marrow infiltration indicates stage IV disease (Table 3.5, p. 106)

Treatment
Regimens are complex and evolving. Specialist oncological advice is recommended. General guidelines are as follows.
- Surgery for:
  - stage IE disease (Table 3.5, p. 106)
  - complications (haemorrhage or obstruction)
- Radiotherapy for stage IIE disease, often with chemotherapy
- Chemotherapy for stage IIIE or stage IVE disease

MALT lymphoma
- B-cell lymphoma due to an immunological response to chronic *H. pylori* infection. Associated with *H. pylori* Cag A strains
- Histological hallmarks are lymphoepithelial lesions due to tissue invasion by atypical lymphocytes, and reactive lymphoid follicles
- After diagnosis, patients are best referred for management to a centre where clinical trials of MALT lymphoma treatment are in progress
- *H. pylori* eradication leads to 70–80% complete remission in patients with stage IE$_1$ low-grade MALT lymphoma. Endoscopic evaluation is repeated at 2 months, then 6-monthly for the first 2 years, and thereafter annually
- Endoscopic mucosal resection, radical gastrectomy, radiotherapy and mono-chemotherapy are alternatives for patients with stage IE$_1$ disease who are *H. pylori*-negative, or who remain persistently *H. pylori*-positive

- Chemotherapy using the CHOP regime (cyclophosphamide, hydroxydaunomycin, Oncovin, prednisone) is used for advanced disease

Polyps

- Hyperplastic or cystic fundal polyps are regenerative and the commonest epithelial lesions (85%). They are of no significance. It is good endoscopic practice to biopsy all mucosal lesions, because early gastric cancer may look insignificant (p. 97).
- True adenomatous polyps are unusual but are premalignant. Endoscopic removal or resection is indicated. They may be associated with colonic polyps, so colonoscopy is appropriate

Gastrointestinal stromal tumours (leiomyomas and leiomyosarcomas)

- Located in the muscularis propria and submucosa. Only 50% have an intragastric component. The defining feature is expression of the c-KIT oncogene, a tyrosine kinase receptor for stem cell factor that regulates the growth of GISTs. Expression is identified on immunohistochemistry
- Common presentations include blood loss due to ulceration, abdominal pain and a mass. Endoscopy characteristically shows an umbilicated, broad-based polyp with central ulceration
- Immunohistochemical staining for c-kit expression is diagnostic
- Slow, indolent nature makes definitions of malignancy inapplicable and necessitates long-term follow-up
- Predictors of malignant potential are size, mitotic count and the presence of a missense mutation in the c-kit gene
- There are no trial data to guide management. Traditionally wedge or radical resection has been carried out. The high rate of recurrence of both benign and malignant lesions has prompted the recent use of adjuvant chemo- and radiotherapy
- Imatinib (Glivec®), an oral monoclonal antibody against the tyrosine kinase receptor, is effective for > 60% malignant GISTs. Specialist advice should be sought

Other tumours

- Submucosal lipomas may reach a large size and bleed. Carcinoid tumours are more common in patients with pernicious anaemia. Secondary deposits and heterotopic pancreas are extremely rare
- 'Microcarcinoids' are a histological description of collections of enterochromaffin cells that occur in some patients on long-term PPIs or pernicious anaemia. They are unrelated to carcinoid tumours and have no clinical significance other than being a trap for the unwary

3.8 Duodenitis

Duodenitis is an endoscopic diagnosis and may not account for the patient's symptoms. If the patient is *H. pylori*-positive, as is commonly the case, it is best regarded as an expression of duodenal ulcer disease.

Causes
- Almost always caused by *H. pylori* colonising islands of gastric metaplasia in the duodenal bulb
- Very rarely due to Crohn's disease, cytomegalovirus, ectopic pancreatic tissue, nematodes or sarcoidosis

Clinical features
- Duodenitis causes variable symptoms that may be provoked by alcohol or drugs. Ulcer-type pain, dysmotility symptoms (p. 79) or no symptoms may be present. Duodenitis never causes anaemia, but is sometimes the only abnormality found at endoscopy for haematemesis
- Recognised endoscopically as patchy erythema or superficial erosions (salt-and-pepper duodenitis) in the first part of the duodenum. The mucosa can be nodular and the second part of the duodenum is normal
- Histology does not correlate with the endoscopic appearance, but biopsies may show *H. pylori*

Management
- *H. pylori*-positive duodenitis should be treated with eradication therapy (Table 3.2, p. 89)
- Treatment of *H. pylori*-negative duodenitis is empirical and frequently disappointing. It depends on the characteristics of the symptoms (Section 3.1, p. 77)

3.9 Duodenal ulcer

Duodenal ulcers (DU) are four times more common than gastric ulcers below the age of 40 years and are more common in men. Overall incidence is falling in the UK and USA due to decreased prevalence of *H. pylori*, but the incidence among women and older people is increasing. The number of DU-related hospital admissions is rising due to NSAIDs. Almost all are caused by *H. pylori* or NSAIDs, but the number of *H. pylori*-negative, non-NSAID DUs has increased in the last decade.

Causes

H. pylori and genetic factors
- *H. pylori*: More than 95% of non-drug related DUs are due to *H. pylori* antritis, causing hypergastrinaemia, high acid secretion and gastric metaplasia in the duodenal cap, which is then colonised by *H. pylori*
- Familial aggregation and twin studies indicate a genetic susceptibility. 20–50% of DU patients have a positive family history of DU compared to 5–15% of non-ulcer subjects
- Blood group O (relative risk 1.25) and non-secretion of blood group substances in saliva are weakly associated with duodenal ulceration

Ulcerogenic drugs
- Drugs (NSAIDs, aspirin and possibly steroids) are associated with bleeding and perforation, but not necessarily with uncomplicated ulcers (Section 1.5, p. 17)
- The elderly are at risk and may be asymptomatic before presenting with a complication

Other factors
- Smoking retards healing and increases the likelihood of relapse. This may reflect the effect of smoking on *H. pylori* (p. 90)
- Stress is said to be related, but cannot be quantified. It may contribute to the non-specific association with chronic renal failure, lung disease and cirrhosis

Clinical features
- Epigastric pain classically occurs before meals (hunger pain), wakes the patient at night and recurs several times a year for a few weeks. It may radiate to the back
- Vomiting and weight loss may indicate pyloric stenosis
- Examination, apart from epigastric tenderness, is unremarkable in the absence of complications
- Symptoms frequently fail to fit this pattern and all conditions that may cause dyspepsia (Table 3.1, p. 77) are included in the differential diagnosis

Investigations

Initial presentation
- Testing for *H. pylori* (p. 86) or endoscopy are appropriate (p. 78). *H. pylori*-induced DUs occur almost exclusively in the cap whereas NSAID ulcers may be found in the 2nd part of the duodenum. Ulcers more than 3 cm beyond the pylorus are atypical (< 2%) and require a search for underlying disease (see below)
- Biopsies should be taken from the antrum to diagnose *H. pylori* infection, and from the ulcer if unusual causes are suspected (Crohn's disease, lymphoma, ectopic pancreatic tissue)
- Blood tests to detect anaemia or hepatic dysfunction should be performed. An elevated ESR does not occur in uncomplicated ulceration and raises the possibility of Crohn's or other disease

Management

H. pylori eradication
- All *H. pylori*-positive DU patients need eradication therapy (Table 3.2, p. 89), prescribed at diagnosis
- Simple DUs need no additional acid-suppressive treatment
- For complicated ulcers (e.g. after a bleed), acid suppression with a PPI (Section 3.5, p. 94) should be continued for 4 weeks. Some gastroenterologists advise continuing treatment until ulcer healing has been confirmed by repeat endoscopy in these patients, but otherwise repeat endoscopy is unnecessary

- Guidelines for gastric ulcers (stopping smoking, reducing alcohol intake, regular meals, p. 94) apply equally to DUs. A summary of the differences between gastric ulcers and DUs is shown in Table 3.4 (p. 93)

Resistant ulcers
- Patients with persistent symptoms after *H. pylori* eradication, or after 4 weeks' acid suppression if *H. pylori*-negative, should be reviewed. Drug compliance, smoking habits or alternative causes of dyspepsia (Table 3.1, p. 77) should be considered
- Repeat endoscopy is necessary to diagnose a resistant ulcer, but a urea breath test performed > 4 weeks after eradication therapy will determine whether treatment has worked (p. 86)
- If there is any doubt about the DU, biopsies must be taken from the ulcer at the repeat endoscopy and fasting gastrin concentrations checked. Acid suppression causes hypergastrinaemia and drugs should be stopped for 2 weeks before the test if clinically possible
- Failure to heal on PPIs suggests poor compliance, or an unusual cause (discussed below)

Subsequent presentations
- Reflux symptoms may only become apparent after *H. pylori* eradication. This has to be distinguished from ulcer relapse
- First recurrence of ulcer-type symptoms, in a patient who has had an endoscopically diagnosed DU, can be treated without further investigation
- Further recurrence and persistent pain are indications for repeat endoscopy and biopsies to exclude unusual causes

H-pylori and NSAID-negative duodenal ulcers
Many of these patients will be labelled as having idiopathic ulcer disease, but consider the following.

Causes of false-negative *H-pylori* tests
- Individuals taking antibiotics, H_2 antagonists or PPIs
- Atrophic gastritis or intestinal metaplasia with reduced density of *H. pylori*
- Unreliability of the rapid urease test (but not other tests) during bleeding due to the buffering action of albumin in blood

To minimise false-negative tests:
- Delay testing for 4 weeks after antibiotics or 2 weeks after PPIs
- Two or more antral biopsies from separate sites
- Alternative tests for *H. pylori* on *H. pylori*-negative patients

Inadvertent aspirin or NSAID ingestion
- Many alternative therapies contain anti-inflammatory agents

Other drug-related ulcers
- Bisphosphonates, mycophenolate, potassium chloride

- Intravenous fluoxuridine
- Crack cocaine, amphetamines

Zollinger–Ellison syndrome
- Gastrin-secreting neuroendocrine tumours present with recurrent, multiple, severe duodenal ulceration typically distal to the duodenal bulb. Patients typically have diarrhoea, due to excess acid and inactivation of pancreatic lipase; 25% have other endocrine tumours as part of multiple endocrine neoplasia type 1
- Gastrin concentrations (p. 432) are high. H_2-receptor antagonists, PPIs and hypochlorhydria may also cause hypergastrinaemia. The secretin test (> 100% rise in gastrin with a gastrinoma) is not always reliable and gastric acid studies (increased basal and peak acid output) can also give false-positive results
- Localisation is difficult because multiple tumours, sometimes in the duodenal submucosa, and metastases are common. Somatostatin receptor scintigraphy (Octreoscan, Fig 7.5, p. 240), endoscopic ultrasound, pancreatic MRI, or selective angiography may be needed
- Referral to a specialist centre is advised. Resection of the tumour is usual. When surgical treatment is inappropriate, PPIs should be used in a sufficient dose to keep basal acid output < 10 mmol/h.
- Octreotide is reserved for incomplete resection
- Outpatients should have their blood pressure, calcium, electrolytes and liver function checked at intervals to detect associated endocrinopathies. Gastrin levels are uninterpretable in patients taking PPIs
- Gastrinomas grow very slowly and prolonged survival is possible even after hepatic metastases have occurred

Rare infectious causes
- *Helicobacter heilmannii* may be transmitted to man from domestic animals. It has a lower pathogenicity than *H. pylori* but may occasionally cause duodenal ulceration. It appears to be sensitive to standard *H. pylori* eradication regimes
- Cytomegalovirus (CMV) is a rare cause of duodenal ulceration in transplant recipients and human immunodeficiency virus (HIV)-positive patients
- Other rare causes include tuberculosis and syphilis

Other disorders
- Systemic mastocytosis causes duodenal ulceration, diarrhoea and skin manifestations. Serum histamine is elevated and mast cells infiltrate affected tissue
- Crohn's disease
- Lymphoma, carcinoma
- Radiation-induced ulceration

Maintenance treatment
- No evidence exists to guide long-term management, but maintenance therapy with PPIs seems logical in drug-related or *H. pylori*-negative 'idiopathic' ulcers, and in those in whom eradication treatment has failed

- Stopping smoking is sensible but unproven
- Patients with severe symptoms sometimes request surgery, but the risk of postoperative sequelae (Section 3.10) including recurrent ulceration below must be discussed

Indications for surgery

Surgery for duodenal ulceration is of historical interest except for complications, including:
- Continuing, recurrent or major haemorrhage (p. 13)
- Perforation (p. 26)
- Pyloric stenosis—profuse postprandial vomiting is characteristic, with an audible succussion splash, but is now rarely due to benign duodenal ulceration. Hypokalaemia is more common than metabolic alkalosis. Antral malignancy must be excluded by endoscopic biopsies. Intravenous fluids and nasogastric suction are required prior to definitive treatment. Endoscopic balloon dilatation for benign pyloric stenosis gives transient relief, but surgery is usually necessary later
- Resistant ulcers, but other pathology (e.g. Zollinger–Ellison syndrome) must first be excluded

3.10 Sequelae of gastric surgery

Gastric surgery was declining before the introduction of H_2-antagonists and has declined further since the introduction of effective *H. pylori* eradication. It is now the province of malignant disease, and the complications of surgery are rarely seen by physicians. Management remains relevant for some older patients and because of decreasing familiarity among surgical colleagues.

Derangement of gastric function causes symptoms in nearly all patients after surgery, but adaptation occurs within weeks. After 6 months only 10–15% have persistent symptoms. A combination of problems is common in those affected, and few are specific to the type of surgery.

Vagotomy and antrectomy have the lowest risk of recurrent ulcers, but other complications are common. Highly selective vagotomy has the lowest rate of complications but a higher incidence of recurrent ulceration (Fig. 3.3).

Table 3.5 Ann Arbor classification of extranodal lymphoma (modified by Musshoff)

	5-year survival (%)
IE Lymphoma restricted to gastrointestinal tract	80%
IE_1 Infiltration confined to submucosa	
IE_2 Infiltration beyond submucosa	
IIE Nodal involvement (infradiaphragmatic)	40%
IIE_1 Regional nodes	50%
IIE_2 Extraregional nodes	35%
IIIE Nodal involvement (both sides of diaphragm)	30%
IVE Involvement of extra-gastrointestinal organs	5%

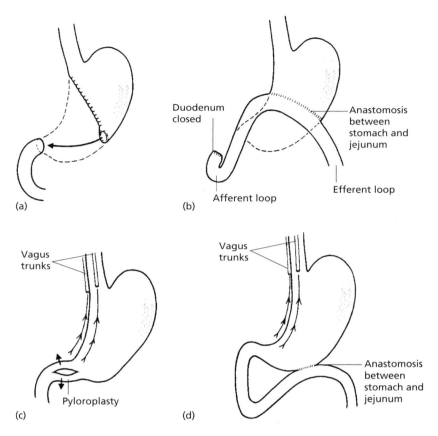

Fig. 3.3 Anatomy of gastric operations. (a) Billroth I partial gastrectomy. (b) Polya gastrectomy. (c) Vagotomy and pyloroplasty. (d) Vagotomy and gastroenterostomy.

Diarrhoea

- More common after truncal vagotomy than gastric resection
- Rapid gastric emptying and fast intestinal transit are the usual mechanisms, but coeliac disease, immunoglobulin deficiency and bacterial overgrowth should be considered
- Treatment with small, more frequent meals, codeine phosphate up to 120 mg/day or loperamide up to 16 mg/day in divided doses is indicated

Gastric stasis

- Persistent postoperative nasogastric drainage, or later postprandial vomiting, may be due to mechanical obstruction or dysmotility
- Barium meal confirms stasis and may give more information than endoscopy. Both investigations are needed to demonstrate patency of the anastomosis and exclude a stomal ulcer
- A prokinetic agent is worth trying for gastric stasis without mechanical obstruction
- Surgical revision is necessary for outlet obstruction

Dumping

Early dumping
- Rapid gastric evacuation results in a hypertonic load to the small intestine, triggering autonomic reflexes
- Characteristic symptoms are epigastric fullness, faintness and palpitations 30 min after eating
- Relieved by fasting
- Helpful advice includes eating smaller meals low in sugar and high in fibre to decrease osmotic load and slow gastric emptying (try Guar gum 5 g with each meal, but difficult to obtain). Drink before or after, rather than during, meals
- Surgical revision is a last resort

Late dumping
- Rebound hypoglycaemia 2–3 h after eating is caused by rapid carbohydrate absorption releasing excessive insulin
- Relieved by eating

The timing of symptoms and effect of eating are the main differences between late and early dumping. Symptoms and management are similar

Recurrent ulcer
- All ulcers should be biopsied
- Gastrin concentrations need checking, but very few are due to Zollinger–Ellison syndrome (p. 105)
- Acid suppression with PPIs followed by maintenance treatment is appropriate. Sucralfate can help. Smoking and NSAIDs should be avoided
- Ulceration may be due to the effect of bile or pancreatic enzymes rather than acid damage

Bilious vomiting
- Free biliary reflux into the stomach is usually asymptomatic
- Burning discomfort with morning bile-stained vomiting can be treated with a prokinetic agent (such as metoclopramide three times daily), cholestyramine 4–12 g/day, or aluminium-containing antacids (aluminium hydroxide mixture, 10–20 mL as needed)
- Severe bilious vomiting may be an indication for surgical revision

Miscellaneous problems after gastrectomy

Anaemia
- Inadequate dietary intake is the most common cause of iron deficiency after gastric surgery. Malabsorption of iron should only be diagnosed after other (colonic) causes have been excluded by barium enema or colonoscopy, which is mandatory to exclude a colonic neoplasm, especially in those aged > 45 years
- Vitamin B_{12} deficiency after partial gastrectomy (usually presenting as macrocytosis) is due to bacterial overgrowth, ileal malabsorption or autoimmune gastritis, since sufficient parietal cells usually remain to produce intrinsic factor

- Osteomalacia due to mild steatorrhoea and calcium chelation is exceptional. Coeliac disease should be excluded

Afferent loop syndrome
- Rapid distension followed by emptying of a kinked afferent loop after a meal causes sudden pain and vomiting. Treatment is surgical after radiological demonstration
- Bacterial overgrowth in the loop after a Polya (Billroth 2) gastrectomy is rare. Metronidazole is indicated, but repeated courses are often needed

Cancer
- The incidence of gastric cancer 15–25 years after resection (but not vagotomy) is increased about fourfold
- Prospective endoscopic surveillance is not indicated, but postoperative dyspepsia needs investigating

3.11 Clinical dilemmas

Persistent dyspepsia despite treatment
Persistent dyspepsia after an identifiable cause has been treated is usually due to a concomitant motility disorder (non-ulcer or functional dyspepsia). A definitive diagnosis of non-ulcer dyspepsia and explanation assists management (p. 79). Treatment aims at symptomatic relief.

First steps
- Careful history and re-examination
- Consider endoscopy but this is not essential in the absence of alarm symptoms

Subsequent investigations
- If the full blood count, ESR and liver function tests are normal, further investigations are not indicated in most patients
- Abdominal ultrasound to exclude gall stones and pancreatic lesions, or small bowel radiology to exclude Crohn's disease, is necessary in a minority
- Dietary modulation and outpatient review is often better than further invasive investigations if the pain persists without other signs
- Oesophageal pH monitoring, or mesenteric angiography (if there is postprandial pain and weight loss), occasionally allow a diagnosis of reflux or mesenteric ischaemia (very rare) to be made in difficult cases

Dyspepsia and NSAIDs
70% of the population of the UK and USA > 65 years take NSAIDs weekly. 15–40% of these patients experience dyspepsia. Symptoms are not a reliable predictor of complications and 50–60% of patients who develop an ulcer or life-threatening complication have no prior warning.

Serious complications occur in 1.5% of NSAID users per year. The relative risk of a serious adverse gastrointestinal event is 3.8% for NSAID users and 1.6% for aspirin users.

The following approach is recommended

- Critically assess the need for NSAIDs. Stop the drug and substitute acetomenophen/paracetamol if possible. Reassess symptoms after 2 weeks (a pain and stiffness chart, scored out of 10 each morning, may help)
- Use the lowest dose for the shortest possible time
- The gastrointestinal risks are cumulative and linear. Review patients regularly to ensure NSAIDs are still required
- Use the least ulcerogenic NSAIDs (e.g. ibuprofen, or prodrugs such as nabumetone)
- Enteric-coated, modified release or rectal administration do not reduce the incidence of peptic ulcer complications, and COX-2 inhibitors cause renal and heart failure as often as unselective NSAIDs
- Use no more than one oral NSAID at a time
- NSAIDs inhibit the antiplatelet action of low-dose aspirin and may increase the risk of ulceration. The combination is best avoided
- Moderate alcohol
- High alcohol intake is a risk factor for serious gastrointestinal complications
- Eradicate *H. pylori* if appropriate
- *H. pylori* probably predisposes to NSAID-induced ulceration, but testing and treating cannot be recommended for all patients prior to starting NSAIDs. Pretreatment is justifiable for patients with a history of peptic ulceration
- Consider gastroduodenal protection
- In high-risk patients give full dose PPI (lansoprazole 30 mg, omeprazole 20 mg). The following patients are at high risk:
  - Age > 60 years (60–69 years, RR = 2.4; 70–80 years, RR = 4.5; > 80 years, RR = 9.2)
  - Past history of PU disease or serious gastrointestinal complication
  - Concomitant oral steroids or oral anticoagulants
  - Comorbidity
  - Requirement for prolonged use of maximal dose NSAIDs
- Both misoprostol 800 µg daily and PPIs are better than H_2 antagonists. Misoprostol may be more effective for *H. pylori*-negative patients, but few patients tolerate this dose without diarrhoea. PPIs are more effective for dyspepsia and less likely to cause diarrhoea
- Consider COX-2 selective inhibitors, if available, but recognise risk of vascular events
- For patients at high risk (above)
- Improved gastrointestinal toxicity is probably due to lack of dual cyclo-oxygenase isoform inhibition (rather than cyclo-oxygenase-1 sparing actions, as previously thought)
- Rofecoxib and celecoxib have been withdrawn in the US, UK and some other countries (2004), because of an increased risk of ischaemic vascular events
- COX-2 inhibitors should be used with caution (or not at all) in patients with cardiovascular or renal disease, or those on aspirin, just as for NSAIDs

4 Pancreas

4.1 Acute pancreatitis

The distinguishing features of acute pancreatitis, predisposing factors, other causes of a raised serum amylase, complications and management are covered in Section 1.6 (p. 27).

Subsequent investigations
- All patients should have an ultrasound scan within 24 h of the diagnosis, to look for gallstones and to assess pancreatic size, although the pancreas may initially be obscured by bowel gas
- Repeat ultrasound should be performed if the first scan did not clearly visualise the biliary tree, and to exclude a pseudocyst if there is persistent pain or pyrexia, or if the amylase has not returned to normal after 5 days
- An ERCP is indicated urgently in the presence of common bile duct (CBD) stones, jaundice, cholangitis, or any patient with severe pancreatitis believed to be caused by gallstones (suspect if ALT > threefold elevated). Sphincterotomy is indicated if CBD stones are found, or if future cholecystectomy is contraindicated by comorbidity.
- A dilated common duct can be caused by pancreatic oedema, as well as by obstructing stories
- ERCP is also appropriate if acute pancreatitis recurs without a provoking factor, but is contraindicated in the presence of a pseudocyst. It appears to be safe to obtain a pancreatogram in acute pancreatitis

Pseudocysts
Pseudocysts complicate acute pancreatitis in < 5% and are not related to the severity of the attack. Persistent pain or elevated serum amylase suggests the diagnosis, but an abdominal mass is palpable in only 50%. Ultrasound is the simplest method of diagnosis, but CT scan is needed if the pancreas cannot be clearly seen due to overlying bowel gas.

Management
- Pain control and nutritional support are initially indicated
- Cysts < 6 cm diameter measured by ultrasound usually resolve spontaneously. Size should be monitored by ultrasound scans every few days during the early stages
- Endoscopic, percutaneous or surgical drainage is indicated if the pseudocyst continues to increase in size, or is associated with persistent pain after 6 weeks, or the development of complications such as obstructive jaundice
- Endoscopic drainage (by inserting a transduodenal or transgastric stent into the cyst to allow internal drainage) is effective in 70–90%. Pancreatic ductal anatomy is defined by ERCP and a transpapillary pancreatic stent closes any communication between the pancreatic duct and the pseudocyst. Contraindications include abscess,

gastric or duodenal varices, coagulopathy and wall thickness > 1 cm. EUS may facilitate safe endoscopic drainage
- Surgery is indicated in the presence of complex duct disruption, if the diagnosis is in doubt (e.g. possible cystic neoplasm), or when the pseudocyst is complex or necrotic (Fig. 4.1)
- Percutaneous aspiration is rarely appropriate, because recurrence is common

Complications
- Jaundice—due to compression of the bile duct
- Infection—abscess may develop spontaneously, or follow ERCP or aspiration

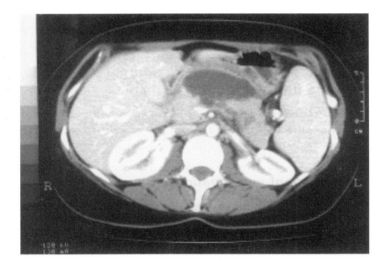

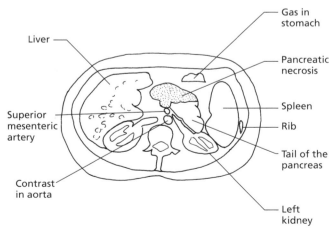

Fig. 4.1 CT scan in acute pancreatitis. Contrast-enhanced scan in a 35-year-old woman showing pancreatic necrosis shortly after developing pancreatitis.

- Haemorrhage into the cyst—causes collapse with an acute abdomen, but may present with haematemesis if the cyst erodes into the stomach, or if blood enters the duodenum through the ampulla
- Painless ascites—high amylase and protein content, exacerbated by hypoalbuminaemia. Leakage of cystic fluid is occasionally chronic
- Rupture—rare but catastrophic

Indications for surgery

Early surgery does not increase survival, but surgery is indicated for gallstones, or local complications that fail to resolve.

Gallstones

- Cholecystectomy is indicated immediately after recovery from the acute attack, preferably on the same admission
- Exploration of the common bile duct is not necessary if an ERCP and sphincterotomy have recently been performed. Whilst retained stones are the most common cause of recurrent pancreatitis after cholecystectomy, these can usually be removed at ERCP
- Cholecystectomy should be performed if pancreatitis is diagnosed during emergency laparotomy for an acute abdomen in the elderly. Peripancreatic drains should be inserted for peritoneal lavage and the abdomen closed

Local complications

- Collections of fluid (pseudocyst), pus (abscess), or necrotic tissue can be visualised by ultrasound and cause persistent pain, elevated amylase, leucocytosis or fever
- Delayed surgical drainage of a collection (6 weeks) is recommended in the absence of fever or jaundice, because 40% resolve and surgery is easier in collections that persist
- Abscesses need early operation if antibiotics (intravenous cefotaxime 1 g and metronidazole 500 mg three times daily) are to be effective
- Cystogastrostomy is most likely to prevent reaccumulation of fluid

Recurrent acute pancreatitis

The first attack of acute pancreatitis is usually the most severe, but 30% of all patients have a recurrent episode. Recurrence is common in alcoholics, or if gallstones have not been treated, but uncommon in idiopathic acute pancreatitis. An ERCP is indicated to exclude or remove retained stones, and diagnose pancreatic or ampullary tumours or pancreatic divisum.

4.2 Chronic pancreatitis

Irreversible glandular destruction may follow episodes of acute pancreatitis, or occur without an identifiable attack. The prevalence is increasing in Europe, where it is more common in men and due to alcohol. Acini are replaced by fibrous tissue causing ductular distortion and later atrophy of the islets.

Causes

- Alcohol—commonest factor (80%)
- Gallstones—very rarely cause chronic pancreatitis
- Genetic:
  - *CFTR* (cystic fibrosis transmembrane conductance regulator) mutations may cause chronic pancreatitis as part of cystic fibrosis (CF; p. 122), but are also associated with acute and chronic pancreatitis in patients who lack pulmonary manifestations of CF. Compound heterozygote individuals who possess both a severe and mild variable CFTR mutation are at greatest risk
  - *SPINK1* (serine protease inhibitor Kazal type 1) reversibly inhibits activated trypsin. The rare N34S variant is associated with chronic pancreatitis
  - PRSS1 (cationic trypsinogen gene) mutations, R122H or N29I are responsible for the majority of cases of hereditary pancreatitis (see p. 122)
- Congenital—pancreas divisum or annular pancreas
- α_1-protease deficiency
- Autoimmune
- Hypertriglyceridaemia
- Hyperparathyroidism
- Malnutrition is no longer thought to be a cause, but the high prevalence among young adults in southern India remains unexplained

Clinical features

Early disease is asymptomatic, but pain, exocrine and endocrine insufficiencies supervene in many patients. 90% loss of exocrine function is necessary before steatorrhoea develops. Acute attacks, with attendant complications, may still occur in chronic disease.

Pain

- Typically short episodes (< 10 days) of anterior pain radiating to the back, followed by long pain-free episodes. The pain may be due to increased intraductal pressure, perineural inflammation or increased visceral nociception.
- Food or alcohol may exacerbate the pain
- Chronic persistent pain suggests complications such as pseudocyst formation, biliary obstruction, or cancer
- Painful attacks resolve as inflammation is replaced by fibrosis, but this takes many years. The pain sometimes becomes continuous, or nearly so, and may become the predominant feature of disease in some patients.
- Painless chronic pancreatitis occurs in a few patients, who present with exocrine insufficiency

Weight loss

Malabsorption and small meals, because of associated pain, lead to malnutrition.

Exocrine insufficiency

- Steatorrhoea (pale, bulky, offensive stools with visible fat globules) occurs when pancreatic enzyme secretion is < 10% normal. It may be masked if patients reduce fat intake, either intentionally or unconsciously.

- Defective secretion of lipase and bicarbonate cause fat malabsorption, but vitamin malabsorption rarely results in clinical osteomalacia or bleeding tendency
- Hypocalcaemia is common, because calcium chelates unabsorbed fat
- Weight loss is exacerbated by protein catabolism, because deficient pancreatic proteases (trypsin) cause protein malabsorption
- Serum B_{12} concentrations are often low because proteases are required to release R-proteins, which bind to B_{12}. Pancreatic enzyme supplements are effective and B_{12} replacement is unnecessary

Endocrine insufficiency
- Glucose intolerance and, eventually, frank diabetes occur in 30%
- Insulin requirements are often low due to the lack of glucagon

Complications of chronic pancreatitis
- Jaundice may be caused by distortion of the common bile duct or associated cirrhosis, but pancreatic carcinoma is a more common cause
- Portal hypertension due to splenic or portal vein thrombosis is rare, but needs to be distinguished from associated alcoholic cirrhosis (about 10% of patients with chronic pancreatitis), because surgical decompression occasionally helps
- The risk of cancer is increased, but can be difficult to distinguish from chronic pancreatitis in the early stages. Rapidly progressive symptoms and weight loss are likely to be due to cancer
- Haemorrhage from associated varices, ulcers or periductular vessels is rare
- Pancreatic duct strictures cause stasis and pancreatic calculi. These can cause recurrent acute pancreatitis, which is difficult to treat. Endoscopic balloon dilatation of strictures and lithotripsy of calculi are potential alternatives to surgery. Referral is advisable
- Duodenal and colonic strictures have been reported in children (very rarely in adults) given high-lipase pancreatic supplements)

Investigations

Blood tests
- Serum amylase may be elevated in acute-on-chronic episodes of pain, but is often normal in between
- Albumin and clotting studies may be abnormal, due to associated cirrhosis or malabsorption. Low calcium or serum B_{12} suggests malabsorption. Elevated ALP reflects biliary obstruction (if the γ-glutamyltransferase is elevated) or, rarely, osteomalacia
- 2 h postprandial blood glucose > 8 mmol indicates impaired glucose tolerance and > 11 mmol is diagnostic of diabetes

Imaging
- Plain abdominal X-ray—30% have pancreatic calcification in the later stages
- Ultrasound—excellent for detecting fluid collections and assessing duct diameter, especially in thin patients. CT or EUS are more sensitive for detecting early disease
- MRCP, with or without secretin stimulation, is a non-invasive alternative to ERCP, which it is likely to replace for diagnostic purposes (Fig. 4.2)

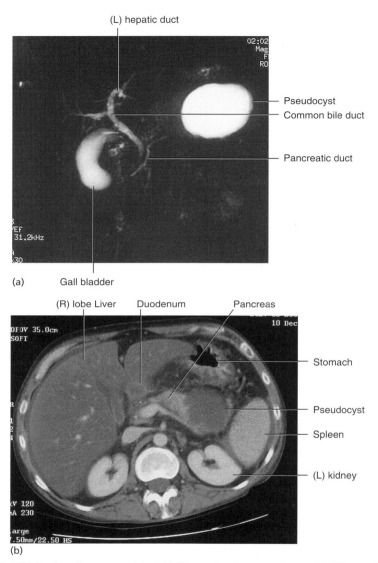

Fig 4.2 MRI in chronic pancreatitis. (a) MR scan showing a pseudocyst. (b) CT scan of the same patient

- ERCP—the previous 'gold standard', revealing duct distortion and side branch dilatation (Fig. 4.3). 'Minimal change pancreatitis' is an indication for pancreatic function tests (see below)

Functional assessment
- Assessment of pancreatic exocrine function is not routinely performed, especially when clinical malabsorption is present because management is rarely altered (p. 429)

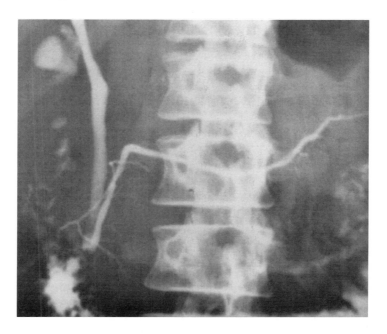

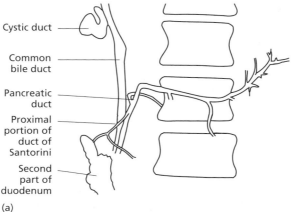

Cystic duct

Common bile duct

Pancreatic duct

Proximal portion of duct of Santorini

Second part of duodenum

(a)

Fig. 4.3 ERCP in chronic pancreatitis. (a) Normal ERCP showing the pancreatic duct, duct of Santorini and the common bile duct entering at the papilla. *(Continued)*

- Faecal pancreatic elastase can be measured in stool using an enzyme-linked immunosorbent assay (ELISA) kit. It is convenient, non-invasive and recommended as a first-line test for pancreatic exocrine insufficiency, although only available in specialist centres
- Function tests (e.g. Pancreolauryl test, p. 430) are indicated to help interpret minimal changes on ERCP, or to assist diagnosis when ERCP is not readily available
- Fat globules in stool indicate malabsorption, but their absence is unhelpful. Quantitative faecal fat measurement (normal < 5 g/day on a 100 g/day fat diet) may

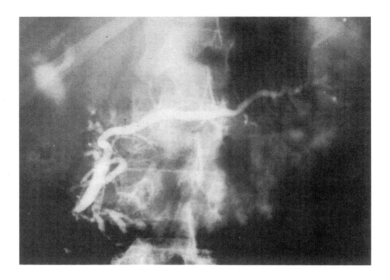

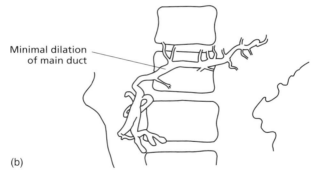

Minimal dilation
of main duct

(b)

Fig. 4.3 *(continued)* (b) ERCP showing moderate chronic pancreatitis (major irregularity of all side branches and minor irregularity of main duct). ERCP is best performed only if diagnostic doubt remains after MR scanning.

help confirm the presence of fat malabsorption. The amount of fat in the stool tends to be higher in patients with pancreatic maldigestion as compared to those with intestinal fat malabsorption
- Direct tests (Lundh test meal with duodenal intubation) are no longer used in clinical practice

Pain control
- Pancreatic enzyme supplements may help, but this is debated
- Avoid alcohol and dietary fat
- Dihydrocodeine 60 mg four times daily is sometimes sufficient
- Opiates (pethidine) are often required during severe pain, but dependence is common, possibly because of a susceptible personality in those who also abuse alcohol

- Repeat ultrasound and ERCP are indicated for persistent pain, because duct strictures or calculi may be the cause
- Coeliac plexus neurolysis with alcohol provides temporary relief, sometimes for months, but results are generally disappointing. Early hypotension and later impotence or total visceral anaesthesia are potential complications. EUS-guided neurolysis with steroids and local anaesthetic may be safer and more effective. Recurrent blocks are often necessary, but relief can sometimes be permanent. Coeliac plexus excision by surgery can be valuable in patients who need recurrent blocks
- The assistance of a psychologist to teach coping strategies for pain is helpful for patients with unrealistic expectations
- Referral to a pain clinic helps both patients and physicians. Gabapentin and SSRIs (e.g. paroxetine) may be helpful
- Surgery is indicated for localised chronic pancreatitis or pancreatic calculi causing severe intractable pain, but should only be performed by an experienced pancreatic surgeon. Total pancreatectomy for diffuse chronic pancreatitis has an unacceptable morbidity and a substantial number still have persistent pain

Exocrine insufficiency
- A low-fat diet (30–40 g/day, p. 391) is important, even with pancreatic supplements. A dietitian's advice is necessary
- Pancreatic enzyme supplements, taken during meals, are a convenient way of replacing deficient enzymes. No one type (Creon, Pancrease) is of proven superiority to another and anything from 5 to 50 capsules/day may be needed. Enzyme preparations are unpalatable when sprinkled on food
- Creon is convenient, because acid suppression is unnecessary unless steatorrhoea persists despite a low-fat diet
- Persistent steatorrhoea may be due to:
  - poor dietary compliance
  - insufficient enzyme supplements
  - taking the capsules at the wrong time (before or after, rather than during, meals)
  - misdiagnosis (consider Crohn's disease, coeliac disease and thyrotoxicosis)
- Medium-chain triglyceride supplements are not very palatable but may help improve fat absorption if a low-fat diet, enzyme supplements and acid suppression fail to control steatorrhoea

Endocrine insufficiency
- Oral hypoglycaemics are ineffective
- Insulin requirements are usually modest, but control is often difficult. 'Brittle' (labile) diabetes needs careful monitoring of blood sugars and close liaison between patient and diabetic team

Indications for surgery
The decision balancing the quality of life with persistent pain against the complications of surgery is always difficult. Surgery is more likely to be successful when ERCP demonstrates localised chronic pancreatitis or focal lesions such as strictures or calculi, and is rarely indicated when there is diffuse disease. Postoperative steatorrhoea and

diabetes that is difficult to control are common, depending on the amount of pancreas resected. An experienced pancreatic surgeon is essential. A joint decision by the physician, surgeons and patient is indicated for:

- Intractable pain
- Pancreatic cysts or pseudocyst
- Recurrent gastrointestinal bleeding

Prognosis
- 80% with alcoholic chronic pancreatitis survive 10 years if drinking stops, but this falls to less than half if drinking continues
- Death occurs from the complications of acute-on-chronic attacks, the cardiovascular complications of diabetes, associated cirrhosis, drug dependence or suicide

Hereditary pancreatitis
- Autosomal dominant with 80% penetrance. The majority of patients have one of two mutations (R122H or N29I) in the cationic trypsinogen gene (PRSS1) (p. 116). These alter a trypsin recognition site preventing deactivation of trypsin within the pancreas, which leads to autodigestion. Although most have a family history, genetic testing is indicated in any patient with 'idiopathic' recurrent acute pancreatitis
- Presentation is usually in childhood, but rarely delayed until 30 years or older. Clinical features and natural history are similar to alcoholic pancreatitis
- Up to 40% of patients will develop pancreatic cancer by the age of 70 years (relative risk 53%). Routine screening is not yet known to have any survival benefit but EUROPAC (European Registry of Hereditary Pancreatitis and Pancreatic Cancer) offers screening by CT, EUS and k-ras analysis of pancreatic juice obtained at ERCP, at 3-yearly intervals as part of a research programme
- Asymptomatic relatives do not need genetic testing, because mutations are not associated with malignancy in the absence of pancreatitis
- Patients should be advised to avoid alcohol and cigarettes

4.3 Cystic fibrosis

CF is the commonest autosomal recessive inherited disorder in Caucasians (1 : 2000 births). Mutations in the *CFTR* gene alter anion transport across epithelia, causing plugs that obstruct pulmonary, pancreatic, biliary and genitourinary glands. The commonest mutation ΔF508 is carried by 70%. A further 850 different mutations are found with varying prevalence among different populations

Clinical features (Table 4.1)
- Respiratory and pancreatic complications are the most important
- Abdominal pain in adolescents with CF may be due to acute or chronic pancreatitis, intussusception, faecal impaction ('meconium ileus equivalent'), gallstones or duodenal ulceration
- Pancreatic exocrine insufficiency varies according to genotype. 99% of patients homozygous for the common ΔF508 mutations have pancreatic exocrine insuffi-

Table 4.1 Clinical features of cystic fibrosis

Infants	Children	Young adults
Meconium ileus	Bronchiectasis	Bronchiectasis
Rectal prolapse	Cor pulmonale	Chronic pancreatitis
Respiratory infections	Pancreatitis	Cholelithiasis
Failure to thrive	acute	Biliary strictures
Steatorrhoea	chronic	Aspermia
Malnutrition	Diabetes	Biliary cirrhosis
	Gallstones	Duodenal ulcer
	Portal hypertension	Intestinal obstruction
	Hypersplenism	
	Heat exhaustion	
	Colonic strictures	
	(high lipase enzyme supplements)	

ciency whilst the majority of patients with one severe and one mild mutation (compound heterozygotes) retain their pancreatic function. Pancreatic insufficiency is seen in > 90% of childhood-onset CF and < 20% of adult-onset CF
- Pancreatic exocrine insufficiency causes steatorrhoea, hyperphagia, deficiency of fat-soluble vitamins (A, D, E, K) in children. Malnutrition is less common in adolescents, but steatorrhoea persists
- Impaired glucose tolerance is common (50%), but rarely causes ketoacidosis
- Hepatic disease due to inspissated secretions blocking bile ductules causes pericholangitis, periportal fibrosis or cirrhosis in 5%

Management (adults)

Diagnosis
- A sweat sodium > 60 mmol/L after pilocarpine iontophoresis is diagnostic in children, but unreliable after adolescence when diagnosis is based upon clinical features and genetic testing
- Low-fat diet—palatability must be maintained (Section 12.5, p. 391)
- Pancreatic enzyme supplements (p. 121) during meals. Excessive enzyme supplementation should be avoided because of the risk of developing colonic strictures due to fibrosing colopathy
- Fat-soluble vitamin supplements are rarely needed if steatorrhoea is controlled
- Nutritional supplements (enteral feeds, medium-chain triglycerides) should be provided according to individual needs. In some health care systems, supplements may be paid for by private insurance or public (e.g. National Health Service, NHS) plans.

Intestinal obstruction
- Gastrografin enema is diagnostic and may be therapeutic for intussusception. Surgery should only be performed in a specialist unit because of respiratory complications

- *N*-acetylcysteine 200 mg three times daily after recovery stimulates secretions and prevents recurrent pain due to faecal impaction

Other aspects
- Joint management with a respiratory physician is essential
- Genetic counselling for parents and young adults is necessary

Prognosis
CF used to be a purely paediatric disease, but 80% now live to be older than 20 years, although all have respiratory complications and 90% have pancreatic exocrine insufficiency. Overall median life expectancy is still reduced to around 30 years.

4.4 Pancreatic cancer

The incidence of pancreatic adenocarcinoma is increasing in Europe. This increase does not appear to be due to better diagnosis. 80% of cases occur between the ages of 60 and 80. Men are more commonly affected than women. Only 3% survive for longer than 5 years. Pancreatic cancer should be distinguished from ampullary carcinoma, which has a much better prognosis (40% 5-year survival).

Causes
- Genetic
  - Hereditary pancreatitis (PRSS1 gene) (p. 116 and p. 122)
  - Pancreatic cancer is a feature of several syndromes, including Peutz–Jeghers syndrome (STK11/LKB1 gene), familial atypical multiple-mole melanoma (FAMMM) syndrome (p16/CDKN2A genes), hereditary non-polyposis colon cancer (HNPCC II—hMLH1 and hMSH2 genes), familial adenomatous polyposis (FAP—APC gene), familial breast cancer (BRCA2 gene), ataxia-telangiectasia (ATM gene) and Li–Fraumeni syndrome (p53 gene)
- Smoking—relative risk 1.3–5.5%. Cancer occurs at younger age in smokers and risk increases with number of cigarettes smoked
- Chronic pancreatitis—cumulative 25-year risk of pancreatic cancer in patients with any form of chronic pancreatitis is 4%. In patients with non-hereditary chronic pancreatitis this risk is controversial and may be due to shared risk factors
- Alcohol—any association is weak, and chronic pancreatitis not related to alcohol does not increase the risk of pancreatic cancer
- Diabetes—association is controversial and may reflect the fact that diabetes is an early symptom of pancreatic cancer rather than a causative factor

Clinical features
- Tumour site determines the presentation
- Cancers of the body or tail cause pain, anorexia and weight loss, and have usually disseminated before diagnosis
- Cancers in the head of the pancreas cause jaundice at an earlier stage
- Multifocal tumours are common

Symptoms
- Mean age 66 years
- Epigastric pain is the presenting feature in 75%. It typically radiates to the back, but may be intermittent, provoked by food and relieved by posture
- Painless obstructive jaundice is the other common presenting feature
- Delayed diagnosis is common because early symptoms are non-specific including anorexia, weight loss, depression or lassitude
- New onset of diabetes is observed in 15–20% of patients, and may present with ketoacidosis
- Recurrent attacks of acute pancreatitis occasionally herald cancer, due to intermittent duct obstruction
- Duodenal obstruction, with nausea and vomiting, is usually a late manifestation

Paraneoplastic features
- Rare
- Tender, subcutaneous nodules (like erythema nodosum) and polyarthritis are due to metastatic fat necrosis. Recurrent venous thrombosis (thrombophlebitis migrans), abacterial endocarditis, hypercalcaemia and Cushing's syndrome are other features
- Local spread to the peritoneum causes ascites. Obstruction of the splenic or renal vein can cause portal hypertension, or nephrotic syndrome

Physical signs
- Usually indicate an unresectable tumour
- The exception is isolated jaundice, which may be due to an ampullary carcinoma (p. 127). Courvoisier's 'law' states that jaundice in the presence of a palpable gall bladder is unlikely to be due to stones
- Exceptions to Courvoisier's law are impacted stones in both the cystic and common bile ducts, or a stone in Hartman's pouch causing oedema of the bile duct (Mirizzi's syndrome)
- Hepatomegaly, splenomegaly, ascites, supraclavicular nodes or an abdominal mass are present in 40% at diagnosis

Investigations
The suggested sequence of investigations is shown in Fig. 4.4.
- Serum CA19-9 to identify early, potentially curable tumours remains unproven. It helps assess prognosis (higher CA19-9 prior to surgery indicates a larger, less resectable tumour) and monitor recurrence following neoadjuvant chemoradiotherapy
- Percutaneous needle cytology is useful in patients with unresectable cancer (to direct palliative chemoradiotherapy) or suspected pancreatic lymphoma
- Laparotomy and biopsy may still be required in younger patients to differentiate chronic pancreatitis from cancer, with the option of palliative or radical surgery at the time
- CT may be required for diagnosis when ultrasound is impracticable (pancreas obscured by bowel gas) or when ERCP or MRCP fails to provide a definitive diagnosis
- Endoscopic ultrasound may be the most sensitive investigation and provide useful information about resectability, but is not widely available and needs to be performed by a skilled operator

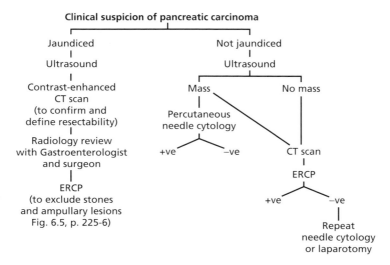

Fig. 4.4 **Investigation of suspected pancreatic cancer.**

Management

Although a cure is impossible in most patients, it is important not to take a despairing approach. There is much that can be offered by expert palliation. The small proportion (< 20%) that might benefit from radical surgery should be identified first.

Radical surgery

Pancreatoduodenectomy (Whipple's procedure) should only be considered by experienced pancreatic surgeons if:
- The patient is fit
- Tumour < 3 cm
- No metastases detected by staging CT and/or EUS

Operative mortality is < 5% in expert hands, but much higher amongst occasional operators. Morbidity after pancreatectomy is substantial.

Chemotherapy

5-Fluorouracil (5FU) or gemcitabine are first-line agents, but the 1-year survival rate is only 20%. They should be considered for adjuvant therapy in those suitable for surgery. Other agents alone, or in combination (carboplatin, cisplatin, marimistat, mitomycin) with 5FU may provide symptomatic benefit, but little survival advantage.

Palliation of jaundice

- ERCP stent insertion by an experienced endoscopist is preferable in the elderly, because the morbidity is lower and hospital stay substantially shorter than after surgery
- A combined percutaneous radiological and endoscopic approach in difficult cases gives a success rate of up to 90%
- Percutaneous drainage alone is unsatisfactory, because the displacement and infection rates are too high

- Recurrent jaundice after stenting is usually due to obstruction by biliary sludge rather than tumour. The stent should be replaced endoscopically as necessary
- Surgery is indicated if there is evidence of duodenal obstruction or if ERCP is unsuccessful. Choledochoduodenostomy and gastroenterostomy are appropriate

Palliation of pain
- Pain can be effectively relieved. It is important to tell this to the patient and family, and to ensure that it is achieved
- Opiate analgesics (start with long-acting morphine sulphate 20 mg twice daily) cannot be introduced too early to relieve pain once the diagnosis is made. The dose is increased by the patient until symptoms are controlled (p. 130)
- Coeliac plexus infiltration with alcohol at the time of palliative surgery should be considered. Percutaneous coeliac plexus block is more difficult and often needs to be repeated after 2 months
- Radiotherapy can relieve intractable pain
- NSAIDs, benzodiazepines and patient-controlled infusions of opiates also have a place (p. 130)

Palliation of other symptoms
- Diarrhoea may be relieved and quality of life improved by pancreatic enzyme supplements (Creon 25 minimicrospheres, dose according to diarrhoea control)
- Nausea and vomiting need proactive treatment by prokinetics (e.g. domperidone), antroduodenal stent insertion (for duodenal obstruction) and a PPI (for reflux caused by vomiting or delayed gastric emptying)

Prognosis
- Median survival after diagnosis is < 6 months
- Overall 5-year survival is 3%
- 5-year survival for the 15% of patients who undergo 'curative' pancreatoduodenectomy is 20%

Ampullary tumours
Any malignant lesion that appears at endoscopy to arise from Vater's ampulla is called an ampullary tumour, but such tumours are rare. They behave very differently from cancer in the rest of the pancreas because they present earlier, but they have no unique histological features.
- 10 times less common than pancreatic cancer
- 90% present with painless obstructive jaundice
- 80% are resectable by local excision
- 5-year survival after local excision is 40%, with an operative mortality of 7%. Proximal pancreatectomy has a similar mortality and probably improves survival

4.5 Neuroendocrine tumours of the pancreas

Neuroendocrine tumours are rare, with an incidence of 1 : 100 000 per year. Tumours are classified as functional or non-functional based upon symptoms due to hypersecretion of hormones, neuropeptides and neurotransmitters. Early diagnosis is mandatory, as the cure rate in sporadic tumours is highly dependant on tumour size. All patients should be referred to a specialist centre for treatment, but outpatient follow-up may be arranged locally. For this reason, management details concentrate on procedure at routine review, rather than definitive treatment. Evidence of recurrent disease is an indication for re-referral

Carcinoid syndrome (Chapter 7, p. 239)

Insulinoma

Syndrome
- Spontaneous hypoglycaemia
- Provoked by fasting or exercise and relieved by eating
- Neuroglycopenia may present with tremor, irritability, hunger, confusion, focal neurological deficit or psychiatric abnormalities
- 90% are solitary and benign

Diagnosis and treatment
- 48–72 h fast under observation in hospital is recommended. A blood glucose < 2.2 mmol/L in the presence of an insulin concentration of > 6 µU/mL confirms the diagnosis in 97% of patients. C-peptide concentration should be > 200 pmol/L. Intravenous glucose must be readily available
- Normal or elevated serum C-peptide concentrations exclude exogenous insulin administration, but not sulphonylurea ingestion
- EUS, CT and MRI help localise tumours and metastases
- Small benign lesions may be treated by simple enucleation. Larger or malignant tumours require pancreaticoduodenectomy
- Nesidioblastosis due to diffuse islet cell hyperplasia should be considered in patients with the clinical and biochemical features of insulinoma in whom a discrete neoplastic lesion cannot be found

Outpatient checks
- Ask about recurrence of presenting symptoms
- Examine visual fields and check calcium levels annually to detect multiple endocrine adenomatosis (MEA type I; pancreatic endocrine tumour, pituitary tumour and hyperparathyroidism)
- Plasma insulin and C-peptide levels do not need checking unless symptoms recur

Gastrinoma (Zollinger–Ellison syndrome) (p. 105)

Glucagonoma

Syndrome
- Necrotising migratory erythema (superficial bullous eruption that moves from one area to another)
- Mild diabetes (insulin secretion compensates for excess glucagon)
- Venous thrombosis

- Wasting
- Neuropsychiatric manifestations
- 80% are malignant

Diagnosis and treatment
- Elevated plasma glucagon levels are diagnostic
- Initial treatment is surgical if the tumour is localised. Octreotide improves the rash and can reverse the catabolic effects of glucagon excess and therefore helps prepare patients for surgery
- Complete resection is possible in only 30%. Hepatic embolisation is the best form of non-surgical palliation
- 5-year survival is 50%

Outpatient checks
- Ask about polyuria, diarrhoea and fatigue
- Examine the skin, check visual fields, serum calcium and glucose (in case of recurrence, or MEA type I)

VIPoma (Werner–Morrison syndrome)

Syndrome
- Watery diarrhoea (profuse, but may be intermittent)
- Hypokalaemia (< 3.0 mmol/L)
- Metabolic acidosis (50% also have gastric anacidity)
- Hyperglycaemia
- Hypercalcaemia

Diagnosis and treatment
- Elevated fasting plasma vasoactive intestinal polypeptide (VIP) concentrations may come from a tumour in the pancreas, or rarely from a retroperitoneal neuroma. VIP secretion may be episodic so several values may need to be measured
- Treatment is surgical but 50% have metastases at presentation. VIPomas are extremely responsive to octreotide, which may result in tumour necrosis and long-term inhibition of tumour growth

Outpatient checks
- Ask about diarrhoea and fatigue
- Measure serum potassium and VIP levels at annual visits

4.6 Terminal care

Terminal care is an important part of management in patients dying from any disease, but especially in pancreatic cancer when the prognosis is so poor. The essential features are symptom control, communication and supportive care.

Symptom control

Pain
- Best relieved by long-acting morphine sulphate. Start at 20 mg twice daily and increase by 20 mg/day until symptoms are controlled. The correct dose is that which controls symptoms
- Breakthrough pain between doses can sometimes be treated by increasing the frequency of doses (three or four times a day) rather than the total amount
- Benzodiazepines (diazepam 2 mg three times daily) or chlorpromazine (25 mg three times daily) have a synergistic effect with morphine for very anxious patients, but excess sedation must be avoided. Anxiety usually has a cause and is aggravated by ignorance or fear
- Fentanyl patches for transdermal delivery are expensive, but are effective and give the patient simple control over their pain
- Bone pain due to metastases often responds to indomethacin 25 mg three times daily, or slow-release diclofenac 100 mg once daily, with or without morphine. Radiotherapy is also effective
- Local pain (arm, leg, chest, abdomen) from metastases may be amenable to anaesthetic nerve blocks, which may need to be repeated
- When oral therapy is no longer possible, subcutaneous morphine by infusion pump (dose/h = oral dose/24) is best combined with methotrimeprazine 100 mg/24 h as an antiemetic. Intramuscular morphine is never justified. Morphine and NSAIDs are available as suppositories

Vomiting
- Consider hypercalcaemia, intestinal obstruction, cerebral metastases and, most important, drug-induced causes
- Standard drugs (p. 83) can be tried. Dexamethasone 2 mg three times daily is frequently helpful
- Methotrimeprazine 100–200 mg/24 h subcutaneous infusion can stop vomiting caused by intestinal obstruction

Irritability
Consider pain, constipation or urinary retention when consciousness is impaired.

Secretions
- Atropine 0.6 mg by intravenous or intramuscular injection (maximum 2.4 mg/day) will dry noisy pharyngeal and bronchial secretions
- Hyoscine patches are useful when managing secretions at home, when a trained nurse is not readily available to give subcutaneous injections

Communication

With the patient
- Discussion of the diagnosis should wait until it has been definitely established and a plan of action made

- Delivering bad news should be done sensitively by a senior doctor, if possible in the presence of a relative or friend and a nurse. Patients (and relatives) frequently have little recall of detailed discussion. Try and arrange a quiet place for discussion, undisturbed by bleeps or telephones. The bedside or corridor of an acute medical ward is less than ideal
- Experience indicates that the best approach involves personal introduction, establishing the extent of individual knowledge, a 'warning shot' about news not being as good as hoped for, explanation of the diagnosis with diagrams if necessary, time for the news to be taken in, expression of sympathy or empathy with emotions where necessary, emphasising what positive features there are, then explanation about the next step
- Not all patients wish to know that they have 'cancer', but the diagnosis should be explained if a direct question is asked
- All patients should be given the opportunity to ask questions, told that symptoms can be treated even if a cure is not possible, and given a contact telephone number (general practitioner, nurse, medical secretary) if there are problems

With the family
- May precede or influence discussion with the patient, but it is always useful to talk to both patient and family together. This avoids future confusion about what has been said to individuals and helps cut down communication barriers within the family
- Explain what support is available in the later stages and whom to call

With the general practitioner
- Telephone prior to discharging the patient from hospital
- Say what the patient/family have been told
- Explain what supportive arrangements have been made
- Offer immediate access to hospital if symptoms become intolerable

Supportive care

Home
Liaise with family, general practitioner, district nurse, palliative care nurses, hospital support team, home help or meals on wheels, as appropriate.

Hospice
- The general practitioner and the patient should agree before a hospice is contacted
- Early referral is advisable. It is poor practice to transfer a patient a few days before death, because the hospice team have no time to apply their skills, or to gain the necessary rapport

5 Liver

5.1 Jaundice

Jaundice is clinically detectable when the serum bilirubin is 50 μmol/L (> 3 mg/dL). Classification into three predominant types (prehepatic, hepatocellular and cholestatic) is convenient, but there is considerable overlap in the clinical and biochemical features.

A basic knowledge of bilirubin metabolism is necessary to understand the investigation of jaundice (Fig. 5.1).

Causes (See Table 5.1)
The predominant type of bilirubin must occasionally be identified before a diagnosis is made. A mixed pattern of conjugated and unconjugated bilirubin is usually present, unless there is an enzyme deficiency or transport defect. Normally about 95% of bilirubin is conjugated.

- Predominant unconjugated hyperbilirubinaemia occurs in adults as:
  - haemolysis
  - Gilbert's syndrome
  - dyserythropoiesis (such as megaloblastic anaemia) or resorption of a large post-traumatic haematoma may cause an elevated bilirubin, but not clinically detectable jaundice

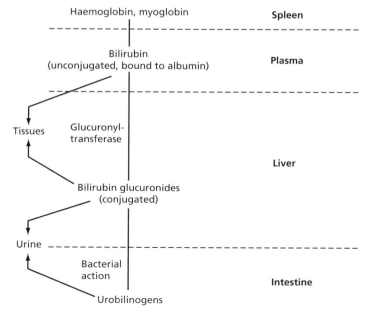

Fig. 5.1 **Bilirubin metabolism.**

5 Liver
5.1 Jaundice

Table 5.1 Causes of jaundice—main types

	Prehepatic	Hepatocellular	Cholestatic
Common	Neonatal	Viral hepatitis Cirrhosis Alcoholic hepatitis	Common duct stones Pancreatic cancer Primary biliary cirrhosis
Uncommon	Haemolysis Gilbert's syndrome	Hepatic metastases Drug-induced Autoimmune hepatitis Liver abscess Hepatoma	Cholangiocarcinoma Sclerosing cholangitis Benign stricture Pancreatitis
Rare	Crigler–Najjar syndrome	Lymphoma Leptospirosis Budd–Chiari syndrome Cardiac failure Pregnancy Postcardiac surgery Wilson's disease Dubin–Johnson syndrome Graft-versus-host disease	Portal lymphadenopathy Chronic pancreatitis Choledochal cyst Benign recurrent AIDS cholangiopathy Biliary atresia Parenteral nutrition Hepatic granulomas

- Predominant conjugated hyperbilirubinaemia occurs as:
  - cholestasis (intra- or extrahepatic; Table 6.3, p. 193; Table 6.4, p. 194)
  - familial hyperbilirubinaemia (rare, normal ALP)
    Dubin–Johnson or Rotor's syndrome

Clinical features
A systematic clinical approach is important.

History
- Occupation (alcohol-related, animal contact, industrial exposure)
- Travel abroad, past or recent (hepatitis-endemic areas, malaria)
- Contact with jaundiced patients
- Injections, especially abroad (drug abuse, transfusions of blood or plasma factors, tattoos)
- Drugs (prescribed, over-the-counter or 'alternative' medicines such as herbal teas, 'Chinese' medicines)
- Sexual relations (hepatitis B)
- Associated symptoms (the time sequence of symptoms is often helpful in distinguishing hepatitis from cholestatic causes):
  - anorexia, nausea, distaste for cigarettes (hepatitis)
  - right upper quadrant abdominal pain (gallstones)
  - weight loss (malignancy, chronic pancreatitis)
  - dark urine, pale stools, pruritus (cholestasis)
  - pyrexia, rigors should always be taken seriously (cholangitis, abscess)

Examination
- The depth of jaundice is not a reliable indicator of the cause
- Look for signs suggesting acute or chronic liver disease (Table 5.2), or cholestasis (Box 6.1, p. 194; Table 6.5, p. 195)

Table 5.2 Physical signs in hepatic jaundice

Acute*	Chronic*	Either
Well nourished	Leuconychia/telangiectasia	Palmar erythema
Tender hepatomegaly	Loss of muscle bulk	Bruising
	Telangiectases (spider naevi)	Splenomegaly
	Splenomegaly	
	Ascites	
	Peripheral oedema	
	Loss of axilliary/pubic hair	
	Testicular atrophy	
	Dupuytren's contracture	
	Small or large liver	

*No clinical sign is invariably associated with either acute or chronic liver disease.

Other signs to be noted:
- Age—young adults may have Epstein–Barr virus (EBV) hepatitis
- Previous biliary surgery—possible obstructive jaundice
- Fever—suspect cholangitis, although hepatitis may cause a low-grade pyrexia
- Palpable gall bladder—more common in malignant obstruction, but 1 in 4 have obstruction due to common bile duct calculi
- Portosystemic encephalopathy—personality change, confusion
- Asterixis—flapping tremor of outstretched hands, with fingers splayed
- Dilated periumbilical veins are rare. They either:
  - flow radiating away from umbilicus (portal hypertension, 'caput medusa'), or
  - flow towards the head only (inferior vena cava obstruction)
- An arterial bruit over the liver is rare—hepatoma or acute alcoholic hepatitis
- Rectal examination for stool colour—pale in cholestatic jaundice

Investigations—all patients

Blood tests
- Typical values that help distinguish different types of jaundice are given in Table 5.3
- Liver enzymes, AST (previously serum glutamic-oxaloacetic transaminase, SGOT) and ALP are markers of liver dysfunction. Alanine transaminase (ALT, previously SGPT) is more specific than AST, but is not as commonly measured by automated assays

Table 5.3 Blood tests in jaundice

Test	Normal	Prehepatic	Hepatocellular	Extrahepatic
Bilirubin (μmol/L)	< 17	50–150	50–400	100–900
Bilirubin (mg/dL)	< 1	3–9	3–20	6–45
AST (IU/L)	< 35	< 35	300–10 000	35–400
ALP (IU/L)	< 120	< 120	< 120–300	> 300
γ-GT (IU/L)	15–40	15–40	15–200	80–1000
Albumin (g/dL)	4–5	4–5	2–5	3–5
Hb (g/dL)	12–16	< 10	12–16	10–16
Reticulocytes (%)	< 1	10–30	< 1	< 1
INR	1.0–1.2	1.0–1.2	1.0–3+	1.0–3.0*
Prothrombin time (s)	13–15	13–15	15–45	15–45*

*Falls in response to parenteral vitamin K 10 mg.

- An AST > 500 is very rare in alcoholic hepatitis and usually indicates coexistent viral infection or drug toxicity (e.g. acetaminophen/paracetamol). Rarely high ALT can be seen in biliary obstruction but biliary pain is a feature
- γ-glutamyl transpeptidase (γ-GT) is elevated when a high ALP is of hepatic, rather than bony, origin. It is an unreliable test for alcohol abuse and a raised MCV is more suggestive. γ-GT will be elevated in liver disease of any cause including non-alcoholic fatty liver disease
- Serum albumin and coagulation (prothrombin time, INR) are better markers of liver function, but serum albumin may also be altered by redistribution of body fluids

Urine
- Urine testing is less commonly performed now that biochemical tests are readily available, but should not be overlooked
- Bilirubin (tested with Ictotest tablets) is absent in prehepatic causes (the urine is clear, not orange, 'acholuric jaundice')
- Urobilinogen (Dipstix testing) is absent in complete cholestasis

Other tests
- Ultrasound—to look for bile duct dilatation or hepatic metastases. Also helpful to assess hepatic size, splenomegaly, the pancreas, portal blood flow, or lymphadenopathy and ascites. It is not a reliable method of detecting cirrhosis, but much depends on the skill of the operator. 'Increased reflectivity' of the liver may represent fatty infiltration or fibrosis
- CT scan—to look for/further evaluate focal liver lesions or pancreatic pathology (Fig. 5.2)
- Chest X-ray—to look for bronchial carcinoma or metastases
- ERCP, MRI, or contrast-enhanced CT scan (p. 191)

Subsequent investigations
Further investigations depend on the type of jaundice, determined from the results of blood tests and ultrasound. Investigation of extra- and intrahepatic cholestatic jaundice is summarised in Figs 6.3 and 6.4 (pp. 190 and 191).

Prehepatic jaundice
- Blood film
- Reticulocyte count
- Direct antihuman globulin (Coombs') test; serum haptoglobins (absent in haemolysis but also low in cirrhosis)
- Discuss with haematologists (bone marrow, or Ham's test to exclude paroxysmal nocturnal haemoglobinuria)

Hepatocellular jaundice
- Viral serology—hepatitis B surface antigen (HBsAg), hepatitis A IgM, hepatitis C virus (HCV) antibody
- Acetaminophen/paracetamol levels on admission sample if drug toxicity possible
- Antismooth muscle, antinuclear and immunoglobulins (IgG), if viral titres are negative, to look for evidence of autoimmune hepatitis
- Monospot (Paul–Bunnell, for infectious mononucleosis) and serum for 'atypical' infections (e.g. *Leptospira* spp., *Mycoplasma pneumoniae*, *Cytomegalovirus*) if viral

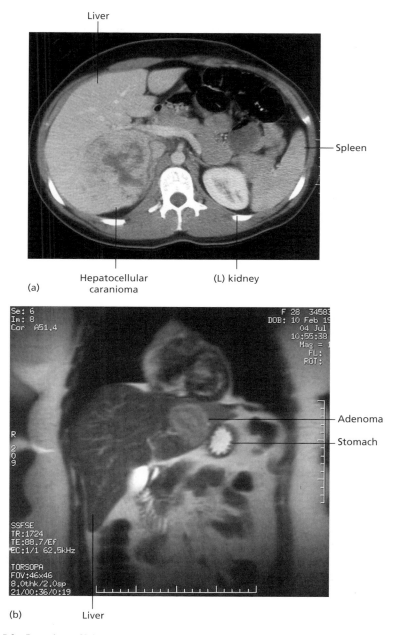

Liver

Spleen

Hepatocellular
caranioma

(L) kidney

(a)

(b)   Liver

Adenoma

Stomach

Fig. 5.2 Imaging of Liver Lesions. (a) CT scan of hepatocellular carcinoma. Resected before biopsy. Histology showed fibrolamellar carcinoma.(b) MR scan of hepatic adenoma, hyperintense mass in the left lobe. Size reduced after oral oestrogens stopped.

serology negative. The presence of renal failure is suggestive of leptospirosis. Consider hepatitis E if recently come from an endemic area (e.g. India)
- Serum copper, caeruloplasmin and 24 h urinary copper (Wilson's disease) if <40 years and viral titres and autoantibodies are negative.
- Serum iron/iron-binding capacity (transferrin saturation) and ferritin (haemochromatosis), α_1-antitrypsin (for protease deficiency) if evidence of chronic liver disease
- Liver biopsy if diagnosis remains uncertain, chronic disease is suspected or hepatic enzymes remain abnormal 6 months after acute viral hepatitis. Biopsies should be stained for iron. Consider sending biopsy for dry-weight copper (Wilson's disease)

Cholestatic jaundice (extra- and intrahepatic)
See p. 193.

Drug-induced liver damage
The list of drugs causing jaundice is long, but drug-induced jaundice is not that common. Drug-induced liver damage usually presents as asymptomatic elevation in liver enzymes (p. 181). Hepatotoxic effects (Table 5.4) can be divided into those that occur in most patients given a sufficiently high dose of the drug (dose-related), and idiosyncratic (dose-independent) reactions.

The diagnosis is suspected from the history of liver dysfunction or jaundice within 3 months of starting any new drug. Occasionally, liver damage can present 1 year or more after starting the drug (minocycline, methotrexate, (α-methyldopa). Peripheral eosinophilia is uncommon, although eosinophils in a liver biopsy raise the possibility of drug-induced damage.

Dose-related hepatotoxicity
- Acetaminophen/paracetamol (> 10 g/24 h, but as little as 6 g/day in those with alcoholic liver disease)

Table 5.4 Dose-independent drug hepatotoxicity

Liver lesion	Common culprits
Hepatitis	Isoniazid
	Sodium valproate
	Rifampicin
	NSAIDs
	Azathioprine
Cholestasis	Co-amoxiclav
	Chlorpromazine
	Prochlorperazine
	Fusidic acid
	Glibenclamide
Chronic hepatitis	Methyldopa
	Nitrofurantoin
	Dantrolene
Alcoholic hepatitis-like	Verapamil
Granulomas	Hydralazine
	Allopurinol
	Phenylbutazone

- Anabolic steroids (should only be used by specialists)
- Halothane-induced liver damage is partly related to dose; it should be avoided for anaesthetics < 6 weeks apart (rarely used now)
- Methotrexate (usually for psoriasis, rheumatoid arthritis) can cause dose-dependent hepatic fibrosis but not jaundice until the terminal stages. Liver function tests are usually normal. Fibrosis is unusual if total dose < 2 g. Toxicity is usually associated with excess alcohol use and routine liver biopsies on treatment are no longer indicated

Dose-independent hepatotoxicity
For a complete list of causes, refer to other textbooks (Appendix 2, p. 442).

Management
- Minor elevations in AST (up to threefold) after starting potentially hepatotoxic drugs (especially isoniazid, rifampicin) are not an indication for stopping the drug, since improvement usually occurs
- Stop all possible drugs if enzymes deteriorate or jaundice occurs
- Exclude other causes of jaundice and liver dysfunction (Table 5.1, p. 136)
- Severe acute liver failure is managed as for other causes (p. 42)
- Monitor liver enzymes until they return to normal—usually over several weeks. Most hepatotoxic effects resolve completely after the drug is withdrawn, unless liver dysfunction is unrecognised for several months (methotrexate, methyldopa). Very rarely persistent loss of small intrahepatic bile ducts (ductopaenia) can occur (persistent elevated ALP)
- Liver biopsy is not necessary if the drug is well known to cause liver dysfunction, unless liver enzymes have not returned to normal after 8 weeks. Liver biopsy is essential if the history is uncertain. Drug reactions may unmask pre-existing liver disease

Prescribing in liver disease
- Most drugs are safe to prescribe in stable liver disease
- High-risk drugs in patients with cirrhosis are:
  - sedatives (including chlormethiazole and benzodiazepines)
  - opiates (decreased first-pass metabolism enhances the effect)
  - diuretics (overdiuresis can provoke hyponatraemia, renal failure and encephalopathy)
  - NSAIDs (renal failure and erosion of varices)
  - drugs known to cause dose-related or dose-independent hepatotoxicity (the threshold for hepatotoxicity is decreased)

Post-operative jaundice
Possible causes are:
- Drugs—scrutinise each prescription. Prochlorperazine is often implicated
- Anaesthetic-repeated exposure to halothane within 4–6 weeks. Enflurane is preferable for repeated anaesthetics
- Septicaemia—cholestatic pattern
- Acute pancreatitis—pancreatic oedema can obstruct the common bile duct
- Latent liver disease—perioperative hypotension may provoke decompensation of cirrhosis

- Hepatitis—transfusion-acquired HCV, or HBV (1–6 months after operation) in countries where blood is not screened, or operation during the incubation period of hepatitis (shorter interval)
- Benign postoperative cholestasis—self-limiting, 1–2 weeks, especially after cardiac surgery
- Resorption of a large haematoma—jaundice only occurs if there is an associated metabolic disorder, such as Gilbert's syndrome
- Biliary surgical mishap:
  - common bile duct stones overlooked (may be associated bile duct leak)
  - inadvertent ligation of common bile duct
  - oedema, or (later) stricture of the common bile duct

Investigations
- Blood cultures—low-grade sepsis may not cause a fever
- Serology—hepatitis B, C and A, as well as antimitochondrial antibodies (AMA)
- Measure unconjugated bilirubin (> 75% suggests haemolysis, or resorption of a large haematoma)
- Ultrasound—look for dilated bile ducts and at the pancreas. If the common bile duct is dilated, ERCP is indicated, whether a stone is visible or not
- Contact blood transfusion laboratory to trace donors if hepatitis is diagnosed; sexual partners should be traced and offered hepatitis B vaccination if appropriate (p. 160)

Jaundice in pregnancy (p. 398)
Specific conditions related to pregnancy are as follows.

First trimester
Hyperemesis gravidarum—jaundice in 10%, especially in those with Gilbert's syndrome. Self-limiting. High serum transaminases are common. Liver failure does not occur.

Third trimester
- Intrahepatic cholestasis of pregnancy—preceded by pruritus. Increased fetal mortality and early delivery often required. Recurs with subsequent pregnancies because of genetic defect in bile transport (p. 193). Ursodeoxycholic acid is used during pregnancy. Resolves within 2 weeks of delivery. Self-limiting
- Acute fatty liver of pregnancy—nausea, abdominal pain, encephalopathy. High uric acid, coagulopathy and acidosis seen. Potentially fatal without prompt delivery
- Pre-eclampsia—often associated with elevated transaminases
- HELLP syndrome—potentially severe liver disease associated with pre-eclampsia, haemolysis, thrombocytopenia and elevated transaminases. Prompt delivery also needed

Any trimester
Any other cause of jaundice (drugs, viral, common bile duct calculi, etc.).

Jaundice with normal liver enzymes
Bilirubin may be disproportionately elevated compared to the AST or ALP when there is very severe liver disease (acute liver failure, alcoholic hepatitis or end-stage cirrhosis), because there are few hepatocytes to produce the enzymes. In these cases the albumin is low and coagulation disordered.

Isolated hyperbilirubinaemia is uncommon. Consider:
- Haemolysis—blood film, reticulocyte count, haptoglobins
- Gilbert's syndrome—unconjugated bilirubin
- Dubin–Johnson or Rotor's syndrome—conjugated bilirubin

Gilbert's syndrome
- Slight elevation of unconjugated bilirubin is common (up to 5% of the population). It is not an indication for ultrasound or other investigations in the absence of symptoms
- Liver enzymes are otherwise normal
- Bilirubin increases on fasting (rarely necessary to establish)
- Jaundice is rare (usually < 70 µmol/L), except in concomitant illness with anorexia
- No treatment other than reassurance is necessary

Crigler–Najjar syndrome
Crigler–Najjar syndrome (glucuronyl transferase deficiency) rarely affects adults, although some with the milder (type II) form survive from childhood.

Dubin–Johnson and Rotor's syndromes
Dubin–Johnson and Rotor's syndromes are very rare causes of isolated conjugated hyper-bilirubinaemia due to genetic defects in bile transport, but can present with jaundice in adults. In Dubin–Johnson the liver has a macroscopically black appearance. Rotor's syndrome is differentiated by a normal-coloured liver and a raised urinary coproporphyrin 1.

Other causes of hyperpigmentation
Very occasionally other causes of diffuse hyperpigmentation (carotenaemia, melanosis) may be confused with jaundice, but these do not cause scleral discoloration and the bilirubin is normal.

5.2 Hepatic decompensation

Hepatic decompensation refers to the onset of one or more of jaundice, worsening coagulopathy, ascites, or encephalopathy in an individual with chronic liver disease (usually cirrhotic). There is often a reversible component and aggressive management is indicated.

An acute exacerbation of chronic hepatic failure is far more common than acute (fulminant) liver failure (p. 42).

Causes
Every patient who presents with decompensation of chronic liver disease should be investigated for a provoking factor:
- Intestinal bleeding from:
  - varices
  - ulcer or erosions
- Infection:
  - urinary tract
  - chest
  - spontaneous bacterial peritonitis (usually *E. coli*) in ascites

- Drugs:
  - excess diuretics (hypokalaemia, hypomagnesaemia or uraemia)
  - sedatives
  - opiates (including codeine)
- Alcohol abuse (coexistent alcoholic hepatitis)
- Progression of underlying disease
- Constipation (causing encephalopathy)
- Hepatocellular carcinoma (p. 178)

Clinical features

Hepatocellular dysfunction
- Jaundice increasing
- Encephalopathy:
  - personality change, inability to draw a five-pointed star, forgetfulness, poor concentration
  - drowsiness, inappropriate behaviour
  - stuporous, inarticulate speech
  - coma
  - the changes in mental state are graded 1–4 (grade 4 means no response to painful stimuli) (Table 1.7, p. 43)
- Asterixis
  - arms outstretched, wrists hyperextended, fingers apart
  - slow (every second), flapping movements at the wrist
- Fever and other signs of infection may be absent

Portal hypertension
- Ascites—develops or increases (p. 146)
- Varices are not a sign of decompensation but of portal hypertension, but bleeding (p. 13) often triggers acute-on-chronic hepatic failure
- Venous hum—heard as a buzzing over the liver. It is rare

Child–Pugh grading
Child–Pugh grading (Table 5.5) may be clinically useful in predicting survival in patients with bleeding oesophageal varices or possibly in patients with cirrhosis under-

Table 5.5 Child–Pugh score

Feature	1 point	2 points	3 points
Bilirubin (mg/dL)	< 2	2–3	> 3 (i.e. jaundiced)
Albumin (g/dL)	> 3.5	2.8–3.5	< 2.8
Ascites	None	Controlled	Poorly controlled
Encephalopathy	None	Grade 1–2	Grade 3–4
Prothrombin time (seconds prolonged)	1–3	4–6	> 6
Child class	A	5–6 points	
	B	7–9 points	
	C	10–15 points	

going surgery. Mortality from variceal bleeding in grade A is 5%, grade B is 20% and grade C is 40%.

Meld Score

This newer scoring system, used to assess the severity of liver disease, incorporates aetiology of liver disease as well as creatinine, bilirubin and INR (see Mathematic Models in Chronic Liver Disease; www.mayo.edu/int-med/gi/model/mayomodl.htm)

Investigations

- Rectal examination for melaena
- Culture urine, blood and sputum if available
- Ascitic tap and urgent white cell count and Gram stain on admission. Neutrophil count in ascitic fluid > 250/mL is an indication for antibiotics, even if no organisms are seen
- Electrolytes, urea, full blood count, coagulation studies
- α-fetoprotein (AFP) for hepatocellular carcinoma
- Abdominal ultrasound for detecting hepatocellular carcinoma and portal vein thrombosis

Management

Acute episode

- Identify and treat the provoking factor, especially infection—intravenous cefotaxime 1 g three times daily is appropriate until the organism is identified. In spontaneous bacterial peritonitis intravenous cephalosporins can be followed by an oral ciprofloxacin/norfloxacin
- Dietary salt restriction:
  - no salt added to food (equivalent to 100 mmol sodium)
- Lactulose starting at 80 mL/day (in divided doses) until mild diarrhoea develops and then reduced, but not stopped (more effective than neomycin 4 g/day, which is now rarely used)
- Magnesium sulphate enema—if constipation is present despite lactulose treatment or unable to tolerate oral lactulose such as after/during an acute gastrointestinal bleed
- Fresh frozen plasma (FFP) is only indicated if there is active bleeding (2–4 units rapidly, repeated after 8 h if bleeding continues)
- Intravenous saline should be avoided once hypovolaemia has been treated, especially in the presence of oedema due to liver disease, because salt (and water) are avidly retained due to secondary hyperaldosteronism. Added salt on food and sodium-containing drugs (many antacids, p. 148) should also be avoided. Avoid 5% dextrose (water) if hyponatraemic as this is due to water retention, which will be exacerbated by dextrose
- B vitamins containing thiamine should be given to alcoholics, who often have dietary deficiency
- A PPI is indicated if varices have been banded
- Monitor:
  - clinical state (encephalopathy) daily
  - daily weight (more accurate than a fluid balance chart)

- daily electrolytes, INR and full blood count
- twice weekly bilirubin, AST, ALP and albumin
- Patients aged < 60 years with acute-on-chronic liver failure not due to alcohol may be suitable for a liver transplant, although this is best deferred until after recovery from the acute episode. Criteria for liver transplantation eligibility will vary somewhat from centre to centre (p. 45)

After recovery
- Discharge the patient only when the weight, diuretic dose and mental state are stable
- Protein restriction should be avoided if possible, because patients are protein-depleted and the diet is unpleasant
- Continue dietary salt restriction (no salt added to food or cooking) to delay reaccumulation of ascites
- Long-term prophylactic antibiotics are required with a quinolone antibiotic (norfloxacin or ciprofloxacin 250 mg twice daily) to prevent recurrent episodes following spontaneous bacterial peritonitis
- Lactulose can be decreased to 10–30 mL at night, before discharge and discontinued in outpatients. A few patients in whom encephalopathy is precipitated by constipation will also need long-term enemas

5.3 Ascites

In cirrhosis it is thought that peripheral vasodilatation is the initiating event, possibly due to impaired hepatic metabolism of endogenous vasodilators. This decreases renal blood flow, which stimulates the renin–angiotensin–aldosterone axis, leading to salt and water retention. Portal venous hypertension is then the driving force that causes fluid to accumulate in the peritoneal cavity. Sodium retention occurs before ascites develops. As liver disease worsens, ascites forms, which eventually becomes diuretic-resistant. This is followed by water retention (through antidiuretic hormone, ADH) leading to hyponatraemia and reduced renal blood flow leading to hepatorenal failure.

This theory does not readily explain ascites in malignant disease, which also responds to aldosterone antagonists.

Causes
- Most cases (90%) are due either to chronic liver disease or carcinomatosis with peritoneal seeding (Table 5.6)
- *Rapid onset of ascites* is a feature of decompensated cirrhosis, malignancy (including hepatoma), portal or splenic vein thrombosis, or Budd–Chiari syndrome
- *Ascites in an alcoholic cirrhotic* with pancreatitis may be due to hepatic decompensation or a pancreatic duct leak from pancreatitis. High ascitic amylase distinguishes pancreatic ascites
- Severe right heart failure, constrictive pericarditis, or hepatic venous outflow obstruction (Budd–Chiari syndrome) can be confused with cirrhosis. The clinical signs (hepatomegaly, elevated jugular venous pressure and ascites) are the same, so a high index of suspicion and echocardiography are indicated if cirrhosis has not

Table 5.6 Causes of ascites

Common	Uncommon	Rare
Cirrhosis	Nephrotic syndrome	Budd–Chiari syndrome (sudden onset)
Carcinomatosis	Cardiac failure	Portal vein thrombosis (if cirrhotic)
		Tuberculous peritonitis
		Chylous ascites
		Pancreatitis
		Biliary ascites
		Constrictive pericarditis
		Meig's syndrome
		Pseudomyxoma peritonei
		Ovarian hyperstimulation syndrome
		Peritoneal mesothelioma

been proven by liver biopsy. Cirrhosis secondary to cardiac failure is extremely rare and if the two conditions coexist, alcohol or haemochromatosis should be considered

Investigations

Examination of ascitic fluid is essential when ascites is first diagnosed, or if the clinical condition changes. The colour, protein content, results of microscopy and culture should be recorded on every sample; other tests are performed as indicated (Tables 5.7 and 5.8). Investigation of the underlying cause is then appropriate.

Consider non-hepatic causes of ascites if liver enzymes and coagulation studies are normal. Pay particular attention to:
• serum albumin (consider intestinal as well as urinary loss)
• urine protein (24 h collection)
• echocardiography (to exclude cardiac causes)

Management

The aim is a gradual, controlled loss of ascitic fluid. Diuretics are usually adequate, supplemented by fluid restriction and a low-sodium diet if ascites becomes refractory. Rigid insistence on fluid and salt restriction at too early a stage merely make the patient's life miserable, but views vary.
• Fluid loss > 500 mL (0.5 kg) each day exceeds the capacity of the peritoneum to absorb ascites and results in hypovolaemia. This rate of weight loss should not be exceeded unless peripheral oedema is present because interstitial oedema fluid can be more rapidly mobilised and excreted
• Other drugs should be reviewed and NSAIDs stopped because they cause fluid retention with deterioration in renal function

Small or moderate amounts of ascites
• Treated as an outpatient, starting with spironolactone 50–100 mg/day and no salt added to the food, rather than a low-sodium diet. Normal or near-normal renal function is required for spironolactone to have any effect on sodium excretion. Amiloride (5–15 mg/day) is an alternative if side-effects of spironolactone (e.g. gynaecomastia) are unacceptable, but is less effective
• Loop diuretics are used to augment response to aldosterone antagonists (Fig. 5.3)

Table 5.7 Ascitic fluid investigations

Condition	Investigation	Interpretation
All ascitic fluid	Colour	Table 5.8
	Protein*	< 25 g/L (2.5 g/dL), transudate (cirrhosis or hypoalbuminaemia)
		> 30 g/L (3.0 g/dL), exudate (malignancy, inflammation or Budd–Chiari), but there is substantial overlap between the two groups
	Culture	Any growth is abnormal
	Gram stain	> 1 bacterium/μL or > 250 polymorphs/μL indicate bacterial peritonitis
	Ziehl–Nielsen	If tuberculosis is suspected
Malignancy	Cytology	Large volume (20–50 mL), fresh specimen necessary. Malignant cells are diagnostic
Pancreatitis	Amylase	Varies between laboratories
Milky (chylous) ascites	Triglyceride	> 5 mmol/L is abnormal; normal in ascites pseudochylous ascites
Ascites from a biliary leak	Bilirubin	Ascitic fluid/serum bilirubin (ratio > 1.0 is abnormal)

*The serum–ascites protein gradient (serum albumin–ascitic albumin) is more accurate than the ascitic protein content alone for identifying the cause of ascites. An exudate (such as malignancy) has a protein gradient < 11 g/L (1.1 g/dL), and a transudate (such as portal hypertension) has a gradient > 11 g/L (1.1 g/dL).

Table 5.8 Colour of ascitic fluid

Pale straw	Haemorrhagic	Turbid	Milky
Cirrhosis	Carcinomatosis	Infection	Chylous
Nephrotic	Pancreatitis	Pancreatitis	Pseudochylous
Cardiac failure	Tuberculous		

- Review and weigh every week (aim for 2–4 kg/week) until ascites disappears
- Increase spironolactone by 100 mg/day every 3–5 days if ascites persists. The half-life of spironolactone is increased in liver disease: more frequent dose increases do not allow a steady state to be achieved

Refractory ascites
- Ensure that all specimens (Table 5.7) have been taken and that the cause of ascites has been established
- Ensure a sodium diet of < 100 mmol (no added salt) and fluid restriction (1000–1500 mL/day)
- Indications for paracentesis include tense ascites causing respiratory distress or discomfort and ascites that persists despite treatment as in Fig. 5.3
- Start therapeutic paracentesis, with intravenous colloid replacement (5–8 g albumin/L removed). This means 100 mL 20–25% human albumin solution for every 5 L drained
- Drain to dryness and remove paracentesis catheter within 6 h to prevent secondary infection
- Colloid replacement is essential to avoid hypotension and hepatorenal syndrome
- Diuretic therapy is usually needed to prevent reaccumulation of ascites

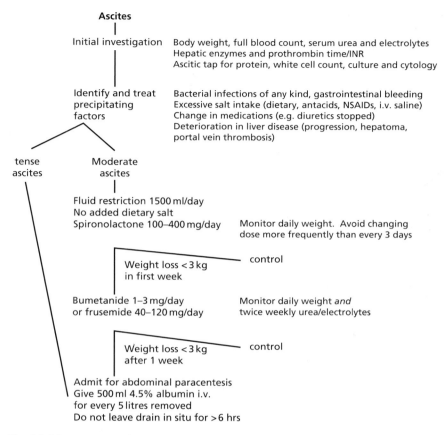

Fig. 5.3 Management of ascites.

- Paracentesis with colloid replacement is appropriate as the initial approach for tense ascites because it provides rapid relief. The risks of infection or rapid drainage causing renal impairment are probably no greater than the hazards of high-dose diuretics (20–70%, including renal impairment, hyponatraemia and encephalopathy)
- Transjugular intrahepatic portal–systemic shunt (TIPSS) has been used for diuretic-resistant ascites requiring repeated paracentesis. Referral to a specialist centre is necessary
- Surgical insertion of a peritoneovenous (LeVeen) shunt is occasionally justified. Blockage of the shunt is common
- Consider liver transplantation

Hepatorenal syndrome

Functional renal failure without any other demonstrable cause in the context of advanced liver disease is intimately related to the renal circulatory changes in cirrhosis and the management of ascites. Renal cortical hypoperfusion appears to be the key event, but renal blood flow and glomerular filtration rate do not correlate with the severity of ascites. A separate defect in tubular sodium handling is likely and hepatovascular natriuretic peptides may play a role.

Features

- Precipitated by excessive diuretic therapy, paracentesis without adequate colloid replacement, hypotension during surgery, and aggravated by sepsis
- Hypovolaemia must be excluded before making the diagnosis of hepatorenal failure
- Hyponatraemia and a high urea are invariable. Urine sodium is low (< 5 mmol/L), but there is little response to fluid challenge
- Sodium is avidly reabsorbed, water retained and ascites becomes refractory, whilst cortical hypoperfusion leads to renal failure
- Hyponatraemia, uraemia and hepatic failure contribute to terminal coma

Management

- Recognise the signs at the earliest stage—increasing urea or creatinine, especially with hyponatraemia—and stop diuretics
- Correct intravascular hypovolaemia with intravenous colloid (e.g. 1 L 4.5% human albumin solution)
- Splanchnic vasopressors (e.g. terlipressin 0.5 mg twice daily) with volume replacement (human albumin solution 1 g/kg, Section 1.9, p. 42) can lead to short-term improvements in renal function and may be appropriate as a bridge to transplantation and/or if reversible component to liver dysfunction (i.e. alcoholic hepatitis)
- Haemodialysis and haemofiltration are ineffective and have no impact on survival. The role of MARS in managing hepatorenal failure in the presence of jaundice is being evaluated
- Liver transplantation is the only treatment to affect survival, but is usually inappropriate by the time hepatorenal syndrome is established
- Prevention is the key, because mortality approaches 100% once hepatorenal syndrome is established. The following decrease the risk:
  - avoid hypotension, inadequate biochemical monitoring of diuretic therapy, excessive paracentesis and nephrotoxic drugs (aminoglycosides)
  - recognise and treat sepsis promptly
- Active measures are inappropriate if the underlying disease cannot be treated

Malignant ascites

The response to aldosterone antagonists, fluid and salt restriction is similar to cirrhotic ascites, but tense ascites is common and best managed by paracentesis. This may need to be repeated frequently. Instillation of cytotoxic drugs into the peritoneum is rarely effective and illogical if chemotherapy has not affected metastatic disease. Specialist advice should be sought. A peritoneovenous shunt may provide relief for some months before it blocks.

Chylous ascites

Chylous ascites is caused by lymphoma or neuroendocrine tumour obstructing lymphatics, surgical transection of lymphatics during aortic aneurysmectomy, lymphangiectasia, or occasionally nephrotic syndrome. Pseudochylous ascites, caused by malignancy or infection, looks the same but has a normal triglyceride content (Table 5.7, p. 148).

Treatment is with diuretics, salt restriction and dietary fat substitution with medium-chain triglycerides. Resection of a localised area of lymphangiectasia may be possible.

150

5.4 Portal hypertension

Portal hypertension usually arises from sinusoidal obliteration due to cirrhosis. Obstruction of the hepatic, portal or splenic veins (Fig. 5.4) may also raise portal venous pressure and cause collateral venous dilatation (varices).

Causes

Three main groups exist: presinusoidal, hepatic (sinusoidal) and venous outflow (postsinusoidal) obstruction (Table 5.9). The distinction is practical because presinusoidal causes have relatively normal hepatocellular function, which means that encephalopathy after a gastrointestinal bleed is less common and the results of surgical decompression are better. Hepatic causes are commonest in the West, but schistosomiasis is commonest worldwide.

Clinical features

The consequences of chronically raised portal venous pressure are varices, ascites, splenomegaly, hypersplenism, or portal hypertensive enteropathy.
- Varices—oesophageal varices are common, gastric and anorectal varices are less common. Umbilical varices (caput medusae) only occur if the umbilical vein remains patent after birth, and are very rare
- Ascites—does not occur if presinusoidal hypertension alone (e.g. portal vein thrombosis, p. 154)

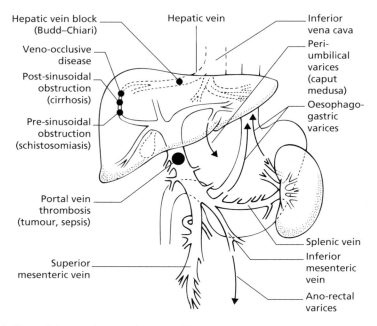

Fig. 5.4 Sites of obstruction causing portal hypertension and varices.

Table 5.9 Causes of portal hypertension

Presinusoidal	Sinusoidal	Venous outflow obstruction
Extrahepatic	Cirrhosis*	Budd–Chiari syndrome
portal vein thrombosis	Congenital hepatic	Veno-occlusive disease
splenic vein thrombosis	fibrosis	
Intrahepatic		
schistosomiasis		
primary biliary cirrhosis*		
sarcoidosis		
myeloproliferative disease		
Nodular regenerative hyperplasia		
(Azathioprine or rheumatoid arthritis)		

*Portal hypertension in cirrhosis is complex and partly due to postsinusoidal obliteration.

- Hypersplenism—recognised by splenomegaly, anaemia, thrombocytopenia and leucopenia
- Portal hypertensive enteropathy may cause mucosal congestion and bleeding from the stomach, small bowel or occasionally the colon. Gastropathy is by far the commonest site and may be becoming more common, due to variceal ligation (p. 15). Enteropathy is usually detected when there is recurrent bleeding of uncertain origin in a patient with portal hypertension who does not have obvious varices

Investigations

The diagnosis is made by finding splenomegaly or varices in the presence of chronic liver disease. Spleen size, however, does not correlate with the degree of portal hypertension and a normal spleen size does not exclude the diagnosis.

- Liver biopsy—histological proof of chronic liver disease should always be established if possible
- Endoscopy is best for detecting oesophageal and gastric varices. Asymptomatic patients with cirrhosis should be endoscoped, because although bleeding only occurs in 30% of patients with known varices, large varices are most likely to bleed and if identified, the risk can be reduced by beta-blocker prophylaxis
- Measurement of portal pressure (indirectly corresponding to *wedged hepatic venous pressure*) and *hepatic venous pressure gradient* (HVPG, wedged minus free hepatic venous pressure) to ascertain the cause of portal hypertension can be performed at the same time as a transjugular liver biopsy in difficult cases (see Table 5.10). The normal portal pressure is 7–12 mmHg and HVPG is 1–4 mmHg. Variceal haemorrhage does not occur with portal pressures < 12 mmHg

Table 5.10 Hepatic pressure gradient measurements in portal hypertension

Type of portal hypertension	Portal pressure (mmHg)	Hepatic venous pressure gradient
Normal	7–12	1–4
Extrahepatic	> 12	1–4
Sinusoidal	> 12	> 10
Presinusoidal	> 12	4–10

Difficulty arises when liver histology is apparently normal in the presence of varices and splenomegaly. This is an indication for:
- Ultrasound—with hepatic and portal vein Doppler studies to look for venous obstruction
- Hepatic venography—largely replaced by Doppler ultrasound, but may be needed if diagnostic uncertainty. Best performed at a specialist referral centre, together with review of liver histology (see portal pressure measurement above)

Management
Treatment of portal hypertension is directed at the complications of bleeding varices (p. 13) or ascites (p. 147). Specific treatment of the underlying disease (such as abstinence in alcoholic cirrhosis, venesection in haemochromatosis or anticoagulation in coagulopathies) is also appropriate.

Variceal prophylaxis
- Variceal banding (p. 14) is not currently indicated unless bleeding has occurred. It must be systematic and done repeatedly to be of value. The highest risk of rebleeding is in the first 6 weeks after the initial bleed
- Varices recur after obliteration in about 40%
- Propranolol 20–40 mg three times daily decreases the risk of bleeding and is indicated following initial variceal banding if varices are not eradicated endoscopically. It is the treatment of choice for portal hypertensive gastropathy. Unfortunately it is not always well tolerated

TIPSS
- Radiological insertion of a stent has transformed the management of refractory variceal bleeding. The technique is demanding and only available at specialist centres (Fig. 5.5)
- Principal indication is active or recurrent, especially gastric, variceal bleeding in spite of sclerotherapy, banding or other medical intervention. It effectively controls bleeding, but is best considered a temporising measure pending transplantation
- It can also be considered in managing refractory ascites (p. 149)
- Early complications relating to insertion are uncommon. Late complications include occlusion (up to 80% at 1 year) and chronic encephalopathy (around 25%). Monitoring patency by Doppler ultrasound and venography is necessary with subsequent stent dilatation. The occlusion rate has been reduced by using covered stents

Indications for surgical decompression
- Surgery (portosystemic shunting, oesophageal stapling or transection) should be considered if there are refractory bleeding varices despite endoscopic eradication (banding/sclerotherapy), and liver function is good (albumin normal, no encephalopathy during bleeding). This usually means patients with presinusoidal portal hypertension (i.e. congenital hepatic fibrosis)
- Orthotopic liver transplant should be considered if there is refractory bleeding in the presence of cirrhosis

Portal or splenic vein thrombosis
- Malignancy, pancreatitis, portal sepsis or haematological disorders (see below) can cause thrombosis of the portal or splenic veins. 50% are idiopathic

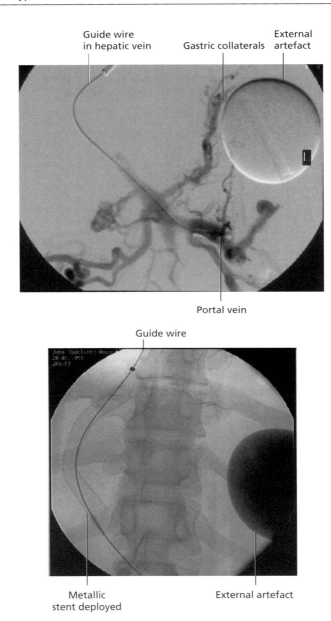

Guide wire
in hepatic vein

Gastric collaterals

External
artefact

Portal vein

Guide wire

Metallic
stent deployed

External artefact

Fig. 5.5 Insertions of transjugular portal shunt. (a) A guide wire is passed from the hepatic to the portal vein. (b) The metallic stent is then deployed.

- The possibility of portal vein thrombosis should always be considered if refractory ascites develops in cirrhosis. Once this occurs prognosis is poor
- Isolated splenic vein thrombosis results in gastric varices. Recurrent bleeding often responds to splenectomy. Splenectomy should be avoided in patients with cirrhosis as it often results in secondary portal vein and mesenteric vein thrombosis

- Treatment is directed at the ascites and underlying cause
- Anticoagulants or thrombolysis are rarely appropriate, because of the risk of variceal bleeding.

Surgery is usually unsatisfactory because the veins used for grafting are thrombosed

Budd–Chiari syndrome

- Hepatic vein obstruction may be caused by haematological disorders (polycythaemia, protein C deficiency, antithrombin III deficiency, paroxysmal nocturnal haemoglobinuria), antiphospholipid syndrome (positive anticardiolipin antibody), malignancy, trauma, or oral contraceptives
- Abdominal pain, tender hepatomegaly and ascites are variable: it may present as a severe, acute condition, or as a mild, chronic illness
- Liver biopsy is diagnostic
- Enlargement of caudate lobe is common but not diagnostic
- Treatment of the underlying disease, anticoagulation or surgical decisions (including transplantation and TIPSS) are best made at a referral centre. Early referral is important

Veno-occlusive disease

Non-thrombotic obliteration of intrahepatic venules is diagnosed by liver biopsy, but may be difficult to distinguish from Budd–Chiari syndrome. Pyrrolizidine alkaloids (*Senecio* ragwort, or comfrey herbal teas), irradiation and cytotoxic drugs are possible causes.

5.5 Hepatitis

Hepatitis involves inflammation of the whole liver. Most episodes are subclinical, detected (if at all) by abnormal liver enzymes, but the spectrum extends to include acute liver failure with jaundice. It may be caused by viral or bacterial infections, drugs, chemicals or toxins (e.g. alcohol).

Causes

(See Table 5.11)
Although identification of hepatotropic viruses appears to be proceeding through the alphabet (hepatitis A, B, C, D, E), almost all cases of transfusion-associated hepatitis can be accounted for by currently known viruses (including CMV, *Herpes simplex* virus, etc.). Hepatitis B, C and D lead to chronic hepatitis.

Clinical features

A high prevalence of asymptomatic hepatitis is suggested by the frequency of patients with antibodies to hepatitis A, B or E without recalling a specific illness.

History

These features are characteristic of viral hepatitis (all types), but are less common in other causes of jaundice.

- Prodrome (2 days to 2 weeks)—malaise, anorexia, distaste for cigarettes, nausea, myalgia, fever
- Jaundice:
  - prodromal symptoms start to resolve

Table 5.11 Causes of hepatitis

Common	Uncommon	Rare*
Hepatitis viruses	Hepatitis viruses	Delta virus[†]
A	C (parenteral non-A, non-B)	CMV
B	E (enteral non-A, non-B)	Hepatitis G
Alcohol	Epstein–Barr virus	Coxsackie A and B
	Drugs (p. 160)	Herpes simplex
	Autoimmune	Echovirus
	Ischaemia	*Mycoplasma*
		Leptospirosis
		Measles
		Arenavirus (Lassa)
		Flavivirus (yellow fever)
		Rickettsia (typhus)
		Chemicals (CCl_4)
		Toxins (mushrooms)

*Consider CMV and Hep E first.
[†]Only with coexisting hepatitis B infection.

- itching is rare (except in alcoholic or drug-induced cholestatic hepatitis)
- dark urine and yellow (not clay-coloured) stools may occur
- Associated symptoms can occur in any viral hepatitis although most commonly reported with acute hepatitis B, including arthralgia, arthritis and an urticarial rash. Membranous glomerulonephritis and nephrotic syndrome have been reported in persistent hepatitis B infection. Cryoglobulin-induced glomerulonephritis occurs rarely with chronic hepatitis C infection.
- Resolution is usual, although some forms progress to chronic disease (Table 5.12)

Examination
- Jaundice (anicteric cases are detected by liver enzyme tests)
- Tender hepatomegaly
- No signs of chronic liver disease (Table 5.2, p. 137) except in alcoholic hepatitis as cirrhosis often coexists, when fever is also prominent
- Splenomegaly is commonly present in alcoholic hepatitis, infectious mononucleosis (EBV) or rickettsial infections. It occurs in about 15% of uncomplicated viral hepatitis

Outcome
- Complete recovery may take several weeks, or occasionally months. Lassitude and anorexia are commonly the most persistent symptoms
- Acute hepatic failure (p. 42) hardly ever occurs in hepatitis A and is exceptionally rare in hepatitis C. It develops in about 1% of symptomatic hepatitis B infections, and is characteristic of hepatitis E acquired during pregnancy
- Chronic liver disease may follow acute viral hepatitis (B and C), but the risk depends on the virus (Table 5.12). This includes all grades and stages of chronic hepatitis (p. 162), cirrhosis (p. 173) and hepatocellular carcinoma (p. 178)
- Relapse, usually with a milder attack, occurs in 2–10%. Recovery may still be complete, or it may indicate progression to chronic liver disease. A characteristic cholestatic (rise in ALP) phase occurs following acute hepatitis A in 10%

Table 5.12 Differences between types of viral hepatitis

	A	B	C	D	E
Incubation (weeks)*	2–6	4–26	6–12	3–20	2–9
Transmission	Faeces Saliva	Blood Semen Saliva Perinatal	Blood	Blood	Faeces
Epidemic	Yes	No	No	No	Yes
Risk factors	Children Institutions Seafood Travel to Middle/Far East Seasonal (winter) Homosexuals	Middle/Far East Drug abuse Homosexuals Haemophiliacs Renal dialysis Neonates of HBV +ve mothers	Drug abuse Haemophiliacs Transfusion	HBV only Drug abuse Homosexuals	Travel to North India/ Middle East/ Mexico Has been reported in UK
Chronic disease	No	5–20%	70%	30–50%	No
Prevention	Immunoglobulin Vaccination	Immunoglobulin Vaccination	Screen blood products	None	None
Carrier	No	Yes	Yes	Yes	No

*The incubation period varies widely.

- Asymptomatic carriers (5–10% following hepatitis B) may have normal liver function or chronic liver disease

Investigations

Liver enzymes
- An AST > 10 times the upper limit of normal is the hallmark of acute hepatitis (Table 5.3, p. 137). The pattern of change in relation to serological markers is shown in Fig. 5.6
- The AST does not always correlate with the degree of liver damage, especially in severe cases or in chronic hepatitis C infection (p. 166)
- Predominant cholestasis is unusual in acute viral hepatitis, but more common in *Leptospira* sp. or alcoholic hepatitis and as a late phase of hepatitis A
- An AST > 700 in alcoholics suggests another aetiological factor, such as acetaminophen/paracetamol toxicity or viral illness

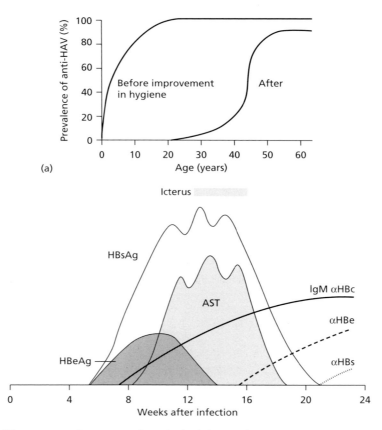

Fig. 5.6 **Time course of enzyme and serological changes in acute hepatitis B.**
(a) Hepatitis A. (b) Hepatitis B. From Sherlock S., Dooley J. Dis Liver Bil Sys.

Other blood tests
- Monospot or Paul–Bunnell test is advisable in adults who are HAV IgM and hepatitis B-negative. EBV DNA or IgM can be measured if there is doubt about the diagnosis, but also consider *Mycoplasma pneumoniae*
- Neutropenia is common in viral hepatitis before jaundice appears. Atypical lymphocytes are seen in infectious mononucleosis, and rarely in cytomegalovirus or toxoplasmosis. Rarely viral hepatitis can be followed by aplastic anaemia. CMV infection can be diagnosed by PCR or a rising antigen titre and should be considered if predominant prodromal symptoms with lymphadenopathy or if immunosuppressed

Serology
- Hepatitis A IgM (anti-HAV IgM) and HBsAg should always be checked
- Hepatitis B e antigen (HBsAg) should be checked if HBsAg-positive, to assess infectivity
- δ-hepatitis (anti-HDV) should be checked if the patient is HBsAg-positive and a drug abuser, homosexual, or unwell
- Antibody tests for hepatitis C are appropriate if anti-HAV IgM and HBsAg are negative
- Autoantibodies (antismooth muscle and antinuclear antigen) should always be checked if tests for hepatitis A, B and C are negative

Polymerase chain reaction
- PCR detects viral DNA (hepatitis B) or RNA (hepatitis C), indicating the presence of active viral infection and replication
- Its main role is in confirming the presence of hepatitis C viral RNA when an HCV antibody test is positive, so that decisions can be made about interferon therapy for chronic hepatitis (p. 162) and the response can be monitored. About 20% will be persistently HCV RNA negative, consistent with viral clearance
- Genotype identification of hepatitis C is also important when deciding about treatment (p. 167). Certain hepatitis B genotypes may also be associated with a more favourable prognosis. Specialist advice is appropriate

Meaning of markers

Hepatitis A
- Anti-HAV IgM antibody indicates recent infection (within 8 weeks) and disappears soon after jaundice appears
- Anti-HAV IgG antibody indicates immunity, appears within 2 weeks of infection and persists for years

Hepatitis B
(See Table 5.13)
- Persistence of HBsAg for more than 6 months defines a carrier
- About 1% per year will subsequently develop antibodies to surface protein
- The complete virus is called the Dane particle. Antihepatitis B core antigen (anti-HBcAg) acts against the core, which is formed in the hepatocyte nucleus

Hepatitis C
- Second-generation ELISA or radioimmunoblot assay (RIBA, 'third generation') against a range of HCV epitopes are more reliable, approaching over 95% positive predictive value

Table 5.13 Serological markers in hepatitis B

Stage	HBsAg	HbeAg	Anti-HBs	Anti-HBe	Anti-HBc (IgG)
Incubation	+	+		−	−
Acute liver failure*	−	−	−	−	+ core IgM
Acute hepatitis	+	+	−	+/−	+ core IgM
Carrier	+	+/−	−	+/−	+
Recovery	−	−	+	+	+
Vaccination	−	−	+	−	−

*In acute liver failure damage is due to immunological response to viral clearance and thus recent HBV infection can only be diagnosed by presence of HBcore IgM (need to request specifically).

- PCR (p. 159) is the only absolute confirmatory test
- HCV antibody develops within 3 months of infection. HCV RNA can usually be detected within 6 weeks of acute infection (e.g. needlestick injury) and often as early at 2 weeks

Management

Acute attack
- No specific treatment is available and most patients will settle with symptomatic treatment
- General or specific immunoglobulin does not alter the outcome of severe hepatitis A or B
- Bed rest is unnecessary. Exercise has no effect on the severity of the attack or relapse rate, but most patients with hepatitis prefer to avoid exercise
- Careful hand washing and a high standard of personal hygiene are essential to prevent transmission
- Admission to hospital is only necessary for severe attacks or if the patient is unwell and lives alone. Isolation is unnecessary, but gloves should be worn when handling all excreta (urine, faeces, vomit) or when taking blood
- It is essential to withdraw drugs or alcohol if these are the causative agent
- Patient preference is the best guide to diet. A low-fat diet is often preferred by patients, but otherwise has no special value
- Every case of acute viral hepatitis requires notification of public health officials (p. 367)

Contacts
- It is usually too late to treat close contacts of hepatitis A (shared bathrooms or kitchens and physical contact) with human normal immunoglobulin (5 mL intramuscular injection) but may be considered in an outbreak
- Sexual partners of hepatitis B patients should be tested for HBsAg and if not immune given recombinant vaccine (p. 161). Hyperimmune HBV immunoglobulin can be given as well if abstinence is impracticable whilst active immunity develops (2–4 weeks)

Follow-up
- Abstinence from alcohol is often recommended until liver function has returned to normal, but moderate drinking (4–8 units/week) is not harmful

- Normal activity, including work, can be resumed as soon as the patient feels ready, but this often takes 2–6 weeks
- Liver enzymes should be checked after 6 weeks and again after 6 months if they have not returned to normal
- Abnormal liver enzymes elevated over twofold after 6 months are an indication for further investigation, including ultrasound and liver biopsy. Minor abnormalities can be observed with repeat blood tests every few months, and only investigated if there is an increasing trend
- Chronic hepatitis (see p. 162)

Immunisation

Hepatitis A

Active immunisation against HAV
Active immunisation with live attenuated and killed vaccines have largely been replaced by recombinant vaccines. It is indicated for:
- Travellers to highly endemic areas (Indian subcontinent, Middle East, South America, Mexico), who will not be staying in hotels
- Close contacts (family, institutional members) of patients with acute HAV who have not previously been exposed, given in a different site to immunoglobulin

Passive immunisation against HAV
Passive immunisation with intramuscular human normal immunoglobulin 5 mL is effective for about 4 months. In many cases it suppresses the clinical manifestations rather than preventing infection. It is indicated for:
- Close contacts of patients with acute HAV (infection risk is 45% in children, 5–20% in adults)
- Travellers to endemic areas leaving too soon to complete a course of active immunisation. It is cheaper to test travellers for antibodies to HAV rather than to give immunoglobulin indiscriminately

Hepatitis B

Active immunisation against HBV
Active immunisation with recombinant HBV vaccine (three doses, 0, 1 and 6 months apart) is indicated for:
- HBsAg-negative close contacts of patients with acute HBV
- Haemophiliacs
- Renal dialysis patients
- Patients requiring repeated transfusion
- Staff of institutions for mentally retarded
- Prisoners and prison staff
- Laboratory staff
- Health care personnel (including doctors, dentists, nurses and students)
- People working abroad in highly endemic areas

161

- Drug abusers, prostitutes and homosexuals should be offered vaccination if the opportunity arises In some jurisdictions universal immunisation of preadolescent teens is performed
- Booster doses are needed every 5–10 years at present

Passive immunisation against HBV
Passive immunisation with two doses of intramuscular hyperimmune HBV immunoglobulin 500 IU 1 month apart should be given to:
- Non-immune staff with needlestick injuries from HBV-infected patients, within 1–7 days, followed by active immunisation after 7 days. For needlestick injuries from HBV-negative patients, active immunisation should be commenced and policy procedures reviewed
- Close contacts of patients with acute HBV
- Neonates born to HBV-positive mothers (200 IU within 12 h of birth and 0.5 mL (10 µg) recombinant HBV vaccine at separate sites. Second and third doses of recombinant vaccine at 1 and 6 months)

Hepatitis C, D, E
Neither passive nor active immunisation is currently effective.

5.6 Progressive liver disease

Classification of chronic hepatitis
Chronic hepatitis is defined as hepatic inflammation continuing for more than 6 months. It is a histological diagnosis and, like cirrhosis, is a stage in the progression of many liver diseases of different aetiology (Table 5.16, p. 165). It is defined histologically according to the grade of hepatic inflammation, the stage of fibrosis (Fig. 5.7) and the cause of the liver disease. There are several histological scoring systems in use, which include the Scheuer, Ishak modified histological activity index (HAI) and the METAVIR systems. The latter was developed for scoring damage in chronic viral hepatitis C (Tables 5.14 and 5.15).
- Classification caters for patients with very active inflammation (grades 3 or 4) who may not yet have developed any fibrosis (stage 0 or 1), and for patients with end-stage, inactive cirrhosis (grade 0 or 1, stage 4)
- Treatment decisions depend primarily on the cause, but grading and staging are useful in deciding thresholds for treatment (e.g. hepatitis C) and response to treatment

Causes
A specific cause can be identified for most (70–85%) cases of chronic hepatitis (Table 5.16, p. 165).

Investigations
- Essential investigations for all patients with progressive liver disease include a meticulous history, hepatitis serology (B, C), liver autoantibodies, immunoglobulins, serum ferritin and iron/total iron-binding capacity ratio and liver biopsy with iron, and periodic acid Schiff (PAS) stains. Wilson's disease, although rare, should be considered in anyone < 40 years with chronic hepatitis

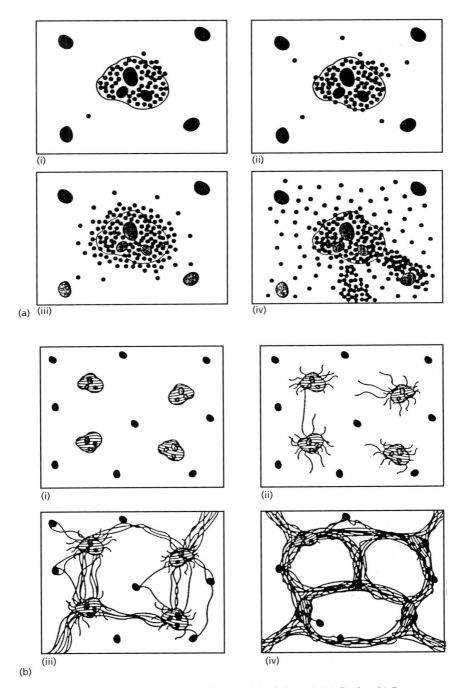

Fig. 5.7 Pathological features of chronic hepatitis (Scheuer). (a) Grades. (b) Stages as explained in Table 5.14. Adapted from Batts and Ludwig, *Am J Surg Path* 1995, 19: 1409–17.

Table 5.14 The Scheuer histological classification of chronic hepatitis

Grade	Lymphocytic piecemeal necrosis	Lobular inflammation and necrosis
0	None	None
1	Minimal, patchy	Occasional spotty necrosis
2	Mild, involving some or all portal tracts	Little hepatocellular damage
3	Involving all portal tracts	Noticeable hepatocellular change
4	Severe, may have bridging necrosis	Prominent and diffuse hepatocellular damage

Stage	Descriptive	Criteria
0	No fibrosis	Normal connective tissue
1	Portal fibrosis	Fibrous portal expansion
2	Periportal fibrosis	Periportal or rare portal septa
3	Septal fibrosis	Fibrous septa with distortion of architecture, no obvious cirrhosis
4	Cirrhosis	Cirrhosis

Table 5.15 Histological scoring systems for chronic hepatitis

Scoring system	Scoring	
	Fibrosis (stage)	Histological activity (grading)
Scheuer	0–4	Portal/periportal 0–4
		Lobular 0–4
Ishak modified HAI	0–6	Periportal hepatitis 0–4
		Confluent necrosis 0–6
		Apoptosis/focal inflammation/necrosis 0–4
		Portal inflammation 0–4
		Total score out of 18
METAVIR	0–4	Piecemeal necrosis + lobular necrosis 0–3

Further details can be found in Brunt, et al. *Hepatology* 2000; 31: 241.

- Table 5.16 emphasises the detail and different investigations necessary for a specific diagnosis. It is always best to have complementary discriminating investigations that confirm the diagnosis, rather than to depend on a single result. Otherwise the unwary will fall into traps such as confusing autoimmune chronic hepatitis with primary sclerosing cholangitis, or missing concomitant haemochromatosis or hepatitis C infection in an alcoholic

Viral chronic hepatitis

Hepatitis B
- Chronic infection is more common in men, infection at a young age, haemophiliacs, Africans and Asians. Up to 60% of chronic HBsAg carriers have little or no hepatic inflammation
- Clinical features vary from mild non-specific symptoms to evidence of severe chronic liver disease. Arthralgia and an urticarial rash can occur, as in acute HBV infection
- Spontaneous improvement occurs in up to 30%

Table 5.16 Diagnosis of specific causes of chronic hepatitis

Viral hepatitis*

B	HBsAg positive. Viral DNA by PCR. Orcein stain positive on liver biopsy
C	HCV antibody by ELISA or RIBA, confirmed by PCR for HCV RNA. Lymphoid follicles characteristic on biopsy
B and D	Antibody to delta virus
Autoimmune	Antismooth muscle antibody titre > 1 : 80, antinuclear antibody > 1 : 80. Elevated IgG titre, female predominance (8 : 1), associated thyroiditis
Metabolic	Serum ferritin elevated and Fe/TIBC ratio > 55%.
Haemochromatosis	HLA-A3 positive. PCR positive (see text) Perl's stain positive on biopsy
Wilson's	Serum caeruloplasmin < 0.2 g/L. Increased urinary copper (> 0.1 mg/24 h). Increased dry weight liver copper
α_1-antitrypsin deficiency	Serum α-antitrypsin < 0.2 g/L, PiZZ phenotype on electrophoresis. PAS-positive globules on biopsy
Alcohol	History, random alcohol, γ-GT, raised MCV, elevated IgA. Fatty infiltration, megamitochondria, Mallory's hyaline on biopsy
Non-alcoholic steatohepatitis	Identical histology to alcoholic hepatitis. Elevated ALT, AST > ALT. Associated increased BMI, hypertension and hypercholesteraemia
Drugs	History. Amiodarone, methotrexate, nitrofurantoin, α-methyldopa, etc. Wide variety of features on biopsy, especially eosinophilic infiltrate
Biliary	
Primary biliary cirrhosis	Antimitochondrial antibody positive, M2 antigen specific. Elevated serum IgM. Bile duct proliferation, lymphoid aggregates and granulomas on biopsy
Primary sclerosing cholangitis	ERCP. Sigmoidoscopy and biopsy (80% associated with ulcerative colitis)
Cryptogenic	All other causes excluded (15–30%). ALP/ALT often only mildly elevated. Possibly represent burnt out autoimmune chronic active hepatitis

*Hepatitis A and other hepatotropic viruses (e.g. Epstein–Barr virus, herpesvirus, arboviruses) cause acute, but not chronic, liver disease. Fe/TIBC; iron/total iron-binding capacity.

- Patients with minimal or mild inflammation on biopsy have an excellent outlook. No treatment is indicated and annual liver function test monitoring can be performed by the family doctor, with referral for review (and possible rebiopsy) if there is a twofold increase in ALT or symptomatic deterioration
- Liver function tests rise in hepatitis B during seroconversion (i.e. spontaneous conversion to e Ab) as well as during flares in hepatitis. Patients with fluctuating transaminases have a worse prognosis
- Patients who are HBeAg-positive (marker of continued viral replication) who have marked activity on liver biopsy should be considered for antiviral therapy and specialist advice sought. Treatment is expensive and local protocols should be used
- Subcutaneous α-interferon 10 MU three times weekly for 4–6 months reduces the ALT level in up to 70% and a sustained loss of viral replication in 30% (becoming HBeAg-negative). Side-effects (malaise, headache, nausea) are almost universal, but usually tolerable. Patients with high transaminases (> 200 IU/L) respond more readily

- Newer antiviral agents include the oral nucleoside analogue lamivudine and adefovir. Both agents are potent suppressors of HBV replication, although the former is associated with the development of HBV DNA polymerase mutations. These agents are particularly effective in decompensated hepatitis B cirrhosis, where α-interferon is contraindicated. Other oral antiviral agents are being developed and may have a therapeutic role in combination with interferon
- Liver transplantation is no longer contraindicated for hepatitis B cirrhosis. Recurrent hepatitis B in the graft can be prevented by prophylactic lamivudine or adefovir, started post-transplantation or shortly before grafting, with or without regular hepatitis B immunoglobulin
- Prognosis is variable. Patients with inactive cirrhosis do well, but in cirrhosis with marked inflammation, 5-year survival is around 50%
- Hepatocellular carcinoma occurs in a small minority of non-cirrhotic hepatitis B carriers and at a rate of 1–3% per year in hepatitis B cirrhosis. It is most common in HBeAg patients and more common in men
- Surveillance for hepatocellular carcinoma with ultrasound every 3–6 months should be considered in cirrhotic patients. Although screening detects smaller tumours, there is as yet no evidence that screening reduces mortality. Alpha fetoprotein is a less useful marker of hepatocellular carcinoma in viral hepatitis, because it rises with active inflammation

Hepatitis C
- Up to 70% develop chronic hepatitis and between 5% and 20% develop cirrhosis within 20 years of infection
- More rapid progression occurs in those with transfusion-acquired hepatitis C, immunosuppressed (renal transplant recipients), infection acquired in later life, and in those drinking excess alcohol
- Symptoms, management and outlook of mild degrees of inflammation are as for HBV (see above). However, transaminases are an inaccurate measure of the degree of inflammation in HCV and cirrhosis may be present with normal liver function tests
- In those with hepatitis C antibodies the presence of HCV RNA should be checked by PCR. Biopsy is usually appropriate if PCR-positive, to assess the degree of fibrosis
- Hepatitis C genotype does not affect disease progression, but does affect response to, and length of, treatment. There are geographical variations in genotype with 70% in the UK being genotype 1. Genotypes 2 and 3 are equally common in the USA
- When there is moderate active inflammation and/or fibrosis, treatment with interferon and ribavirin should be considered. Treatment guidelines have been published by the National Institute for Health (NIH in the USA), European Association for the Study of the Liver (EASL) and NICE (in the UK)
- Long-acting pegylated α-interferon (once weekly subcutaneous injection) with oral ribavirin is associated with an overall 55% cure. Cure is defined as absence of HCV RNA in serum 6 months after treatment has finished and is durable. This equates to a 70–80% cure rate for genotype 2/3 and a 45% for genotype 1. Treatment is given for 6 months (genotype 2/3) or 12 months (genotype 1)

- Response to treatment can be predicted by PCR testing for HCV RNA at 3 months into treatment. Treatment should be discontinued in genotype 2/3 who remain PCR-positive at 3 months or those with genotype 1 who remain PCR-positive and who have not achieved a 2 log fall in HCV RNA over the first 3 months of treatment
- Screening by ultrasound for hepatocellular carcinoma should be considered in cirrhotic patients who would be candidates for potentially curative therapy (ablative local treatment, chemotherapy or transplantation)
- Liver transplantation should be considered in end-stage cirrhosis. However, hepatitis C recurrence is universal and as many as 10–15% will develop cirrhosis within the graft within 5 years of transplantation

Autoimmune chronic hepatitis

Autoimmune chronic hepatitis (previously termed 'chronic active hepatitis') is classically divided into two types, although the type does not alter treatment and has little influence on prognosis.

- Type 1, the most common form, is identified by antinuclear or antismooth muscle antibodies (70–100%). 10% also have weakly positive AMA
- Type 2 has antiliver kidney microsomal antibodies (100%) and may more commonly progress to cirrhosis
- A minority only have antibodies to soluble liver antigens or characteristic histology and no identifiable autoantibody. The term 'lupoid' hepatitis has been abandoned and has nothing to do with systemic lupus erythematosus

Clinical features

- 80% women, most commonly aged 10–30 or > 50 years (men are usually in the older age group)
- Malaise, arthralgia, anorexia or an urticarial rash may precede jaundice by several months. Onset is abrupt in one-third, but others may have mild symptoms and be identified on investigation of abnormal liver function tests
- A minority (up to 30%) have associated autoimmune thyroiditis, diabetes, pleurisy/pericarditis, glomerulonephritis, ulcerative colitis or haemolytic anaemia
- Signs of chronic liver disease (Table 5.2, p. 137) are common, but patients often look remarkably well. Cushingoid features may reflect steroid treatment

Investigations

- ALT is elevated 2–20 times and reliably reflects the degree of hepatic inflammation. Albumin is normal or low. Leucopenia and thrombocytopenia, due to hypersplenism, indicate severe disease. Serum IgG is usually elevated
- HLA-B8 is present in 30–80%, being more common in younger patients and those with more aggressive disease. Tissue typing is indicated if there are unusual features (e.g. males, or outside normal age range)
- Autoantibody tests (see above) and liver biopsy are diagnostic, but confidence in the diagnosis is increased if the IgG is also elevated
- Histology shows a mononuclear infiltrate of the portal and periportal areas, plasma cells, piecemeal necrosis and fibrosis, or cirrhosis. Iron and copper stains should always be performed and be negative

- ERCP is indicated if the ALP is disproportionately elevated (> threefold), because the histology of primary sclerosing cholangitis can occasionally be mistaken for autoimmune hepatitis

Treatment
- Treatment is with prednisolone 30 mg daily. Response is monitored by serial ALT measurements and the dose decreased by 5 mg daily every 2–4 weeks once the ALT has been < twofold elevated for 4 weeks. A dose of 5–10 mg daily is usually necessary indefinitely
- If steroid-induced side-effects are prominent, or it is not possible to reduce the steroids to < 10 mg, azathioprine can be introduced as a steroid-sparing agent. Some do this routinely within 4 weeks and rapidly reduce the dose of prednisolone to 10 mg daily
- Steroids can sometimes be stopped after 1–2 years, but active disease frequently recurs, sometimes in a severe, rebound attack of hepatitis
- Repeat liver biopsy to assess progress is not usually justified if the clinical and biochemical response has been good

Prognosis
- In patients without cirrhosis, about one-third will develop cirrhosis even with treatment after 5 years but this only very rarely leads to decompensated liver disease
- The 5-year survival rate even after cirrhosis has occurred exceeds 90%
- Liver transplantation is appropriate if decompensation occurs in spite of immunosuppression

Primary biliary cirrhosis
- Interlobular and septal bile ducts are destroyed by chronic granulomatous inflammation of unknown cause
- Increasing cholestasis leads to biliary cirrhosis and the complications of portal hypertension. Synthetic liver function (albumin and prothrombin time) is preserved
- AMA are almost invariably present

Clinical features
- 90% women
- Age 40–60 years
- Incidental detection of an elevated ALP is now the commonest presentation. Most (80%) asymptomatic patients have progressive disease and will develop symptoms, although this may take up to 10–20 years
- Pruritus almost always precedes jaundice by 6 months to 2 years and lethargy is common
- Skin pigmentation, xanthelasma, xanthomas, hepatomegaly and a palpable spleen are characteristic signs. Malnutrition and ascites are very late signs because hepatocellular function is relatively preserved, although oesophageal varices are common
- Osteoporosis is common

Investigations
- Elevated ALP (5–20 times normal). This is initially the only biochemical abnormality and hepatic origin is confirmed by an elevated γ-glutamyltransferase. ALT may be slightly elevated, but albumin remains normal until late

- M2 AMA are present in high titre in 98%. These are specific to primary biliary cirrhosis, although M4 AMA may occur in autoimmune chronic hepatitis. Patients with positive AMA and normal liver function tests are likely to develop primary biliary cirrhosis over the course of 10 years
- Serum IgM and cholesterol are usually elevated. Although there is no increased cardiovascular mortality
- Ultrasound (to exclude other causes of cholestasis; Table 5.1, p. 136)
- Liver biopsy demonstrates chronic inflammation around the bile ducts, with granulomas and cirrhosis. Unlike viral hepatitis the disease is patchy and a liver biopsy can underestimate the extent of fibrosis. In the precirrhotic stage it can occasionally be difficult to distinguish from other forms of chronic hepatitis or primary sclerosing cholangitis, but autoantibodies, other serological tests and ERCP should be discriminating
- Autoimmune cholangitis (or AMA–negative primary biliary cirrhosis) is a condition with the biochemical and histological features of primary biliary cirrhosis together with high antinuclear antibody titres, but negative AMA

Management
- As for other causes of cirrhosis, the aim should be to assess hepatic function, specific treatment, treatment of complications and consideration of liver transplantation
- The results of liver enzymes should be recorded at each outpatient visit. The bilirubin level is predictive of outcome
- Treatment with ursodeoxycholic acid 12–15 mg/kg/day daily improves ALP and bilirubin, some aspects of liver histology and results in a trend towards improved survival with a decrease in liver transplantation. Since it is usually well tolerated, treatment should be started early. Other drugs (steroids, azathioprine, penicillamine, colchicine, cyclosporin, methotrexate) have not been shown to work in controlled trials
- Symptoms of pruritus often respond to cholestyramine 4–12 g/day. Other effective antipruritic agents include rifampicin and naltrexone
- Complications of portal hypertension are treated in the standard way for ascites (Fig. 5.3, p. 149) and variceal bleeding (p. 13). Encephalopathy is rare
- Patients may want to get in touch with the Primary Biliary Cirrhosis Support Group (Appendix 1, p. 440)
- Hepatic transplantation is curative and should be considered for patients < 60 years, with jaundice (bilirubin 100 µmol/L), uncontrolled pruritus, or complications of portal hypertension. The earlier the referral, the better the results of transplant, and when clotting is disordered or ascites develops, time is short (p. 182)

Prognosis
- Mean survival in asymptomatic patients is 12 years, but some patients have rapidly progressive disease
- Once jaundice develops, survival is < 2 years
- 5-year survival following transplant is 80–90% and is improving. Although recurrence does occur in the graft, it does not impact on 5–10-year survival rates.

Haemochromatosis
- Autosomal recessive metabolic disorder causing inappropriate intestinal iron absorption and tissue damage from iron deposition ('bronze diabetes')

- Uncommon (3–8 : 10 000 population), but increasingly recognised and an iron stain should be performed on all liver biopsies that reveal chronic hepatitis or cirrhosis
- Caused by an amino acid substitution (cysteine for tyrosine at amino acid 282) in about 90% of cases in the HFE gene. DNA analysis by PCR is both sensitive and specific
- The mechanism of increased iron absorption is complex and contains other genes involved in iron absorption across the enterocyte, including divalent metal transporter (DMT1)

Clinical features
- Many patients now present as relatives of an index case, during investigation of an incidental finding of abnormal liver function tests or with elevated ferritin
- Non-specific malaise and abdominal pain are the commonest symptoms

Classical signs
Classical signs include:
- Age 40–60 years, usually male, because menstrual loss protects premenopausal women
- Arthropathy—earliest or only sign, as a symmetrical polyarthropathy in metacarpophalangeal (always look for evidence of arthritis in the first and second metacarpophalangeal joints) and larger joints. Chondrocalcinosis may be visible on X-rays
- Hepatomegaly—with signs of chronic liver disease (Table 5.2, p. 137). The liver may be tender. A bruit suggests a hepatoma, which develops in 10% or more of those with established cirrhosis
- Diabetes—but exocrine pancreatic malfunction is rare
- Pigmentation—from a 'winter tan' to slate-grey
- Testicular atrophy and loss of libido, pubic and axillary hair are due to impaired pituitary function caused by iron deposition, as well as chronic liver disease affecting hormonal metabolism
- Cardiac failure (dilated cardiomyopathy) is now rarely due to iron deposition, but should always be considered in patients who have both cardiomyopathy and cirrhosis. Alcohol usually only affects one organ or the other, but alcohol abuse is also more common in patients with haemochromatosis

Investigations
- Abnormal liver enzymes depend on the amount of liver damage
- Serum iron is high and total iron-binding capacity is low, with a high saturation (often > 80%). Ferritin is markedly elevated when cirrhosis is present, but may only be at the upper limit of normal in earlier stages. Ferritin is an acute phase protein and is elevated in inflammatory conditions as well as in alcoholics
- Now that PCR for the specific mutation is available, this is likely to become the initial investigation of choice when iron overload is suspected, or in investigating the families of index cases
- Liver biopsy is diagnostic. However, fibrosis is unlikely with a ferritin < 1000 μg/L. In the presence of homozygosity for the HFE, a liver biopsy is indicted in the presence of abnormal liver biochemistry or a ferritin > 1000 μg/L. All biopsies should routinely be stained for iron (Perl's stain). Alcohol, chronic haemolysis (with or without repeated transfusion), hepatic prophyria or excess iron ingestion may cause hepatic siderosis to a lesser degree

Management
- Venesection to a haematocrit < 0.50% and total iron binding capacity > 50 μmol/L (saturation < 40%, or ferritin < 100 μg/L) is the best treatment. This initially means weekly venesection.
- Outpatient checks:
  - ask about fatigue, dyspnoea, arthritis and control of diabetes
  - check liver enzymes, iron and iron-binding capacity and glycosylated haemoglobin (if diabetic)
  - deterioration in liver enzymes despite normal iron studies suggests a hepatoma
- Screen *first-degree relatives* by PCR analysis if available, or HLA typing if not. If the HLA type (usually A3) is the same as the index case, the risk of haemochromatosis is about 95%. However, incomplete gene penetrance means that not everyone with the genetic abnormality will develop iron overload. Screening by total iron-binding saturation is less sensitive and if normal should be repeated in 5 years. No substantial iron overload is likely if > 60%.
- *Homozygote relatives* should then be screened with total iron-binding saturation measurements every 12 months if initially normal, because there is incomplete gene penetrance. Venesection is indicated if saturation increases to > 45%
- *Heterozygote relatives* should only have a liver biopsy if liver enzymes are abnormal or iron-binding saturation is > 45%. Follow-up is unnecessary if enzymes and saturation are normal
- Oral iron-chelating agents are not yet available

Prognosis
- Liver histology improves with effective venesection. Although cirrhosis is irreversible if present, portal hypertension may improve
- Cardiac failure is a poor sign
- Survival is normal if the diagnosis is made before irreversible liver damage or diabetes has occurred
- Once cirrhosis has developed, 10-year survival is around 70% and 20-year survival around 50%
- About one-third of those with established cirrhosis will die from hepatocellular carcinoma, sometimes a decade after initial venesection is completed

Wilson's disease
- The metabolic defect of copper metabolism causing copper deposition in the liver and brain (hepatolenticular degeneration) is the result of an autosomal recessive genetic defect of the ATP7B gene, which is responsible for the transmembrane transport of copper. Reduced function of this gene impairs hepatocellular excretion of copper into bile
- Prevalence may be as high as 30 per million population

Features
- Neuropsychiatric features usually precede hepatic disease in young adults, although the converse is true in children
- Chronic active hepatitis, cirrhosis or, rarely, acute hepatic failure may be the presenting feature

- Kayser–Fleischer rings at the periphery of the cornea are diagnostic, but can only be detected by slit lamp examination and may be absent in acute liver failure
- Haemolytic anaemia may be the presenting feature, with normal LFTs. The ALP is often only mildly elevated and cirrhosis is usually present by the time the diagnosis is made in adults

Management
- Diagnosis is established by the combination of low serum caeruloplasmin (< 0.2 g/L) and high serum copper (reference range from the laboratory), increased urinary copper excretion (> 1.0 µmol/24 h) and excess dry weight hepatic copper in a liver biopsy. All young patients with chronic active hepatitis should have these tests
- Penicillamine must be given for life. Referral to a specialist centre is advisable. There is a risk of acute liver failure if penicillamine is stopped suddenly. Trientine, zinc or tetrathiomolybdate are alternatives if the patient cannot tolerate penicillamine
- The family should be screened (serum caeruloplasmin, serum copper and 24 h urinary copper), but liver biopsy is not needed if these tests are negative. Genetic counselling should be offered to relatives

Non-alcoholic fatty liver disease and non-alcoholic steatohepatitis
Non-alcoholic fatty liver disease (NAFLD) is now recognised as a common cause for referral with abnormal liver function tests, and a proportion go on to develop hepatic fibrosis and cirrhosis. The increasing incidence is probably related to increases in body mass index (BMI) in developed countries. The definition comprises:
- *Simple fatty liver.* Often associated with a raised ALT < 100 IU/L and/or an isolated elevation in γ-GT and appearance of hepatic fat on ultrasound. It does not progress
- *Non-alcoholic steatohepatitis* (NASH). This is histologically indistinguishable from alcoholic hepatitis and associated with fibrosis or progression to cirrhosis in up to 25% within 8 years
- NASH is associated with insulin resistance and diabetes, although it is unclear whether this is cause or consequence
- Although histologically identical to alcoholic hepatitis (including Mallory's hyaline, neutrophil infiltration and pericellular fibrosis), jaundice is not a clinical feature and most individuals are asymptomatic. The distinction from alcoholic hepatitis is the credibility of the history
- Predictors of NASH include BMI > 28 kg/m² (see Appendix 3, p. 450), truncal obesity, hypertension, diabetes mellitus or insulin resistance, ALT > twice upper limit of normal, AST > ALT (i.e. AST/ALT ratio > 1.0) and triglycerides > 1.7 mmol/L
- A liver biopsy is the only way to confirm the diagnosis and should be considered in those with some if not all of the above predictors
- Treatment should be primarily directed at weight reduction, including physical exercise, dietary restriction and management of hyperlipidaemia. Treatment of hyperinsulinaemia with metformin or glitazones is being evaluated: liver biochemistry improves, but the effect on fibrosis is unknown
- Recurrence has been reported following liver transplantation and there is an increased risk of hepatocellular carcinoma once cirrhosis is present

Hepatic granulomas
- Granulomas on liver biopsy are usually an unexpected finding and often increase rather than resolve diagnostic confusion (Table 5.17)
- Granulomatous hepatitis is a misnomer, because neither the histological nor biochemical picture is that of hepatitis. In contrast, the ALP is usually raised
- Symptoms are non-specific, or those of the underlying disease

Differential diagnosis
- The usual dilemma is to distinguish sarcoidosis from tuberculosis, because steroids for the former would be totally wrong for the latter. Sarcoidosis is usually distinguished by chest X-ray (hilar lymphadenopathy, middle zone infiltrates), elevated serum angiotensin-converting enzyme, negative Mantoux tests, but these do not always resolve the dilemma. A trial of antituberculous chemotherapy and rebiopsy is then the safest course of action
- Idiopathic hepatic granulomas have a good prognosis. Occasionally there is a prolonged febrile illness, sometimes with acute abdominal pain and arthritis. Prednisolone 30 mg/day is then indicated, but only after investigation has excluded other (particularly infective) causes

5.7 Cirrhosis

Cirrhosis means loss of normal hepatic architecture due to fibrosis, with nodular regeneration. It implies irreversible liver disease and is the final stage of chronic liver disease from a variety of causes (Table 5.18).

Causes
(See Table 5.18)
Most (70%) are due to alcohol, hepatitis B or hepatitis C (Section 5.5). Up to 20% are of unknown cause (cryptogenic).

Clinical features
Presentation varies from asymptomatic abnormal liver function tests to end-stage liver disease. A long period of compensated cirrhosis, when the patient feels well, is common. The equilibrium is easily upset (p. 143) as hepatic reserve dwindles, leading to:

Table 5.17 Causes of hepatic granulomas

Common	Uncommon	Rare
Sarcoidosis	Brucellosis	Histoplasmosis
Tuberculosis	Drugs	Coccidioidomycosis
Primary biliary cirrhosis	hydralazine	Blastomycosis
Idiopathic (20–40%)	allopurinol	Berylliosis
	many others	Crohn's disease
	Q fever	Whipple's disease
		Hodgkin's disease
		Syphilis
		Leprosy
		Schistosomiasis
		Ascariasis

Table 5.18 Causes of cirrhosis

Common	Uncommon	Rare
Alcohol	Primary biliary	Haemochromatosis
Hepatitis B	Autoimmune	Wilson's disease
Hepatitis C (parenteral non-A, non-B)	Cryptogenic	α_1-antitrypsin deficiency
Non-alcoholic fatty liver	Primary sclerosing cholangitis	Secondary biliary (strictures, sclerosing cholangitis, atresia, cystic fibrosis) Cardiac (chronic right heart failure) Budd–Chiari syndrome Drugs (methotrexate)

- Hepatocellular failure (p. 144):
  - encephalopathy
  - bleeding disorder
  - cutaneous signs (Table 5.2, p. 137)
  - altered drug metabolism (p. 141)
  - malnutrition (loss of muscle bulk)
- Ascites (p. 146)
- Portal hypertension (p. 151):
  - splenomegaly
  - hypersplenism
  - bleeding varices

Other features include:
- Increased risk of hepatocellular carcinoma (p. 178) (largely related to male gender and the cause of cirrhosis)
- Tendency to infections (especially spontaneous bacterial peritonitis)
- Osteoporosis
- Increased mortality following surgery (hepatorenal syndrome, p. 171)

Diagnostic pitfalls
Some of the clinical features of cirrhosis may be simulated by portal or splenic vein thrombosis, Budd–Chiari syndrome, or constrictive pericarditis (p. 146).

Investigations
A clinical diagnosis should usually be confirmed by liver biopsy, because biochemical tests correlate poorly with histological changes and treatable causes may be overlooked, even in alcoholics.

Blood tests
- Liver enzymes may be normal in the compensated phase. Marked elevation of the AST or ALP occurs in alcoholic hepatitis or biliary cirrhosis, until the terminal stages when the levels fall (no functioning hepatocytes, no enzymes)
- HBsAg, HCV antibodies, AMA, antinuclear and antismooth muscle antibodies and serum ferritin should be measured even if the cause appears alcohol-related

- Elevated serum IgA, IgM or IgG are common in alcoholic, primary biliary and autoimmune diseases, respectively, forming part of the pattern of features (including history, other serological tests and liver histology) that confirm a specific diagnosis
- Thrombocytopenia and leucopenia are features of hypersplenism. Coagulation should be normal (INR < 1.3, prothrombin time < 4 seconds prolonged) before percutaneous liver biopsy

Liver biopsy
- Biopsy can usually be delayed until after recovery from an acute presentation
- Ascites and disordered clotting should be treated before biopsy, because the risk of haemorrhage (normally < 1 : 100) is increased
- Transjugular liver biopsy is safe for decompensated cirrhotics, in experienced hands, if the diagnosis needs to be established despite coagulation that cannot be corrected or presence of ascites
- Histological features include fibrosis and nodular regeneration; special stains (such as Perl's for iron, PAS for α1-antitrypsin deficiency) contribute to a specific diagnosis

Management
Cirrhosis need not be progressive.

General measures
- Alcohol—complete abstinence is essential if the aetiology is alcoholic, but is otherwise unnecessary, although restricted intake (< 10 units/week) is sensible advice
- Nutrition—a normal diet is possible in compensated cirrhotics. Salt should not be added to food if ascites develops (p. 150)
- Drugs—NSAIDs, sedatives and opiates should be avoided (p. 141)
- Complications (portal hypertension, ascites) are treated in the standard way (pp. 151 and 146), whatever the cause

Specific treatment
- Alcoholics—abstinence alters the prognosis from 30% to about 70% survival at 5 years
- Hepatitis B and C—interferon and ribavirin can be used in hepatitis C Child Grade A cirrhosis. Oral nucleoside analogues are useful in hepatitis B Child Grade B and C cirrhosis (p. 144)
- Primary biliary cirrhosis—ursodeoxycholic acid may be of value (p. 201), pending a decision about transplantation
- Haemochromatosis—venesection may improve liver histology (p. 169), although established cirrhosis is irreversible
- Wilson's disease—penicillamine (p. 171)

Alcohol and the liver
- Four pathological types of alcoholic liver disease are recognised: fatty liver, acute hepatitis, chronic hepatitis and cirrhosis
- The reasons why some (especially women, Asians and Afro-Caribbeans) are susceptible to liver disease and others develop cerebral, pancreatic or cardiac disease remain unknown

- The amount of alcohol consumed is not directly related to the degree of damage, but the WHO recommendations are < 28 units/week for men and < 21 units/week for women (1 unit is equivalent to one glass of wine, one pub measure of spirits or half a pint of beer)
- Alcohol abuse does not exclude less common causes of chronic liver disease, including viral or autoimmune chronic hepatitis or haemochromatosis

Fatty liver
- The mechanism is complex. Ethanol oxidation to acetaldehyde increases hydrogenated nicotinamide adenine dinucleotide (NADH), which favours triglyceride accumulation by decreasing fatty acid metabolism
- A palpable liver, increased MCV (> 98 fL) and mildly disordered liver enzymes are usually the only features, but these may also be the only signs of established cirrhosis
- Fatty change is rapidly reversible upon abstinence from alcohol
- Liver biopsy is necessary to confirm the diagnosis and exclude irreversible disease. It may also reinforce the need for abstinence. It is reasonable to recheck liver enzymes after 2 months of complete abstinence in alcoholic patients without signs of chronic liver disease, and only to biopsy those whose enzymes remain abnormal
- Obesity, diabetes and parenteral nutrition are other causes of fatty liver

Acute hepatitis
- Jaundice, fever, signs of alcohol withdrawal (tremor, agitation, perspiration), tender hepatomegaly and biochemical changes of hepatitis (Table 5.3, p. 137) are characteristic. A cholestatic picture is more common than in viral hepatitis, as is a polymorphonuclear leucocytosis
- A heavy binge is usually the provoking factor, often in addition to established liver disease. The mortality is high (30%)
- Hepatic failure is not uncommon and the risk is increased by even moderate doses of acetaminophen/paracetamol (4–6 g)
- The *Maddrey Discriminant Function Index* (DF) helps predict outcome. DF = (prothrombin time (in seconds) − control) + (bilirubin (in μmol/L)/17.1). Mortality is approximately the index in %. If the index exceeds 32 (mortality 30%), alcoholic hepatitis is severe and steroids may be considered
- Steroids (40 mg daily for 6 weeks) have been shown to reduce early mortality, excluding patients who were bleeding from varices or septic, but remain controversial. Their use is associated with a high incidence of bacterial sepsis

Chronic hepatitis
- The clinical and biochemical features are the same as in other types of chronic hepatitis (p. 185), so other causes should be excluded, even in drinkers
- Progression to cirrhosis is almost certain without abstinence, particularly in the presence of pericellular and perivenular fibrosis

Cirrhosis
- Telangiectases and Dupuytren's contracture are more common findings in alcoholic cirrhosis than in other types, but other clinical features are similar (Table 5.2, p. 137)

- A micronodular cirrhosis is usual
- Management is directed at complications (ascites, portal hypertension, encephalopathy). Abstinence may still alter the course of end-stage alcoholic cirrhosis: it is never too late to stop drinking

General points on management
- Detoxification is trying for everybody. However, it is easier to prevent delirium tremens than to treat it! A suggested protocol is shown in Fig. 5.8
- Adequate control of agitation is essential if seizures are to be avoided. Nursing staff must be advised to give 'as required' sedation readily if there are any signs of agitation
- Lorazepam (2 mg intravenously) to control seizures should they occur
- Haloperidol can be considered when withdrawal symptoms or delirium tremens are not responding adequately to benzodiazepines
- Vitamins A, C and B_1 and folate are commonly deficient. Intravenous vitamins should be given every day for 3 days to all alcoholic patients admitted to hospital
- Alcoholics with a high MCV (sometimes as high as 115 fL) should still have folate, B_{12} and thyroid function checked
- Careful examination of peripheral nerves, coordination, eye movements, short-term memory and mental state is often rewarding. Wernicke's encephalopathy (confusion,

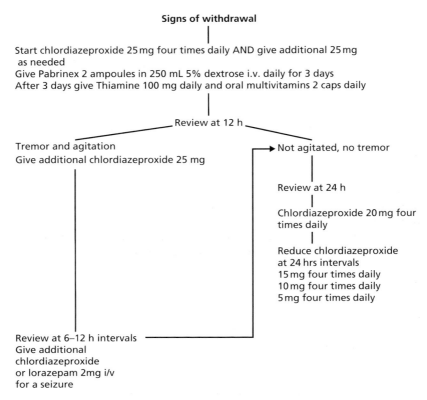

Fig. 5.8 Detoxification of alcoholics.

nystagmus, cranial (VI) nerve palsy, ataxia) is a medical emergency and reversible in the early stages with high-dose thiamine. The signs of Wernicke's, or those of Korsakoff's, psychosis (short-term memory loss and confabulation) can be overlooked by the unwary. Treatment is an emergency, with high-dose thiamine (e.g. Pabrinex 1 + 2 vials three times daily for 3 days)

- Counselling services and psychiatric intervention have variable results. They should be discussed with the patient and arranged if the patient is willing to cooperate (Appendix 1, p. 435). Whilst there are some striking successes, there are more recidivists. Family involvement is as important as organised care
- Chlormethiazole/chlordiazepoxide should not be prescribed to outpatients, because it is often sold or abused

Prognosis
- 10% of alcoholics develop cirrhosis over 10 years
- The Child–Pugh classification (Table 5.5. p. 144) is useful for comparing the outcome of variceal bleeding or surgery in groups of patients with cirrhosis, but is not helpful for predicting the course in an individual
- 5-year survival in alcoholic cirrhotics is 50% overall, 30% for continued drinkers and 70% for abstainers

5.8 Tumours

Hepatocellular carcinoma (HCC)
Primary hepatocellular carcinoma is the most common malignant tumour in the world, although rare in the West. The incidence is around 2 : 100 000 in the USA and Europe, but 85 : 100 000 in Taiwan. 80% of all patients have pre-existing cirrhosis and most are male. All types of cirrhosis predispose to HCC, although hepatitis B is the commonest cause worldwide.

Causes
- Hepatitis B or C
- Alcoholic cirrhosis
- Haemochromatosis
- Aflatoxin (fungal infection of groundnuts) and Thorotrast (radiological contrast medium used until 1950) are now rare causes

Clinical features
- Rapid development of ascites, increasing liver size or jaundice in a patient with known cirrhosis should always suggest HCC
- A hepatic arterial bruit or rub are highly suggestive but rare. A bruit can also sometimes be heard in acute alcoholic hepatitis

Investigations
- Elevated AFP (> 20 ng/mL) occurs in 80% but this is not specific and is often normal in the presence of small tumours (< 3 cm) detected by ultrasound screening. Other causes of a raised AFP include hepatitis, testicular, ovarian or pancreatic

tumours, hydatidiform mole and pregnancy. In patients with an AFP > 400 ng/mL, 97% have a hepatoma

- Ultrasound is as sensitive as CT scanning for detecting hepatic tumours and should be the first imaging technique. CT scanning or MRI should be performed to confirm size and exclude multicentricity
- Liver biopsy should be avoided if the tumour appears confined to one lobe in a cirrhotic, and resection or liver transplantation is being considered. Tumour may seed down the biopsy track, rendering the tumour inoperable. However, in multifocal lesions, biopsy under ultrasound control is necessary for a histological diagnosis. A rare, fibrolamellar type of hepatoma occurs in non-cirrhotics and has a better prognosis following surgical resection
- Angiography is needed for therapeutic embolisation or intra-arterial chemotherapy
- Screening cirrhotics for HCC by ultrasound +/− AFP measurement every 6 months should be considered in cirrhosis due to hepatitis B or C, haemochromatosis and α_1-antitrypsin deficiency if curative treatment is an option in the event of detecting HCC

Management
- Surgical resection should be considered for fibrolamellar tumours. It is occasionally possible in cirrhotics with good liver function (Child–Pugh grade A) but does not reduce the risk of a new tumour occurring in the remaining liver. The tumour must be confined to one lobe of the liver, without extrahepatic spread. Referral to a specialist centre for preoperative assessment is recommended
- Liver transplantation should be considered in cirrhotics with single tumours < 5 cm. Cure can be achieved with single tumours < 5 cm or three tumours < 3 cm
- Chemotherapy (mitozantrone, adriamycin, or multiple drugs) is unsatisfactory at present with only a 10–30% response rate. Transcatheter arterial chemoembolisation (TACE) may have a role in selected patients with good liver function. Patients should be discussed with a specialist centre and a multidisciplinary approach to management undertaken (surgical/oncological/hepatological)
- Local ablative therapy is probably as effective as surgical resection in cirrhotics. Approaches include percutaneous ethanol injection, cryoablation therapy and high-frequency ultrasound
- Prevention by hepatitis B vaccination has reduced HCC in Asia and parts of Africa

Prognosis
- Median survival for tumours detected because of symptoms is 12 weeks after diagnosis. However, the 5-year survival for tumours < 3 cm detected through screening may be as high as 50%. Death then usually occurs because of liver failure, rather than metastatic disease
- In the minority who have surgical resection, 1-year survival may be 60% and 5-year survival 25–40%

Metastases
In Europe 90% of liver tumours are metastatic. Colorectal, breast, lung, gastric or pancreatic cancers are the common primary sites. Metastases are said not to occur in

cirrhotic livers. Median survival after diagnosis of hepatic metastases is 2–4 months. Earlier diagnosis by ultrasound is increasing this period (the 'lead time'), although prognosis remains unchanged.

Single hepatic metastases from colorectal cancer should be considered for resection at a specialist centre, in patients aged < 50 years. More than 2-year survival has been reported. Chemotherapy and arterial embolisation offer no better results than for primary liver tumours.

Benign tumours

Haemangiomas are usually found incidentally on ultrasound or CT scan. They may be confused with metastases (although the density is different) and present a hazard at liver biopsy, but are otherwise unimportant. Focal nodular hyperplasia may also present as an incidental mass on ultrasound scanning. No treatment is needed and the diagnosis can often be confirmed by MRI obviating the need for a biopsy. Hepatic adenomas are very rarely associated with the oral contraceptive pill and these are best resected. A liver biopsy is indicated if there is any doubt about the diagnosis. Histological differentiation of focal nodular hyperplasia, hepatic adenoma and a well-differentiated hepatocellular carcinoma can sometimes be difficult.

5.9 Abscesses and cysts

Hepatic abscess (often multiple) may be occult and surprisingly difficult to diagnose.

Pyogenic

- Cholangitis, diverticulitis or following abdominal surgery are now the usual causes, as opposed to appendicitis, but often no cause can be found
- Fever (90%), weight loss and malaise are non-specific. Hepatomegaly and right upper quadrant pain occur in about 50%. Jaundice is a bad prognostic sign
- Blood cultures are negative in 50%. If *Streptococcus milleri* has grown, it is almost invariably due to a liver abscess
- Ultrasound of the liver is always indicated for patients with fever and mild derangement of liver enzymes. CT scanning is more sensitive for lesions near the diaphragm
- Needle aspiration under ultrasound control identifies the organism in 90%. Mixed aerobes and anaerobes are usual
- Percutaneous drainage of a single abscess and one or two largest cavities of multiple abscesses should be performed urgently by a radiologist. Surgical drainage is now rarely indicated
- Intravenous metronidazole 500 mg and cefotaxime 1 g three times daily should be given for 2 weeks, followed by oral antibiotics for 6 weeks, depending on the sensitivity of the organism

Amoebic

- Very rare in those living in Europe, but patients may present years after living in the tropics
- 80% are aged < 40 years

- Pain is more common and systemic features less common than in pyogenic abscesses. Point tenderness is typical and hiccups herald impending rupture, but dysentery is unusual
- Ultrasound and markedly elevated serum antibodies to *Entamoeba histolytica* are diagnostic in > 90%. Hot stools should be examined for trophozoites (p. 388), which are highly suggestive of the diagnosis. Aspiration of thick, pink-brown 'anchovy sauce' pus is characteristic, but not indicated unless the diagnosis cannot be confirmed in other ways
- Metronidazole 800 mg three times daily for 10 days is effective in most patients, but should always be followed by diloxanide 500 mg three times daily for 10 days to prevent recurrent invasive disease
- Drainage is needed only for impending rupture, indicated by severe or pleuritic pain, or hiccups. Recurrent fever may be due to secondary bacterial infection

Hydatid cysts
- Symptomless hepatomegaly in those from the eastern Mediterranean or South America or in Welsh farmers is occasionally due to cysts of *Echinococcus granulosus*
- Liver function is usually normal, eosinophilia often absent and serological tests may be only weakly positive. Ultrasound presents a characteristic appearance of multiple 'daughter' cysts, with clearly defined walls. Hydatid complement fixation tests should be checked before aspiration of any hepatic cysts in patients from endemic areas
- Hydatid cysts are often best left alone if asymptomatic. Albendazole (800 mg daily for 28 days) may be effective and is an adjunct to surgery for symptomatic disease. Surgery is indicated for increasing size, complications of local pressure or secondary infection and is usually undertaken while on oral therapy. Alternatively aspiration of the cyst followed by injection of ethanol/hypertonic saline can be undertaken after treatment with albendazole (percutaneous aspiration, injection and reaspiration, PAIR)

Polycystic liver disease
Occasional cysts in the liver are a common finding on ultrasound and of no significance, but multiple cysts indicate polycystic liver disease with autosomal dominant inheritance. Associated polycystic renal disease often dominates the clinical picture, but polycystic liver disease may occur in isolation. Cysts may be massive (> 15 cm diameter) and gross hepatomegaly can cause discomfort. Haemorrhage into a cyst or rupture presents as an acute abdomen. Surgical exploration and marsupialisation of the affected cyst(s) are then indicated. Portal hypertension or hepatic failure is rare and transplantation is then possible

5.10 Clinical dilemmas

General advice is given in Appendix 4 (p. 455).

Asymptomatic abnormal liver function tests
Elevated liver enzymes or serum bilirubin are an increasingly common incidental finding due to automated biochemical tests. Normal ranges (Table 5.3, p. 137) represent the

95th centile of a selected healthy population. At best this leads to earlier diagnosis of treatable disease, but at worst it exposes the patient to the complications of ill-advised investigations. The following plan is recommended.

- Ask about:
  - alcohol intake
  - drug treatment or abuse
  - previous jaundice
  - family history of hepatic or chronic disease
  - recent viral illness
  - overseas travel
- Examine for:
  - hepatomegaly and splenomegaly
  - signs of chronic liver disease (Table 5.2, p. 137)
  - lymphadenopathy
  - urticarial rash or arthritis (associated with chronic hepatitis)
- Then investigate (Fig. 5.9)

Liver transplantation (See Box 5.1)

Indications for liver transplant in acute liver failure are given in Table 1.8 (p. 43) and relative contraindications in Box 5.2. The timing of transplantation in chronic liver disease is difficult, so early discussion with a referral centre is advisable. Different systems apply in different countries. In the UK, waiting lists are short because the timing is based on clinical severity alone and matched availability. In the USA, length of time on the waiting list counts in addition to the model end-stage liver disease (MELD) score (p. 145), so patients are placed on the list early and waiting lists are long.

The other side of the coin is that every hospital has a responsibility to face the difficult task of finding donors.

Timing

- End-stage liver disease—histological evidence of irreversible liver damage (fibrosis), with
  - jaundice (bilirubin > 100 µmol/L (6 mg/dL) in primary biliary cirrhosis), or
  - ascites refractory to both spironolactone and a loop diuretic, or
  - after two separate episodes of variceal haemorrhage, or
  - recurrent or chronic encephalopathy, or
  - one episode of documented spontaneous bacterial peritonitis
- The timing is simplest in primary biliary cirrhosis, because once the bilirubin is > 100 µmol/L (6 mg/dL), the prognosis is usually < 1 year
- The prognosis in the later stages of primary sclerosing cholangitis or other types of cirrhosis is much more difficult to predict
- The patient and family should understand the irreversible nature of the disease, the likely delay of weeks (or months) whilst a matched donor is found, and the prognosis

Post-operative implications

- Hospital stay is usually 2–3 weeks

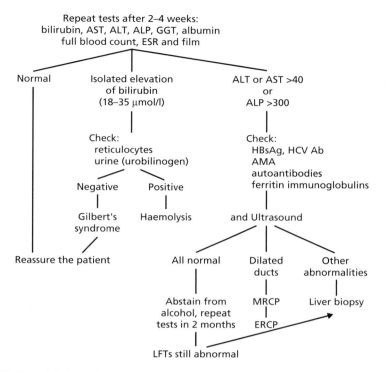

Fig. 5.9 Investigation of asymptomatic abnormal liver function tests.

Box 5.1 Diseases potentially curable by transplant (adults)

Primary biliary cirrhosis
Cryptogenic cirrhosis
Postviral cirrhosis
Alcoholic cirrhosis (if abstinent)
Autoimmune chronic hepatitis
Primary sclerosing cholangitis
Budd–Chiari syndrome
Hepatocellular carcinoma (< 5 cm)
Acute liver failure (Section 1.9, p. 42)
Metabolic disorders: Wilson's disease, others (usually children)

Box 5.2 Relative contraindications to liver transplant

Malignancy (including cholangiocarcinoma)
Recent or continued alcohol abuse (abstinence for < 6 months)
Psychological inability to comply with post-transplant treatment and monitoring (involving regular medication, weekly blood tests, and liver biopsies)
Age > 60 years (but carefully selected older patients up to the age of 70 have done well)
Previous upper abdominal surgery
Portal vein thrombosis
Extrahepatic malignant tumours
Cardiorespiratory or renal disease

- Frequent blood tests are necessary (weekly for several months and then less frequently) to measure ciclosporin/tacrolimus levels, biochemical and haematological tests, in addition to outpatient visits
- Drug compliance must be good
- Early graft rejection is common and responds to high-dose steroids. Chronic rejection is uncommon. Re-transplantation is necessary in 10%
- Late graft loss (several years later) is usually due to recurrent disease, usually in hepatitis C
- The focus of long-term management is reducing complications from immunosuppressive agents. Attention is focused on blood pressure control, weight, hyperlipidaemia as cardiovascular risk factors and minimising nephrotoxicity from the calcineurin inhibitors (tacrolimus or ciclosporin)

Prognosis
- 80–90% 5-year survival in primary biliary cirrhosis, but results are constantly improving. After 1 year, the outlook is excellent. Primary biliary cirrhosis and autoimmune liver disease have very occasionally recurred in the transplanted liver
- 50–80% 5-year survival in primary sclerosing cholangitis or cryptogenic cirrhosis

6 Gall Bladder and Biliary Tree

6.1 Clinical anatomy of the biliary tract

The biliary canaliculi adjacent to each hepatocyte drain into interlobular, then septal, bile ducts, which combine to form intrahepatic ducts visible on cholangiography. The right and left hepatic ducts join at the porta hepatis to form the common hepatic duct, which unites with the cystic duct from the gall bladder to form the CBD. This enters the duodenum through the head of the pancreas (Fig. 6.1).

Gall bladder contraction is stimulated by cholecystokinin (secretin) after meals. Biliary flow is controlled by a pressure gradient between the CBD and duodenum, as well as the peristaltic pump action of the sphincter of Oddi, which is also influenced by cholecystokinin.

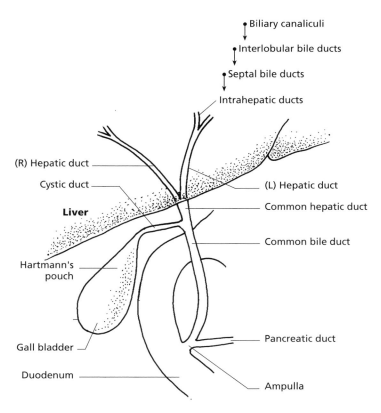

Fig. 6.1 Biliary tract anatomy.

Anatomical anomalies of pathological importance

- Opening of the CBD onto a duodenal diverticulum (cannulation of the papilla is difficult and ERCP/sphincterotomy potentially dangerous, due to risk of perforation)
- Accessory artery superior to the ampulla of Vater in 1% (sphincterotomy can lead to major haemorrhage)
- Separate exit points into the duodenum of the CBD and main pancreatic duct (endoscopic cannulation is difficult)
- Cystic duct fails to join the common hepatic duct in 20% (both the duct and its union must be identified before ligation or stapling, especially at laparoscopic cholecystectomy)
- Cystic artery may arise from the left hepatic or gastroduodenal arteries, rather than the right hepatic artery
- Choledochal cysts occur in 1 : 15 000 in Western countries (more common in Japan). Classified into five types. The commonest type is a fusiform dilation of the CBD, usually presenting with jaundice and abdominal pain in children, but sometimes (10–20%) in adults. Associated with malignant transformation
- Congenital, segmental, saccular dilatation of the intrahepatic bile ducts is termed Caroli's disease. It may be associated with renal tubular ectasia

6.2 Gallstones

Bile is concentrated in the gall bladder, which acts as a reservoir between meals for bile acids (cholic and chenodeoxycholic acid), which are essential for emulsifying lipids prior to digestion and absorption. Bile acids form the outer, hydrophilic layer of micelles, which contain lipid-soluble cholesterol in the centre. Phospholipids insert into the micellar wall to increase the micellar capacity for cholesterol.

Insufficient bile acids (e.g. caused by failure of enterohepatic recycling in terminal ileal disease) or imbalance between cholesterol and phospholipid concentrations in bile, will lead to precipitation of cholesterol crystals from the supersaturated bile, which then form the nucleus for gallstone formation (lithogenic bile). Incomplete gall bladder emptying allows crystals to grow into gallstones. There are proteins that either promote or inhibit nucleation and the balance between these factors may be the key determinant in an individual's susceptibility to form gallstones.

Pigment stones are caused by bilirubin forming insoluble calcium precipitates in bile. Black, brittle pure pigment stones account for 70% of radio-opaque gallstones. Brown pigment stones are soft, often intrahepatic and unusual (Fig. 6.2).

Prevalence

On ultrasound studies of a normal population, 7–15% people have gallstones, which become more common with age. Conditions predisposing to gallstones are shown in Table 6.1.

Symptoms

Most gallstones remain 'silent' in the fundus of the gall bladder. Migration to the cystic duct and impaction causes acute or chronic cholecystitis, which resolves when disimpaction occurs, or progresses to complications (Fig. 6.3).

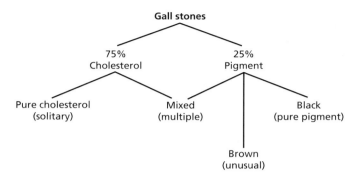

Fig. 6.2 Types of gallstones.

- Silent stones—complications develop in 1–2% per year, or in 3% per year in those with mild symptoms at presentation
- Acute cholecystitis—persistent, severe right upper quadrant pain, fever and leucocytosis (p. 24). Acalculous acute cholecystitis is rare and caused by bacterial infection, polyarteritis or trauma
- Chronic cholecystitis—recurrent biliary colic, dyspepsia, fat intolerance and non-specific features
- CBD stones—jaundice, abdominal pain (p. 193)
- Cholangitis—jaundice, fever, abdominal pain (p. 200), usually due to stones in the CBD
- Gangrenous gall bladder and empyema—septic, and severe illness, with local peritonism
- Mirizzi's syndrome—obstructive jaundice due to external compression of the common hepatic duct by a stone impacted in the cystic duct, often associated with cholangitis
- Biliary fistula—from a chronically inflamed gall bladder eroding into the small intestine or colon, resulting in air in the biliary tree, resolution of symptoms or, very rarely, impaction at the ileocaecal valve and gallstone ileus
- Perforation—local or diffuse peritonitis after acute cholecystitis

Table 6.1 Conditions predisposing to gallstones

Cholesterol	Black pigment	Brown pigment
Gender (2F : 1M)	Chronic haemolysis	Sclerosing cholangitis
Obesity	sickle cell	Oriental
Diet (low fibre)	spherocytosis	biliary parasites
Race (Europe, USA,	prosthetic valve	
American Indians)	Cirrhosis	
Cirrhosis (30%)	Biliary infection	
Terminal ileal	*E. coli*	
Crohn's resection	*Clostridium* spp.	
Drugs		
oral contraceptive clofibrate		

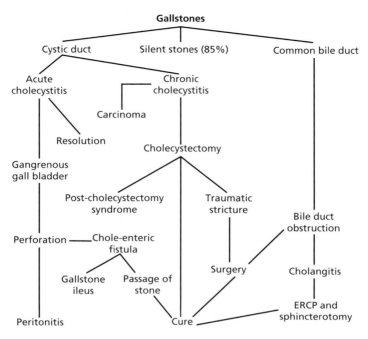

Fig. 6.3 Consequences of gallstones.

- Carcinoma of the gall bladder or bile ducts—jaundice, weight loss, pain (p. 202). More common in patients with gallstones, but does not justify prophylactic cholecystectomy
- Intrahepatic gallstones (hepatolithiasis) is common in the Far East. Often associated with *Clonorchis* sp. infection, it can present as cholangitis, multiple liver abscesses, secondary biliary cirrhosis or cholangiocarcinoma. Hepaticocutaneous jejunostomy allows repeated access to the biliary system for stone removal

Investigations

Ultrasound
- Most effective non-invasive method of detecting stones, but often finds incidental, silent stones. Stones may occasionally be missed, even in experienced hands. In some patients the gall bladder cannot be identified because of gas or unusual anatomy
- Also useful for diagnosing biliary obstruction, acute or chronic cholecystitis
- If the gall bladder wall is of normal thickness, gallstones are likely to be incidental to symptoms of abdominal pain

Blood tests
- All are normal in chronic cholecystitis or silent stones. They can be normal in the elderly with dilated CBD, stones and cholangitis

- Elevated ALP and γ-GT suggests CBD stones. Leucocytosis and/or elevated CRP (C-reactive protein) occurs in acute cholecystitis or cholangitis. Elevated transaminase levels (usually < 1000 IU/L) can be seen with acute biliary obstruction, pain is usually present.
- Serum cholesterol is unrelated to biliary cholesterol, but is elevated in intrahepatic cholestasis such as primary biliary cirrhosis

Other tests
- Plain abdominal X-ray—mandatory in acute abdominal pain. May occasionally show calcified stones
- ERCP—for diagnosis and treatment of biliary obstruction, but priority is changing (Fig 6.4). Non-invasive imaging by CT or MR are best performed *before* ERCP after dilated ducts are identified, to help plan optimal endoscopic or surgical intervention
- MRCP—non-invasive way of detecting CBD stones. Increasingly used before ERCP if available, because avoids risks of ERCP if biliary tree is normal
- Contrast-enhanced spiral CT scan—alternative to MRCP depending upon availability
- Percutaneous transhepatic cholangiogram (PTC)—indicated when dilated intrahepatic ducts are detected on ultrasound and ERCP is not technically possible (p. 196)

Indications for surgery
Most decisions are straightforward. Difficulty arises in deciding whether gallstones in patients with non-specific symptoms are the cause or merely incidental (Table 6.2). Remember that 85% of asymptomatic gall bladder stones remain asymptomatic for over 15 years.

Laparoscopic cholecystectomy
Laparoscopic surgery through a periumbilical incision and two upper quadrant punctures for instrument manipulation is standard and safe in experienced hands. Previous upper abdominal surgery or gross obesity make it more difficult and conversion to open cholecystectomy is necessary in 1–5% of all procedures.

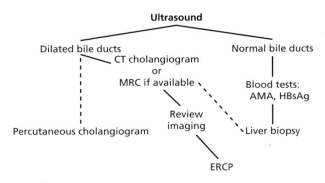

Fig. 6.4 Sequence of investigations in cholestatic jaundice.

Table 6.2 Symptomatic or incidental stones?

	Symptomatic	Incidental
Pain	Acute episodes < 60 s	Constant dull ache
	Like labour contractions	Variable
	1–72 h duration	Most days, or continuous
Pain-free interval	Several weeks/months	Rare
Fat intolerance	Common	Common
Flatulence	Common	Common
Bloating	Less common	Common
Physical signs	RUQ tenderness or none	RUQ tenderness or none
Ultrasound	Gallstone(s)	Gallstone(s)
	Thickened wall	Normal gall bladder wall

RUQ, right upper quadrant.

The risk of bile duct injury is similar (0.25%) to standard cholecystectomy; if a postoperative bile leak occurs from the cystic duct, sphincterotomy or stent placement at ERCP are usually effective. The stent can be removed at 3 months. Advantages over standard cholecystectomy are a short hospital stay (< 48 h), limited postoperative pain and early return to work (< 1 week). Bile duct stones can be removed at the time of laparoscopic surgery, but are usually more easily removed by ERCP.

Mini-laparotomy cholecystectomy
Surgery through a 4–5 cm incision is an alternative favoured by some surgeons. Standard cholecystectomy is now largely confined to patients in whom laparoscopic surgery is not possible, or when exploration of the CBD is necessary, usually for very large calculi that it has not been possible to extract at ERCP.

Absolute indications for cholecystectomy
- Acute cholecystitis—optimum treatment is urgent surgery during the same admission (p. 25)
- Chronic cholecystitis—typical history of biliary colic and a contracted or non-functioning gall bladder shown by ultrasound
- CBD stones—age < 70 years, after ERCP and sphincterotomy. In patients > 70 years or those at poor operative risk, endoscopic sphincterotomy alone has a lower mortality, although a low risk of recurrent biliary colic remains
- Gangrenous gall bladder—emergency cholecystostomy is often safer than cholecystectomy. Later elective cholecystectomy or spontaneous closure is then possible
- Gallstone ileus—to relieve intestinal obstruction, with later cholecystectomy
- Elective cholecystectomy is indicated if gallstones are considered to be the cause of abdominal pain
- Gallstone pancreatitis—early cholecystectomy after recovery from pancreatitis is essential if recurrent pancreatitis and complications are to be avoided
- IBS, peptic ulcer, chronic pancreatitis or renal tract disease may produce similar symptoms to chronic cholecystitis and should be excluded if doubt exists

Non-surgical options

These options must be balanced against safe operations (mortality 0.1% age < 50 years, 0.5% > 50 years) that remove all gallstones without recurrence, although retained stones occur in about 2% and other complications (including postcholecystectomy syndrome) in 10%.

In elderly frail patients with CBD stones a biliary stent inserted at ERCP will relieve symptoms. Stent patency is often longer than when stents are placed for strictures, but patency may be less important than mechanical prevention of stone impaction.

6.3 Cholestatic jaundice

Cholestatic jaundice is due to interruption of bile flow anywhere in the biliary tree. The site of obstruction is either extrahepatic, when there is mechanical obstruction to the main bile ducts, or intrahepatic, when the obstructing lesion is usually not visible (except with intrahepatic strictures, stones or tumour). 'Obstructive jaundice' usually applies to extrahepatic causes. About 20% of patients with clinical or biochemical features of cholestasis have hepatocellular disease.

Causes

Extrahepatic obstruction
About 70% of cholestatic jaundice is due to extrahepatic obstruction. Extrahepatic ducts dilate in distal obstruction, as caused by pancreatic carcinoma, before intrahepatic duct dilatation, which occurs early in high obstruction (at the porta hepatis), and is readily detected by ultrasound.

Intrahepatic obstruction
- Drug-induced cholestasis and primary biliary cirrhosis are the commonest causes
- Jaundice in Hodgkin's disease is usually extrahepatic, due to lymph nodes obstructing the porta hepatis. Intrahepatic cholestasis with jaundice due to tumour infiltration in non-Hodgkin's lymphoma is usually preterminal
- Septicaemia or total parenteral nutrition can cause cholestatic jaundice, usually in a patient with multi-organ failure
- Rarer familial causes of intrahepatic cholestasis due to mutations in canalicular membrane transporters are also being identified now:

Table 6.3 Causes of extrahepatic cholestasis

Common	Uncommon	Rare
Common duct stones	Portal lymph nodes	Pseudocyst
Pancreatic cancer	Pancreatitis acute chronic	Choledochal cyst
	Post-traumatic stricture	
	Cholangiocarcinoma	
	Ampullary carcinoma	

Table 6.4 Causes of intrahepatic cholestasis

Common	Uncommon	Rare
Drugs phenothiazines many others	Viral hepatitis (hepatitis A)	Benign recurrent
	Alcoholic hepatitis	Hodgkin's disease
	Primary sclerosing cholangitis	Intrahepatic stones
Primary biliary cirrhosis	Cholangiocarcinoma	Hepatic granulomas
	Metastases	Familial
	Septicaemia	
	Total parenteral nutrition	

- FIC1 is a P-type ATPase. Mutations in this gene lead to progressive familial intra-hepatic cholestasis type 1 (PFIC1) in childhood (Byler's disease), or benign recurrent intrahepatic cholestasis (below)
- BSEP is a bile salt export pump. Mutations result in progressive familial intrahepatic cholestasis type 2 (PFIC2), associated with a normal γ-GT and cirrhosis in childhood
- MDR3 protein transports phospholipid. Mutations result in progressive familial intrahepatic cholestasis type 3 (PFIC3), associated with an elevated γGT and cirrhosis in childhood. Mutations have also been identified in adults with idiopathic intrahepatic cholestasis, gallstones, or intrahepatic cholestasis of pregnancy
- MRP2 mutations cause Dubin–Johnson syndrome
- MDR1 is an organic anion transporter that transports drugs such as ciclosporin
- Benign recurrent intrahepatic cholestasis (BRIC) presents as recurrent cholestatic jaundice lasting for several weeks, for which no cause can be found. It is associated with mutations in the FIC1 gene. Liver biopsy shows bland cholestasis without fibrosis, unlike Byler's disease

Clinical features
- Jaundice appears slowly, usually preceded by pruritus
- Itching and pale stools are characteristic of both intra- and extrahepatic cholestasis (Box 6.1)
- Dark urine also occurs in hepatocellular (but not prehepatic) jaundice, but urobilinogen is only absent in complete bile duct obstruction
- Extrahepatic cholestasis due to stones may be associated with pain and fever, indicating cholangitis (Table 6.5). Urgent culture, antibiotics and drainage are then indi-

---

Box 6.1 Physical signs in cholestatic jaundice

Pale stools
Dark orange urine
Scratch marks (excoriation)
Polished nails (itching)
Xanthelasma (eyelids)
Xanthomas (rarely palmar creases, tendons)
Hepatomegaly (alcohol, malignancy)
Palpable gall bladder (especially carcinoma)

Table 6.5 Differences between extra- and intrahepatic cholestasis

	Extrahepatic	Intrahepatic
History	Abdominal pain Fever Middle age/elderly Previous biliary surgery	Anorexia, malaise Drug exposure or abuse
Examination	Fever Abdominal tenderness Palpable gall bladder	Ascites Stigmata of liver disease (Table 5.2, p. 137) Encephalopathy

Biochemistry	Concomitant elevation of
	  bilirubin and alkaline
	  phosphatase
	Prothromin time corrects
	  with vitamin K
		High alkaline phosphatase
		  without elevated bilirubin
		
		Concomitant elevation of
		  transaminases

cated (p. 200). This is rare in intrahepatic cholestasis unless there has been a previous ERCP (i.e. in primary sclerosing cholangitis, PSC)
- If the gall bladder is palpable in the right upper quadrant, then jaundice is unlikely to be due to stones (Courvoisier's sign). By implication, it is more likely to be due to malignancy

Investigations

Confirmation of cholestasis
- ALP is markedly elevated (> three times, often 10 times, normal), associated with an elevated γ-GT
- Bilirubin concentrations reflect the duration of cholestasis. The highest levels are reached in complete obstruction by carcinoma or end-stage intrahepatic disease such as primary biliary cirrhosis
- An isolated high ALP without elevated bilirubin suggests intrahepatic disease (primary biliary cirrhosis or PSC)—as long as Paget's disease is excluded!
- ALP isoenzymes are very rarely indicated and only when there is real doubt about the origin of the ALP

Identifying the cause
The aims are to distinguish intra-from extrahepatic cholestasis and to plan endoscopic or surgical procedure appropriate to the individual patient. The sequence of investigations is shown in Fig. 6.4.

Ultrasound
- Ultrasound is not good at identifying CBD stones, although it will reliably detect a dilated CBD (diameter > 7 mm)
- Endoscopic ultrasound reliably detects CBD calculi in experienced hands, but is operator-dependent and availability is limited. Centres with access to biliary EUS often have access to magnetic resonance cholangiography (MRC), but the choice depends on local availability

ERCP
- ERCP should be rapidly arranged if intrahepatic ducts are dilated. If available, high-resolution MRC or EUS should be considered before ERCP, to select only those with CBD calculi or strictures for ERCP and reduce the risks (Table 1.6, p. 32)
- A dilated CBD without an obstructing lesion occurs shortly after an obstructing stone has passed (air may also be seen in the biliary tree)
- Or after cholecystectomy (persists for years, but rarely > 9 mm diameter)

PTC
PTC is indicated if:
- ERCP-directed cannulation of CBD is not achieved
- Therapeutic stenting of a high, tortuous stricture is necessary (for percutaneous insertion of a self-expanding metal stent or, less commonly, in conjunction with ERCP)

Indications for ERCP

As non-invasive biliary imaging techniques become available (CT and MRC), efforts are being made to avoid the risk of ERCP (p. 419). Previously, ERCP was the next step for any patient with dilated ducts. Non-invasive imaging best precedes ERCP, and if surgery (e.g. cholecystectomy or resection) is going to be necessary, then surgery and CBD exploration or definitive surgery can be performed without ERCP. Much depends on local expertise and joint decision-making between radiologist, surgeon, endoscopist and patient.

Diagnostic
- Jaundice with dilated intrahepatic ducts—after CT or MR scan and if surgery is inappropriate
- Cholangitis (urgently, within 48 h)
- Jaundice or elevated ALP with normal calibre intrahepatic ducts in the presence of typical biliary pain and gall bladder stones. Incomplete obstruction of the CBD may not cause dilation. High-resolution MRC, if available, is preferable in the first instance
- Jaundice or elevated ALP with normal calibre intrahepatic ducts, when liver biopsy does not establish a diagnosis and especially if the patient has ulcerative colitis (high chance of PSC)
- Recurrent acute or chronic pancreatitis (Fig. 4.3, p. 120), after MRC
- Post-cholecystectomy pain (p. 203), but after MRC

Therapeutic
- Sphincterotomy for CBD stones (Fig. 6.5)
- Stenting of malignant strictures (Fig. 6.5)
- Acute pancreatitis if ultrasound identifies stones in the gall bladder

Management
Joint decision-making between specialists and patient about appropriate procedures should precede ERCP (above). Precipitate ERCP may restrict options and carries risk

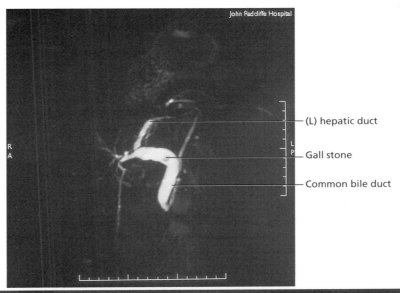

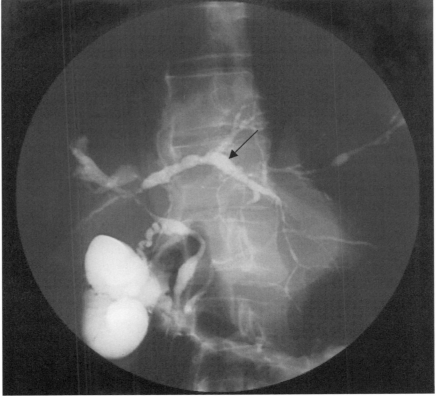

Fig. 6.5 **Radiology in biliary obstruction.** (a) Magnetic resonance cholangiography (MRC)—non-invasive procedure, best performed if diagnostic doubt persists about cause of biliary obstruction after transabdominal ultrasound, before ERCP. (b) ERCP showing primary sclerosing cholangitis (PSC). *(Continued)*

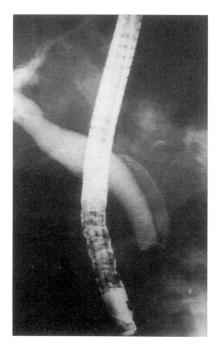

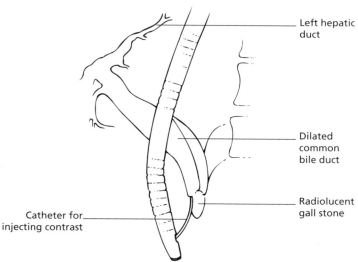

Left hepatic
duct

Dilated
common
bile duct

Radiolucent
gall stone

Catheter for
injecting contrast

Fig. 6.5 (*continued*) (c) ERCP—classical method of defining CBD calculi, but carries 5% risk of serious morbidity (p. 32), so is best performed only when a therapeutic procedure is necessary.

(p. 419). Metal stents, for instance, should only be inserted once a decision not to proceed to surgery has been made.

Common bile duct stones

Patients > 70 years
- Endoscopic sphincterotomy (8–15 mm incision through the ampulla) allows the stones to be extracted by trawling the CBD with a balloon cannula or basket. It may be possible to crush large calculi with a lithotripter to aid extraction. Whilst duct clearance at the initial ERCP is optimal, small residual stones can be allowed to pass spontaneously
- Subsequent cholecystectomy is not required in 90%
- If large calculi cannot be extracted, or if the patient is very frail or sick, insertion of a large (11 French gauge) stent is effective at preventing recurrent jaundice or cholangitis

Fit patients < 70 years
- Endoscopic sphincterotomy is usually performed first
- Early cholecystectomy with peroperative cholangiography is then necessary, to remove the source of stones and confirm clearance of the bile ducts. Some surgeons prefer to perform cholecystectomy and exploration of the bile ducts as a single procedure, without first doing an endoscopic sphincterotomy

Retained stones after cholecystectomy
- ERCP is diagnostic and therapeutic (sphincterotomy)
- Acute cholangitis or acute pancreatitis with CBD stones at any age are indications for urgent sphincterotomy within 48 h

Malignant biliary strictures
- Endoscopic insertion of a stent is indicated, pending a decision about surgery. Brushings for cytology and sometimes biopsies can be taken at ERCP to confirm malignancy, although false-negative results are common
- Curative surgery should be considered if the patient is young (< 60 years) and fit, with a pancreatic tumour < 2 cm on CT scan. Palliative surgery (gastrojejunostomy) is indicated if there are signs of duodenal infiltration
- The success rate of stent insertion (85%) is similar to palliative surgery (choledochojejunostomy), but complications and hospital stay are appreciably reduced
- Duodenal obstruction by tumour following stent insertion (which might have been avoided by surgery) is unusual (17% in one controlled trial)
- Repeat ERCP for blocked stents is required in 20% with malignant obstruction, after 3 months. Most stents block in time and replacement is usually straightforward when jaundice recurs
- High or tortuous strictures are best stented by percutaneous radiological insertion of a self-expanding metal stent or a joint percutaneous and endoscopic procedure. If this fails, jaundice can sometimes be relieved by segment III biliary diversion in expert hands

Benign biliary strictures
- Single benign strictures (often post-traumatic) are best treated surgically at a specialist referral centre, although balloon dilatation at ERCP may be possible
- Surgical treatment usually involves biliary drainage through a Roux loop. A loop of jejunum leading to the anastomosis can be left with a radio-opaque marker, so that percutaneous dilatation under fluoroscopy can be performed if (or when) the stricture recurs

Surgery in cholestatic jaundice
- Mortality and complications are common—up to 50% if the patient has underlying cirrhosis
- Contributing factors are the age of the patient (often elderly), sepsis (especially cholangitis), cause of jaundice (cirrhosis or malignancy) and predisposition to renal failure (hepatorenal syndrome, p. 149)

6.4 Cholangitis

Bacterial cholangitis
Ascending infection in the biliary tree occurs when the main bile ducts are obstructed, usually by stones. Surgery or endoscopic procedures can introduce infection.

Features (Charcot's triad)
- Jaundice
- Pain—usually central, severe and colicky, but may also be minimal
- Fever—may be minimal in the elderly, those on steroids and the immunosuppressed
- A high index of suspicion is needed in any patient with fever and cholestatic liver function tests. In the elderly biliary sepsis may be a cause of confusion and liver function tests may be normal, particularly if the CBD is very dilated and thus not completely obstructed

Management
- General—blood cultures, intravenous fluids, analgesics (e.g. pethidine/mepiridine)
- Antibiotics—intravenous third-generation cephalosporin or quinolone (e.g. ciprofloxacin)
- Ultrasound—to look for a dilated common duct (> 7 mm), although obstructing stones are rarely seen
- Drainage—urgent (< 48 h) ERCP and sphincterotomy if CBD stones are present, whatever the age. Mortality is 5–10%
- Emergency surgery and exploration of the common duct has a mortality of 30% in poor-risk patients

Primary sclerosing cholangitis
All parts of the biliary tract may be involved in a fibrosing process that ultimately leads to biliary cirrhosis. The cause is unknown. 75% have associated ulcerative colitis and 20–30% subsequently develop cholangiocarcinoma.

Clinical features
- 70% are male
- Asymptomatic elevation of ALP in a patient with ulcerative colitis (rarely Crohn's disease) is highly suggestive. Patients are usually male (3 : 1), with quiescent pancolitis
- Pruritus, jaundice, right upper quadrant pain and weight loss occur in 75%
- Bacterial cholangitis and oesophageal varices due to portal hypertension occur less commonly than in other types of progressive liver disease
- Rapid deterioration may be due to a cholangiocarcinoma in later stages, which is more common in those with ulcerative colitis

Investigations
- ALP is elevated together with γ-GT. AMA is negative
- Ultrasound excludes other causes of cholestasis (gallstones are also more common in ulcerative colitis)
- ERCP is diagnostic. It demonstrates irregular stricturing and dilatation (beading) of intrahepatic ducts. 30% have a stricture of an extrahepatic bile duct. Diffuse cholangiocarcinoma can rarely cause this appearance
- Liver biopsy may be characteristic (periductular onion skin fibrosis), but the diagnosis must be confirmed by ERCP. Histological appearances can be confused with autoimmune chronic hepatitis, but an unusually high ALP in these patients is an indication for ERCP. Small duct PSC is recognised with characteristic liver biopsy findings but a normal ERCP. This condition has a better prognosis than classical PSC
- Sigmoidoscopy and rectal biopsy should be performed in all patients who have not previously been diagnosed as having ulcerative colitis

Management
- There is no specific treatment, although ursodeoxycholic acid, at 15–20 mg/kg, improved liver biochemistry. Higher doses are under trial. Symptomatic treatment is the same as for primary biliary cirrhosis (p. 169)
- Itching that does not respond to cholestyramine or rifampicin often responds to naltrexone, but this may be associated with side-effects particularly early in the course of therapy
- Colonoscopy and serial biopsies are appropriate to exclude colonic dysplasia, since colorectal cancer complicating ulcerative colitis appears to be more common (Table 9.5, p. 310)
- Early colectomy for severe ulcerative colitis is probably warranted in PSC. There is an increased risk of both colonic carcinoma pre and post transplantation.
- Hepatic transplantation should be considered in patients with end-stage disease (jaundice, ascites), although the timing is more difficult and the outcome less effective than for primary biliary cirrhosis (p. 183)

Prognosis
- Mean duration from the onset of symptoms to death is 7 years, but the time is variable and most are now detected at the asymptomatic stage during investigation of cholestatic liver function tests
- 5-year survival after transplantation is 50–70% and is improving

Secondary and autoimmune cholangitis
- Very rarely, an identical picture to PSC can be caused by long-standing biliary obstruction due to a benign stricture or common duct stones. *Cryptosporidia* sp. infection (associated with HIV disease and common variable immunodeficiency) is also associated with intrahepatic sclerosing cholangitis
- Autoimmune cholangitis, or AMA-negative primary biliary cirrhosis, is a condition with cholestasis, high titres of antinuclear antibodies, but negative AMA. The clinical features and histological appearance are identical to primary biliary cirrhosis (Section 5.6, p. 168)

6.5 Cholangiocarcinoma

Carcinoma may arise anywhere in the biliary tree. The site determines the presentation—distal tumours obstruct main ducts and present early; intrahepatic tumours present late and may be mistaken for hepatomas. There is a high prevalence in Thailand and the Far East, possibly due to liver fluke (*Clonorchis sinensis*) infection.

Clinical features
- Age typically > 60 years
- Associated with PSC
- Jaundice, followed by pruritus (pruritus precedes jaundice in PSC). Carcinoma of the pancreas or ampulla is a more common cause. The jaundice occasionally fluctuates, which can be deceptive. Cholangitis does not occur except after ERCP or secondary bile duct stone formation
- Pain—epigastric and mild
- Weight loss and diarrhoea, due to fat malabsorption
- Rapid deterioration in a patient with PSC
- Hepatomegaly or a palpable gall bladder is common, but splenomegaly and ascites are rare

Diagnosis
- Investigations for cholestatic jaundice (ultrasound, MR scan, CT scan or ERCP; Fig. 6.5, p. 197) are complementary diagnostic techniques
- Blood tests show a cholestatic picture. AFP is normal
- Ultrasound identifies dilated ducts, but only occasionally detects a tumour mass
- CT scan and/or MRC may show a mass
- ERCP often shows an abrupt or irregular obstruction to contrast, usually at the hilum. A percutaneous transhepatic cholangiogram is then indicated to define the extent, if intervention to relieve jaundice is considered feasible

Difficulties
- Histological confirmation. Liver biopsy rarely shows tumour even in intrahepatic lesions
- Brush or bile cytology should be obtained at ERCP (30% positive)
- Distinguishing distal lesions from pancreatic cancer. CT scan may show the site of the main bulk of the tumour

- Widespread intrahepatic cholangiocarcinoma looks like PSC. The clinical course over a few weeks indicates the diagnosis
- There are rare but well-documented cases of intraductal hepatocellular carcinoma

Management
Cure is rarely possible unless a tumour is found incidentally at hepatic transplant for PSC.

Resection
Surgery should be considered for distal, localised tumours in young patients who present with jaundice early. Referral to a specialist centre is advisable.

Symptomatic treatment
- Endoscopic stenting of distal strictures to relieve jaundice and itching. This may be difficult, because most tumours are at the porta hepatis (p. 193)
- Cholestyramine 4–12 g/day or naltrexone (50 mg/day) for pruritus; naltrexone may be associated with loss of pain control
- Analgesics for pain
- Low-fat diet for diarrhoea

Prognosis
- In contrast to pancreatic cancer, the tumours are slow-growing
- Mean survival is 14 months, but may be up to 5 years

6.6 Clinical dilemmas

Post-cholecystectomy symptoms and biliary dyskinesia
Recurrent symptoms occur in 15% patients who have an elective cholecystectomy. Most are attributed to ill-defined motility disorders (IBS or biliary dyskinesia), but there are several other important causes.

Causes
- Retained CBD stone
- Duodenal or gastric ulcer
- Chronic pancreatitis
- Renal tract disease (including pelviureteric junction obstruction)
- Irritable bowel syndrome
- Biliary dyskinesia (sphincter of Oddi dysfunction (SOD), or post-cholecystectomy syndrome)

Biliary dyskinesia and sphincter of Oddi dysfunction
Biliary dyskinesia or SOD describes recurrent colicky pain, fat intolerance, often with diarrhoea and dyspepsia, without a retained stone or other cause. It often predates a cholecystectomy that was done to relieve the symptoms.
- Three types have been described that influence treatment:
  - I—biliary pain, twofold elevation of ALP or AST on two occasions and dilated CBD > 12 mm or delayed biliary drainage at ERCP)

- II—biliary pain and one of the objective criteria of biliary obstruction)
- III—biliary pain and none of the criteria of biliary obstruction)
- Endoscopic manometry of the sphincter of Oddi shows increased baseline pressure (> 40 mmHg for 30 s) in about 60%, but even without manometry, the classification helps management (see below). An 8–31% risk of acute pancreatitis following biliary manometry is reported in large series

Management

Careful history
To identify differences from pre-cholecystectomy symptoms and associated features of other diseases.

Initial investigation
- Blood tests for ALP, γ-GT (elevated in retained stones or biliary dyskinesia) and full blood count
- Urine for blood, protein, bilirubin and urobilinogen
- Abdominal ultrasound (the CBD is usually slightly dilated after cholecystectomy, 7–9 mm). Repeating the ultrasound after a fatty meal may show duct dilatation, consistent with sphincter of Oddi spasm
- If these tests are normal, IBS is the likely diagnosis

Subsequent investigations and treatment
Indicated if severe symptoms persist, or if initial investigations are abnormal:
- Upper gastrointestinal endoscopy
- High-resolution MRCP *before* ERCP, to look for evidence of a retained stone or chronic pancreatitis
- ERCP is more often complicated by pancreatitis (5–10%) than normal and should only be performed when there is objective evidence of obstruction
- Sphincterotomy is indicated for retained calculi, for type I and occasionally for type II biliary dyskinesia (above). In prospective studies, long-term symptomatic relief occurred in 90% of type I and 60–70% of type II, but < 10% with type III obstruction. The risk of pancreatitis is much higher following sphincterotomy for biliary dyskinesia (up to 40%) than for CBD stones (5–8%, Table 1.6, p. 32)
- A long cystic duct remnant is not an indication for surgery
- Pharmacological therapy is sometimes helpful, with nifedipine (5–10 mg twice daily) or tricyclic antidepressants (e.g. amitryptiline 10–30 mg) and reassurance that the symptoms do not represent anything serious. The many alternatives (aluminium-containing antacids, cholestyramine, treatment for non-ulcer dyspepsia (p. 90), other antidepressants, laxatives, exclusion diet) indicate how difficult it can be to treat effectively
- Referral for sphincter of Oddi manometry is indicated for type II SOD (typical biliary pain and one objective criterion of biliary obstruction) that persists despite pharmacological therapy. Sphincterotomy is justified and usually effective if basal pressure is > 40 mmHg

7 Small Intestine

7.1 Diarrhoea

Food, fluid and intestinal secretions amount to 7 L/day. Normally 5 L is absorbed by the small intestine and 1.5–2 L by the colon. The residual 100–200 mL (or 100–200 g when solid) is excreted as faeces. Consequently a 10% decrease in fluid absorbed by the colon will double the stool volume. There is, however, considerable reserve colonic absorptive capacity, which compensates for increased ileal effluent volume in osmotic or secretory conditions (Table 7.2, p. 208), until that capacity is exceeded, when diarrhoea develops.

Diarrhoea means increased stool water. Chronic diarrhoea may be defined as the abnormal passage of three or more loose or liquid stools per day for more than 4 weeks and/or a daily stool volume of > 200 mL/day (weight > 200 g/day). Patients may describe increased stool frequency alone, a single loose motion or even rectal discharge as diarrhoea.

- Prevalence in Western populations is 4–5%
- A careful history is essential. Diagnosis initially depends on excluding colonic causes and identifying common conditions

Table 7.1 Causes of diarrhoea

Common	Uncommon	Rare
Gastroenteritis viral (rota, echo) bacterial (*Salmonella, Campylobacter* spp.) parasitic (*G. lamblia*) toxin (*E. coli, Shigella* spp.)	Coeliac disease	Autonomic neuropathy
	Hypogammaglobulinaemia	Tropical sprue
	Bacterial overgrowth	Ischaemic colitis
	Microscopic colitis	Whipple's disease
	Chronic pancreatitis	Collagenous colitis
Irritable bowel syndrome	Thyrotoxicosis	Addison's disease
Drugs (many, alcohol)	Pseudomembranous colitis	Hypoparathyroidism
Colorectal carcinoma	Laxative abuse	Amyloidosis
Ulcerative colitis or Crohn's disease	Food allergy	Behçet's disease
Hypolactasia	Ileal/gastric resection	Intestinal vasculitis
		Gastrinoma
		Mastocytosis
		Carcinoid
		VIPoma
		Medullary thyroid cancer
		Pellagra
		Zinc deficiency

Causes
Common causes of recurrent or persistent diarrhoea are shown in Table 7.1. Diarrhoea has traditionally been classified into osmotic, secretory, motility and combined types (Table 7.2). Although this is seldom of practical use, it may aid diagnosis in patients with difficult diarrhoea (p. 211).

Osmotic diarrhoea
- Due to malabsorbed, osmotically active substances such as carbohydrate and peptides, which retain water in the intestinal lumen. Diarrhoea occurs when the extra ileal effluent exceeds colonic absorptive capacity, and may be intermittent (if the colon compensates for the fluid load), or may only present when there is associated colonic disease (such as hypolactasia with Crohn's colitis)
- Characterised by an osmotic gap > 125 mOs/kg and by cessation of diarrhoea on fasting
- Faecal osmotic gap = $290 - 2x([Na^+]_{faeces} + [K^+]_{faeces})$. Faecal sodium and potassium concentrations are measured in stool water after homogenisation and centrifugation. A gap > 125 mOs/kg indicates the presence of other osmotically active electrolytes (usually Mg^{+++} or short chain fatty acids)
- Laxative abuse with magnesium-containing medicines or lactulose should always be considered

Secretory diarrhoea
- Secretion, stimulated by a toxin (such as cholera toxin) or peptide (such as vasoactive intestinal polypeptide, VIP), is mediated by cyclic nucleotides. 'Traveller's diarrhoea' is usually due to *E. coli* enterotoxin (Table 7.2)
- Characterised by stool volume > 200 mL and an osmotic gap < 50 mOs/kg when fasting (Fig. 7.2, p. 212)

Deranged motility
- Both enhanced (causing rapid transit) and decreased motility (predisposing to bacterial overgrowth) may cause diarrhoea
- Faecal osmotic gap and response to fasting are unhelpful in diagnosis

Table 7.2 Mechanisms of diarrhoea

Osmotic	Secretory	Motility	Combined
Hypolactasia	Toxins	Irritable bowel	Inflammatory bowel disease
Drugs (lactulose, magnesium salts)	*E. coli* *Vibrio cholerae* *Staphylococcus aureus* *Clostridium perfringens*	Drugs (senna, phenolphthalein)	Coeliac disease
		Post vagotomy Post cholecystectomy	Carcinoid
	Tumours VIP		Malabsorption
	Villous adenoma of rectum Zollinger–Ellison syndrome Bile acid malabsorption	Post gastrectomy Irritable bowel syndrome	
			Post ileocaecal resection

Combined mechanisms

- Diarrhoea is frequently due to multiple factors
- The diarrhoea of ulcerative colitis, for example, is caused by disordered motility, altered mucosal permeability, prostaglandin or short-chain fatty acid–induced changes in ion transport, decreased capacity of the rectal reservoir and loss of blood or mucus into the lumen

Clinical features

History

- Duration > 4 weeks (or less in the very young or old, dehydrated or debilitated) needs investigation
- Factors that strongly suggest organic pathology include duration < 3 months, continuous (as opposed to intermittent), nocturnal diarrhoea, or weight loss
- Morning diarrhoea is a feature of alcohol abuse and IBS, but may indicate more serious pathology (such as inflammatory bowel disease)
- Weight loss despite a good appetite is typical of thyrotoxicosis
- Blood (altered or fresh) indicates a colonic cause
- Fat globules in the pan after flushing suggests steatorrhoea
- Colour of diarrhoea, undigested food, odour, abdominal cramps, bloating, flatulence and audible borborygmi are non-specific

Specific factors in the history

Also ask about:

- *Family history*—particularly of neoplastic, inflammatory bowel or coeliac disease
- *Previous surgery*—gastrectomy, cholecystectomy, terminal ileal resection
- *Previous pancreatic disease*
- *Systemic disease*—thyrotoxicosis, parathyroid disease, diabetes, scleroderma
- *Extra-intestinal manifestations*—arthritis, skin rashes (erythema nodosum, dermatitis herpetifomis), iritis
- *Alcohol*—increases intestinal transit, decreases disaccharidase activity and may cause pancreatic dysfunction
- *Drugs*—account for about 5% of chronic diarrhoea, including antibiotics, magnesium-containing antacids, PPIs, β-blockers and NSAIDs
- *Recent travel*—or other potential sources of infectious diarrhoea
- *Recent antibiotics*—in case of *Cl. difficile* infection

Examination

- Look for dehydration, weight loss, skin rashes and abdominal surgical scars. Clubbing sometimes occurs in active Crohn's disease
- Feel for an enlarged thyroid, or an abdominal mass, which may indicate colonic carcinoma or Crohn's disease
- Rectal examination, sigmoidoscopy and rectal biopsy are essential for chronic diarrhoea or bloody diarrhoea

Initial investigations

Appropriate for all patients with chronic diarrhoea (> 4 weeks), or for diarrhoea in the very young, very old, dehydrated or debilitated.

Stool sample
- Microscopy for *Giardia lamblia* (other parasites and ova when from endemic areas), and cysts of *Cryptosporidium* spp. if immunodeficient. ELISA for *G. lamblia* if stool microscopy negative and strong index of suspicion
- Culture for *Salmonella*, *Shigella*, *Campylobacter*, *Yersinia* spp.
- *Cl. difficile* toxin assay when antibiotics have been recently taken
- Electron microscopy (for viruses) only in children, or during an epidemic or outbreak

Sigmoidoscopy
- Record the distance reached, stool and mucosal appearance (p. 270)
- Always take a biopsy of any identifiable lesion and a representative area, because 10–20% of patients with Crohn's disease have microscopic changes even when the mucosa looks normal. Histology provides an independent record of the sigmoidoscopic findings, but microscopic colitis may still be missed on a rectal biopsy (p. 272)

Blood tests
- Microcytic anaemia suggests a carcinoma or inflammatory bowel disease
- Macrocytosis may be due to coeliac disease, distal ileal Crohn's disease, or alcohol
- A high CRP indicates active inflammatory bowel disease, carcinoma or occasionally infective causes. The CRP is more sensitive than the ESR, but both Crohn's disease and carcinoma can occur with a normal ESR and CRP
- Low potassium (< 3.5 mmol/L) occurs in any severe diarrhoea. Also consider laxative abuse, villous adenoma and VIPoma
- Thyroid function tests are best checked at the first or second visit, so that they are not overlooked
- Serological tests for coeliac (antiendomysial antibodies or tissuetransglutaminase (tTG) antibodies) should be checked at the first visit together with serum immunoglobulins (see p. 222)

Imaging the colon
- Always investigate the colon if sustained diarrhoea develops for the first time over the age of 50 years
- Colonoscopy and ileoscopy is the best investigation if there is visible blood in the stools, chronic watery diarrhoea (to exclude microscopic colitis), for young patients (to avoid X-ray exposure) and if inflammatory bowel disease is suspected (to obtain biopsies)
- Flexible sigmoidoscopy (p. 417) can be rapidly performed and is a useful investigation when there is fresh rectal bleeding
- Abdominal CT scan (especially spiral imaging, p. 399) to exclude colonic carcinoma is useful in the frail or elderly (p. 399), because it avoids the need for bowel preparation
- If < 50 years, carcinoma is unlikely. IBS is the most likely diagnosis if other tests are normal and infective causes excluded. Review after treatment is often more appropriate than invasive investigation

Subsequent investigations
If malabsorption is suspected, subsequent investigations should be directed as indicated in Section 7.2. The following plan is recommended if the results of initial

investigations do not establish a diagnosis or suggest malabsorption, and symptoms justify invasive investigation (Fig. 7.1).

Difficult diarrhoea

If the cause of diarrhoea remains obscure after outpatient investigation (Fig. 7.1), admission may be necessary to distinguish between organic disease and a motility disorder (Fig. 7.2). Diarrhoea due to organic disease has a stool volume > 200 mL/day, which usually does not settle on admission. Functional diarrhoea (due to an irritable bowel) often disappears on admission and the stool weight is usually < 200 g/day (volume < 200 mL/day).

General points

- Faecal calprotectin (a neutrophil protein that is stable for up to 7 days in faeces at room temperature) has been advocated as a non-invasive way of discriminating between functional and inflammatory or malignant bowel disease. It is expensive, not widely available and needs better validation before it replaces other investigation
- Stool electrolyte assay and osmolality needs to be discussed with the biochemistry laboratory. Don't bother sending solid stool.
- Planned admission for stool weight and frequency measurement on a normal diet for 48–72 h, then (if stool weight exceeds 200 g/24 h) on intravenous fluids for 48–72 h is a simple way of discriminating functional, osmotic and secretory causes of intractable diarrhoea

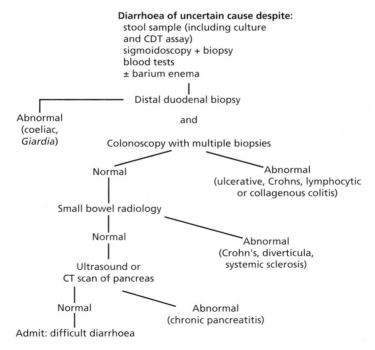

Fig. 7.1 Outpatient investigation of diarrhoea.

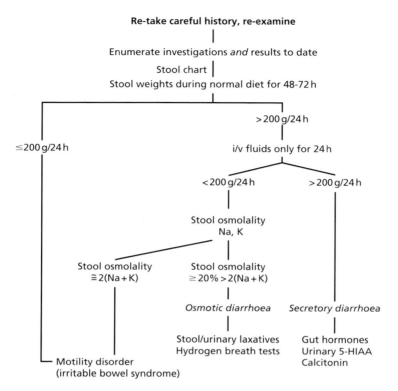

Re-take careful history, re-examine

Enumerate investigations *and* results to date

Stool chart

Stool weights during normal diet for 48-72 h

≤200 g/24 h

>200 g/24 h

i/v fluids only for 24 h

<200 g/24 h

>200 g/24 h

Stool osmolality Na, K

Stool osmolality ≅2(Na + K)

Stool osmolality ≥20% >2(Na + K)

Osmotic diarrhoea

Secretory diarrhoea

Stool/urinary laxatives
Hydrogen breath tests

Gut hormones
Urinary 5-HIAA
Calcitonin

Motility disorder (irritable bowel syndrome)

Fig. 7.2 **Investigation of difficult diarrhoea.**

- Lactulose or glucose breath tests are non-invasive methods of detecting bacterial over-growth, but limited by low sensitivity and specificity (p. 427). Breath H_2 normally rises as the lactulose (or any carbohydrate load, including glucose) reaches the colon, but when lactulose is broken down by small intestinal bacteria, this rise occurs < 2 h after ingestion
- Lactose breath test is a non-invasive method of detecting lactase deficiency (p. 219). Hypolactasic subjects exhale more H_2 than normal (> 20 ppm.) after 2 h. Subjects with normal lactase levels produce little or no H_2. False-negative rate is 25%, so a negative result does not exclude the diagnosis. A trial of a lactose-free diet (p. 390) should be considered if clinical suspicion is high.
- Xylose absorption is an unreliable screening test for carbohydrate malabsorption. Distal duodenal biopsy or dual sugar tests (p. 429) are preferable
- ^{75}Se-HCAT test is used to identify bile acid malabsorption; a positive test is indicated by < 15% retention of the synthetic radiolabelled analogue of taurocholic acid at 7 days (p. 228)
- Peroral pneumocologram (discuss with radiologists) gives the best views of the cae-cum and terminal ileum if they are not clearly seen by other methods
- A laxative screen should include detection of anthraquinones, bisacodyl, and phe-nolphthalein in urine, and magnesium and phosphate in stool. 4% of patients with chronic diarrhoea visiting gastroenterology clinics have factitious diarrhoea. This figure rises to 20% in tertiary referral centres. Establishing laxative abuse may be

difficult and methods once used, such as examining the patient's personal belongings, may not be allowable under privacy legislation

Management

- The cause of diarrhoea should be identified and treated if possible
- Oral rehydration solution (sodium chloride 3.5 g, sodium citrate 2.9 g, potassium chloride 1.5 g and glucose 20 g in 1 L, WHO formula), or commercial preparations (such as Dioralyte, Pedialyte or Gastrolyte) are indicated for severe diarrhoea in the young or elderly
- Codeine phosphate 30–60 mg/day is the first choice when stool frequency needs to be controlled
- Loperamide 4 mg, then 2 mg after each loose stool can be used for acute gastroenteritis or motility disorders. Although drugs are best avoided if possible, there is no convincing evidence that clearance of intestinal pathogens is delayed. It should not be used in children, because fatal paralytic ileus has been reported
- Amitriptyline 10–25 mg at night may be effective for motility disorders, because of anticholinergic effects
- Antibiotics are only indicated for a few infections (*G. lamblia*, *Yersinia enterocolitica*, severe shigellosis, or bacterial overgrowth; p. 227). Excretion of *Salmonella* spp. is prolonged by inappropriate antibiotics and increases the risk of a carrier state

Post-infectious diarrhoea

Persistent diarrhoea after acute gastroenteritis may be due to persistent infection (especially *G. lamblia*), acquired hypolactasia, hypogammaglobulinaemia, unrecognised disease (coeliac, ulcerative colitis) or postinfectious IBS, which is the commonest reason (p. 214).

Traveller's diarrhoea

Enterotoxigenic *E. coli* cause most acute, self-limiting episodes of diarrhoea in travellers (Box 7.1). *Cryptosporidium* spp. and *Cyclospora* spp. are other causes.

- Budget travellers, particularly those aged 20–29 are at greatest risk
- Incubation is 1–5 days
- Sudden onset of severe diarrhoea with abdominal pain is only serious in the young, debilitated or elderly
- Resolution within 48–96 h is usual; < 5% persist for > 4 weeks and then need investigation to exclude underlying disease
- *Symptomatic treatment* is indicated and drugs avoided if possible. If the patient's job is affected and rapid control of symptoms needed, a single dose of ciprofloxacin 750 mg is usually effective
- *Preventive advice* includes avoiding salads, uncooked vegetables, shellfish, ice cream and unsterilised water (including ice) in uncertain areas. Chemoprophylaxis with antibiotics (cotrimoxazole 2 tablets twice daily or ciprofloxacin 500 mg once daily) offers 70–95% protection against traveller's diarrhoea but should be considered only in high-risk short-term travellers. Sulphonamides can produce sensitivity to sunlight
- For severe symptoms in the absence of adequate microbiological facilities, empirical treatment with ciprofloxacin followed by cotrimoxazole (2 tablets twice daily for 1–2

> **Box 7.1 Differential diagnosis of diarrhoea after foreign travel**
>
> Traveller's diarrhoea (enterotoxigenic *E. coli*)
> *G. lambia**
> Infective diarrhoea
>   *Salmonella* spp.
>   *Shigella* spp.[†]
>   *Campylobacter* spp.[†]
>   *Cyclospora* spp.
>   *Y. enterocolitica*
>   *E. coli* 0157[†]
>   rotavirus
> Post-infective irritable bowel syndrome
> Post-infective hypolactasia* (when drinking milk)
> Latent disease revealed by infection*
>   ulcerative colitis[†]
>   coeliac disease
>   Crohn's disease
>   ileocaecal tuberculosis
> Other infections
>   *Strongyloides stercoralis*[†]
>   hepatitis A, B or E (community acquired non-A, non-B)
>   acute falciparum malaria
>   *Cryptosporidium* spp.
>   amoebic dysentery (*Entamoeba histolytica*)
>   fasciolopsiasis,* capillariasis*
>   schistosomiasis,[†] enterobiasis,[†] trichuriasis[†]
> Tropical sprue*
>
> ---
> *Usually chronic diarrhoea.
> [†]Often bloody diarrhoea.

weeks) in the case of *Cyclospora* sp. infection, then metronidazole 750 mg three times daily for 3 days in case of *G. lamblia* is reasonable

- *Persistent diarrhoea* may be due to postinfectious IBS, persistent infection (consider *Cyclospora* spp., *G. lamblia*), hypolactasia, or unmasked latent disease (Fig. 7.3), and is investigated in the same way as for other causes (p. 209; Fig. 7.1, p. 211)

7.2 Malabsorption

Defective luminal digestion, mucosal disease, or structural disorders are the mechanisms of malabsorption. Fat, carbohydrate, protein, vitamin or mineral malabsorption may predominate, but combined deficiency is usual except in metabolic defects.

Causes

- Knowledge of the mechanism is more useful for deciding about investigations than for classifying causes (Table 7.3). More than one mechanism commonly operates. Mucosal disease may be associated with defective digestion and sometimes with structural change as well

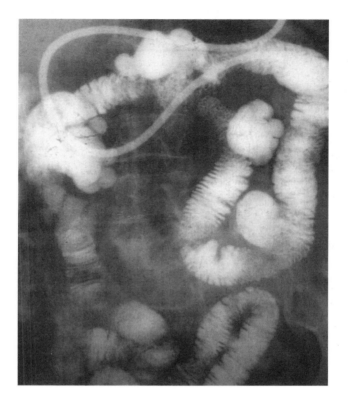

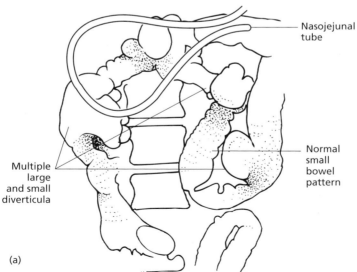

(a)

Fig. 7.3 **Small bowel radiology and malabsorption.** (a) Small bowel enema showing multiple jejunal diverticula, causing malabsorption due to bacterial overgrowth. *(Continued)*

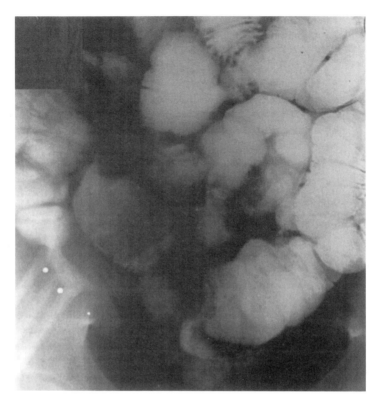

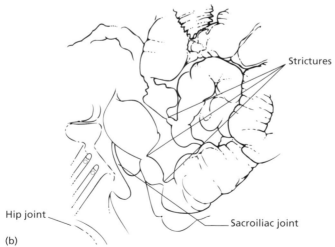

(b)

Strictures

Hip joint

Sacroiliac joint

Fig. 7.3 *(continued)* (b) Small bowel study in a patient with malabsorption due to extensive Crohn's disease, causing multiple strictures.

216

Table 7.3 Causes of malabsorption

Common	Uncommon	Rare
Coeliac disease	Pancreatic cancer	Small bowel lymphoma
Chronic pancreatitis	Parasites (*G. lamblia*)	Lymphangiectasia
Crohn's disease	Bacterial overgrowth	Whipple's disease
Postinfective	Drugs	Thyrotoxicosis
Biliary obstruction	Short bowel syndrome	Zollinger–Ellison syndrome
Cirrhosis	Resection	Metabolic defects
	gastric	Mesenteric ischaemia
	terminal ileal	Mastocytosis
	pancreatic	Amyloidosis
		HIV enteropathy
		α-chain disease
		Tropical sprue
		Starvation

- Hypoalbuminaemia and vitamin K or D deficiency in cirrhosis may be due to liver disease as well as malabsorption
- Crohn's disease causes malabsorption from distal ileal disease (vitamin B_{12} and bile salts), duodenal–jejunal mucosal disease (fat malabsorption, iron and folate deficiency), disaccharidase deficiency, enteroenteric fistulae, bacterial overgrowth, or a short bowel (p. 231)
- Other causes are discussed below

Clinical features

Diarrhoea
- Steatorrhoea is due to defective digestion of fat, resulting in malabsorption. Pancreatic exocrine insufficiency (p. 116) is the usual cause, and severe steatorrhoea is rare in mucosal or structural disease. It is characterised by pale, bulky, malodorous motions with oily globules in the pan after flushing
- Stool bulk is increased more than frequency, unlike the diarrhoea of colonic disease
- Malabsorption occasionally occurs without diarrhoea. Intestinal causes (coeliac disease, bacterial overgrowth) are then likely

Weight loss
Weight loss occurs whatever the cause of malabsorption, but may be minimal during malabsorption of specific nutrients (such as B_{12} malabsorption from bacterial overgrowth).

General symptoms
Lassitude, anorexia, abdominal bloating, discomfort and borborygmi may be inappropriately dismissed as an irritable bowel.

Specific features (See Tables 12.2–12.4, pp. 371–372)
- Hypoalbuminaemia causes dependent oedema or, rarely, ascites when severe
- Hypocalcaemia and hypomagnesaemia cause paraesthesiae and tetany if severe

- Vitamin deficiencies can cause cheilitis (riboflavin), glossitis (B_{12}), bruising (K), bone pain or myopathy (D), night blindness or xerophthalmia (A), dermatitis (niacin), neuropathy or psychological disturbance (thiamine or E)
- Mineral deficiencies can cause muscle weakness (calcium, magnesium), skin rashes, anaemia or leucopenia (zinc, copper). Deficiencies are rare, but often multiple

Investigations
Once malabsorption has been documented, the site and severity must be established.

Documentation
- The combination of diarrhoea, documented weight loss and abnormal blood tests (full blood count, INR, calcium, haematinics, or albumin) are sufficient to document malabsorption and identify the need for further investigation
- Full blood count, folate and B_{12} estimation (anaemia and folate deficiency are common in mucosal disease and B_{12} deficiency in terminal ileal disease or bacterial overgrowth)
- Prothrombin time or ratio (INR) may indicate vitamin K deficiency and is necessary before invasive tests
- Albumin, calcium and ALP. Hypoalbuminaemia indicates severe malabsorption. Osteomalacia causes hypocalcaemia or an elevated ALP. Serum magnesium should be measured if symptoms of hypocalcaemia respond slowly to treatment, since it may be low (< 0.7 mmol/L)
- 3–5-day faecal fat estimation is effectively obsolete. It is rarely helpful and not diagnostically discriminating
- Stool sample for fat globules (which are rarely present except in malabsorption) is a qualitative method of documenting malabsorption, but false-negative results are common and is not recommended
- Pancreatic elastase in stool (using an ELISA kit, but may not be locally available) is recommended as a first-line test for pancreatic insufficiency, since it is reliable, convenient and non-invasive
- Xylose test to assess carbohydrate absorption has a 25% false-negative rate and is not recommended (p. 428)
- Enteric protein loss can be documented by assessing faecal radioactivity after intravenous ^{131}I-albumin injection. It is rarely necessary and is best done at a specialist referral centre

Identify the site
- Jejunal biopsy is the definitive investigation for mucosal lesions and small bowel radiology for structural causes. Defective luminal digestion may (rarely) be confirmed by lactose breath test or mucosal enzyme assay
- Distal duodenal biopsies (D3, beyond the papilla) at endoscopy are usually adequate for detecting villous atrophy, but normal villi may appear flattened over duodenal glands. Causes of villous atrophy are shown in Box 7.2
- Aspiration of jejunal juice may detect *G. lamblia* that are not visible on distal duodenal biopsy
- Small bowel radiology will usually identify distal ileal disease, diverticula, strictures, systemic sclerosis or tumours. Small bowel enema (enteroclysis fig 7.3) demonstrates

---

Box 7.2 Other causes of villous atrophy

G. lamblia	Whipple's disease
Acute infectious enteritis	NSAIDs
viral	Recent chemotherapy
bacterial	Graft-versus-host disease
Hypogammaglobulinaemia	Zollinger–Ellison syndrome
Bacterial overgrowth	Radiation
Tropical sprue	HIV enteropathy
Cows' milk intolerance*	Starvation
Soya protein intolerance*	Chronic ischaemia
Lymphoma	

*Children only.

---

the mucosal pattern better than a barium follow-through (p. 458). Flocculation, thickened folds and slight dilatation are all non-specific. MR enteroclysis (Fig. 7.4) is an evolving technique

Radiolabelled white cell scans (Tc-HMPAO) offer a relatively non-invasive way of detecting active small bowel Crohn's disease and may be particularly useful in children (Table 14.1, p. 427)

- Lactose breath test is the most convenient non-invasive way of confirming hypolactasia, but it is usually simpler to document symptoms before and after stopping milk and milk products (p. 390) for 1 week. Enzyme assay is usually impracticable and unnecessary
- Ultrasound of the pancreas offers a sensitivity of 50–60% and CT 75–90% for detecting chronic pancreatitis. ERCP is the current gold standard, but is invasive and

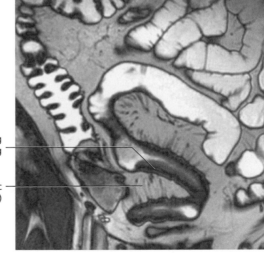

TrueFISP image demonstrating wall thickening

Increased mesenteric vascularity (comb sign)

Courtesy: N. Gourtsoyiannis, MD, University of Crete

Fig. 7.4 MR Enteroclysis. MR enteroclysis in Crohn's disease. This technique is not yet widely available and the technique is evolving, but it images both intestinal and surrounding structures.

219

carries appreciable (5%) risk. It is likely to be replaced by MRP for diagnostic purposes, possibly with secretin enhancement to evaluate dynamic function. The role of endoscopic ultrasound is still being defined

Assess severity
- Document weight and height (BMI; Appendix 3, p. 453) and laboratory evidence of malabsorption
- Formal nutritional assessment by dietitians is appropriate for patients with a BMI < 19 (p. 371)

Coeliac disease
- Coeliac disease (gluten-sensitive enteropathy, coeliac sprue) is defined as small intestinal villous atrophy (Fig. 7.5) that resolves when gluten is withdrawn from the diet. It results from an inappropriate T cell–mediated immune response against gluten in genetically susceptible individuals
- Gluten is a group of proteins derived from wheat, barley and rye but not oats, rice or maize; α-gliadin is the most important toxic moiety. Digestion of dietary α-gliadin in the gut leads to the production of a stable 33-mer peptide containing a PQPQLPY central motif. This peptide is absorbed intact into the lamina propria where exposure to tissue transglutaminase (released by damaged epithelium) results in deamidation of the glutamine residues. This modification enables binding to the HLA-DQ2 molecule and activation of a pro-inflammatory T-cell response
- Prevalence: 1 : 120–300 persons in Europe and N. America. Rare in Afro-Caribbean, Japanese and Chinese
- Female preponderance
- 20% of adult patients are > 60 years at diagnosis

Genetic susceptibility
- 10% prevalence in first-degree relatives. Greatest risk in siblings (relative risk 30%)
- 90–95% carry HLA-DQ2 (HLA-DQA1*0501 and DQB1*0201). The remainder carry DQ8 (HLA-DQA1*03 and DQB1*0302 in cis or trans). This information is useful if there is diagnostic doubt after biopsy (e.g. partial villous atrophy with negative endomysial antibody serology)

Disease presentation
- Coeliac disease may present at any age
- Infant disease presents between 4–24 months (after the introduction of cereals) with impaired growth, diarrhoea, vomiting, abdominal distension
- Older children may present with anaemia, short stature, pubertal delay, recurrent abdominal pain, or behavioural disturbance
- Adult disease usually presents with:
  1. Chronic or recurrent iron-deficiency anaemia
     - 50% of patients now present with isolated asymptomatic iron-deficiency anaemia
  2. Specific symptoms

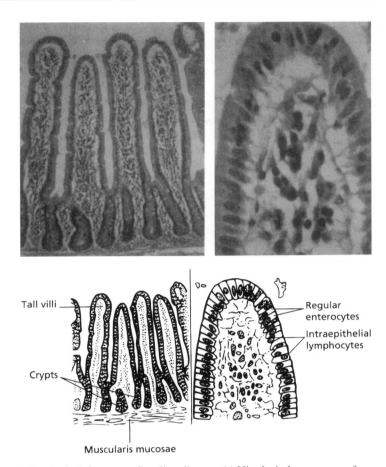

Tall villi

Regular enterocytes

Intraepithelial lymphocytes

Crypts

Muscularis mucosae

Fig. 7.5 Histological features of coeliac disease. (a) Histological appearance of normal jejunal mucosa. Tall villi (left, × ~ 70). The villus height: crypt depth ratio is at least 3 : 1. Tip of a villus showing a few intraepithelial lymphocytes (right, × ~ 320). Haematoxylin and eosin stain. (b) Subtotal villous atrophy showing total absence of villi and a corresponding increase in depth of the crypts, producing an apparently increased mucosal thickness, but insufficient magnification to see the characteristic increase in intraepithelial lymphocytes. Haematoxylin and eosin stain, × ~ 70.

- lethargy, bloating, flatulence, abdominal discomfort may be present for many years and attributed to IBS
- 50% of adult patients have no diarrhoea. Constipation may coexist with coeliac disease
- symptomatic disease may be provoked by infection, pregnancy or surgery
3. Isolated nutritional deficiency
- megaloblastic anaemia, myopathy and bone pain may occur, especially in the elderly
4. Reduced fertility, recurrent abortion, or amenorrhoea
- obstetricians are frequently unaware of the associations

5. Bone fractures
   - patients with osteoporosis not explained by other causes (steroids, rheumatoid arthritis, inflammatory bowel disease) should have their endomysial antibody serology checked
6. Unexplained elevated AST or ALT
   - 10% of patients with isolated hypertransaminasaemia may have coeliac disease
7. Neurological or psychiatric symptoms
   - examination is often normal. Aphthous ulcers are common, but signs of nutritional deficiencies (p. 371) through severe malabsorption are now rarely seen

Associated disorders
- Dermatitis herpetiformis (intensely itchy vesicular papules on the elbows or buttocks)—up to 90% have villous atrophy. Most respond to a gluten-free diet (GFD) (even those without villous atrophy). Dapsone is an alternative
- Autoimmune disease—type I diabetes (3–8% have coeliac disease), thyrotoxicosis, Addison's disease
- Arthritis—rheumatoid or seronegative arthritis are unusual associations
- Pericarditis, spinocerebellar degeneration, pancreatic insufficiency and primary biliary cirrhosis are very rare associations

Diagnosis and investigations in adults
- Deficiencies of iron, folate, calcium and Vitamin D are common. Vitamin B_{12} deficiency is rare as the enteropathy rarely extends to the ileum. Hyposplenism (Howell–Jolly bodies, target cells) may be detected on the blood film, especially in older patients. ALT and AST may be raised. A prolonged prothrombin time due to vitamin K deficiency is rare
- *Serological tests* facilitate diagnosis, although coeliac disease can be present despite negative serology. If there is low clinical probability of disease, negative serological tests may be used to exclude diagnosis. All patients with positive serology and patients with high clinical probability of coeliac disease need confirmation by duodenal histology
- IgA antiendomysial antibodies detected by immunofluoresence have a reported 85–98% sensitivity and 97–100% specificity
- IgA tissuetransglutaminase (tTG) antibodies detected using an ELISA assay are cheaper, easier to perform, more sensitive, but less specific (particularly in Down's and autoimmune disease)
- IgA antigliadin antibodies have moderate sensitivity but poor specificity. Their use is limited to the evaluation of symptomatic children < 2 years of age since levels are easiest to quantify
- Serological results should not be interpreted without knowledge of IgA status as 2–5% of coeliac patients have selective IgA deficiency. In IgA-deficient individuals, diagnosis should be made or excluded by duodenal histology
- Serological tests should be used to screen all first-degree relatives, although no cost-benefit analyses have yet been carried out
- The gold standard remains a *small intestinal biopsy* (D3, beyond the papilla) and should still be performed to confirm the diagnosis before committing a patient to a

lifelong GFD (Fig 7.4). Histological features are villous atrophy, crypt hyperplasia and increased intra-epithelial lymphocytes. At least four biopsies should be taken, as villous atrophy is occasionally patchy

Other causes of villous atrophy

Subtotal villous atrophy is almost always due to coeliac disease in European adults. Partial villous atrophy has other (rare) causes (Box 7.2, p. 219).

Management

- *Gluten-free diet* (p. 389) for life, with advice *and continued support* from a dietitian. There is now good evidence that this decreases the risk of small intestinal malignancy.
- Symptomatic improvement is reported in 70% of patients within 2 weeks
- *Continue dairy products* even though 50% of coeliac patients have secondary hypolactasia at diagnosis. Dairy products are a crucial source of calcium intake and are often inappropriately restricted
- 85% respond, although histological resolution may take 3–12 months. *A second biopsy* after 3–6 months on a GFD to confirm histological recovery can be considered, but some gastroenterologists depend on seroconversion (from positive to negative endomysial antibody serology) and reserve biopsy for patients who have an unsatisfactory response
- Gluten rechallenge is unnecessary in adults, but may be useful in patients diagnosed in childhood (since a number of transient childhood enteropathies can mimic coeliac disease) or patients who have initiated a diet on their own accord without a firm diagnosis
- Iron and folate supplements are needed if anaemic, until recovery. Specific deficiencies may need treating (hypocalcaemia: effervescent calcium 6–12 tablets daily, but serum calcium must be checked monthly)
- Osteoporosis is common, occurring in up to 50% of patients on a GFD. Bone loss is secondary to calcium malabsorption, and secondary hyperparathyroidism. A recommended strategy for the prevention and treatment of osteoporosis in coeliac disease is given in Box 7.3. However, despite the high prevalence of osteoporosis, the real risk of hip fracture differs little from the general population
- Annual outpatient review is advisable when stable, to confirm adherence to the diet and detect complications. Relapse or poor compliance is most readily detected by anaemia or folate deficiency, followed by repeat distal duodenal biopsy
- The Coeliac Society, the Celiac Sprue Association in the USA and the Canadian Celiac Association (Appendix 1, p. 437) provide useful advice, food and drink lists, recipe books, support and motivation for patients

Poor responders

If there is no clinical or histological improvement after 3 months (less if the patient is unwell), the possibilities are as follows

Poor compliance

- Failure to adhere meticulously to a strict GFD. Also the most common cause of recurrent symptoms after an initial response

---

Box 7.3 Strategy for the prevention and treatment of osteoporosis in coeliac disease

---

General advice
- Strict gluten-free (wheat, rye and barley, but not oats)
- Adequate dietary calcium; add calcium tablets if necessary to ensure daily intake 1500 mg
- Exercise, no smoking, no alcohol excess
- Seek and treat Vitamin D deficiency
- Measure bone mineral density (BMD) at diagnosis; if low reinforce above advice

Postmenopausal women and men > 55 years
- Measure BMD when first seen
- If osteoporotic, offer bisphosphonate

All with fragility fracture
- Measure BMD
- If osteoporotic, offer bisphosphonate

Duration of drug treatment
Bisphosphonate or calcitonin:
- Measure BMD annually
- If BMD falls > 4% per year in 2 successive years, change to other drug
- If no fall, continue drug for at least 3 years, possibly longer
- Restart drug if, on stopping, annual BMD falls > 4%

- Review by a dietitian for further guidance/input on hidden or obscure sources of gluten should be arranged
- Persistent positive endomysial antibody serology strongly suggests poor compliance, but negative serology is poor at confirming compliance

Concomitant associated conditions
- Hypolactasia (due to mucosal atrophy)
- Microscopic colitis (up to 10%)
- Pancreatic insufficiency (rare)
- Endocrine disease (hypothyroidism or Addison's disease—often insidious and not considered)

Untreated nutritional deficiency
- Folate or B_{12} (autoimmune pernicious anaemia is more common in coeliac disease)
- Iron
- Calcium
- Magnesium
- Other deficiencies, less commonly

Complications
- Malignancy—small intestinal T-cell lymphoma develops in < 5%. Other types of small intestinal lymphoma originate from B cells. Small intestinal adenocarcinoma is also more common. Recrudescence of symptoms, abdominal pain or deterioration despite a GFD should suggest the diagnosis. Oesophageal and possibly colorectal malignancy is also more common

- Coexistent malignancy should be considered when coeliac disease is diagnosed in the middle-aged or elderly. An elevated CRP may be the only indicator that there is underlying lymphoma
- A long-term follow-up study (Appendix 2, p. 445) has shown that meticulous adherence to a GFD reduces the risk of malignant complications
- Ulcerative jejunitis (ulceration and strictures in the small intestine) is rare, but may cause pain, persistent anaemia or bacterial overgrowth. A small bowel enema is diagnostic, but resection may be necessary to exclude lymphoma or multifocal adenocarcinoma

Refractory sprue
Symptomatic severe enteritis that has not responded to 6 months of GFD, having ruled out other causes of villous atrophy and malabsorption.

Unrelated conditions
- *G. lamblia*
- Irritable bowel syndrome

Management of poor responders
- Emphasise the importance of complete gluten exclusion and ask the dietitian to review dietary compliance carefully. Check that contact with the Coeliac Society in the UK, Celiac Sprue Association in the USA or the Canadian Celiac Association has been established. Give support, encouragement and motivation
- Advise a low-lactose diet (up to 10 g/day can often be well tolerated) in case of secondary hypolactasia and reassess in 4 weeks
- Check that *G. lamblia* has been excluded (p. 226), and that hypogammaglobulinaemia or nutritional deficiencies have been corrected. Give an empirical single dose of tinidazole 2 g, even if *G. lamblia* has not been identified
- Check CRP, perform small bowel radiology and obtain jejunal biopsies using a paediatric colonoscope or enteroscope, to exclude lymphoma, Crohn's disease, diverticula or adenocarcinoma
- Start prednisolone 20 mg/day, but only after other causes of a poor response have been rigorously excluded. Enteropathy associated with hypogammaglobulinaemia often responds to steroids
- Rebiopsy to assess response after 3 months on steroids. Some still do not respond and should be referred to a specialist centre

Prognosis
- Gluten sensitivity persists for life
- Children with coeliac disease often have quiescent symptoms as young adults, but symptoms or complications develop later if the diet is not continued (p. 222)
- Life expectancy is normal on a gluten-free diet

Tropical sprue
Post-infective tropical malabsorption may affect adults of any race who have lived in India, Asia or Central America, but is rare in Africa. Tropical sprue is a disease of res-

idents rather than visitors and is now exceptionally rare. The cause of mucosal damage is uncertain although secondary bacterial overgrowth and hypolactasia commonly exacerbate the malabsorption.

Clinical features
• Malabsorption (p. 217) in a person who has recently lived in the tropics (rarely in the subtropics or several years previously)

Investigation
Diagnosis is established by a consistent history, partial villous atrophy and response to tetracycline. Other causes of tropical malabsorption should be considered (Box 7.4).
• Jejunal biopsy reveals partial villous atrophy (total atrophy is rare), but unlike coeliac disease the changes are more severe in the terminal ileum. Jejunal juice should be examined for *G. lamblia*
• Stools should be examined for parasites
• Small bowel radiology is non-specific, but helps exclude intestinal tuberculosis

Management
• Tetracycline 250 mg four times daily for 4 weeks
• Folic acid 5 mg three times daily for 2 months

Giardiasis
200 million people throughout the world are infected with the flagellated protozoan *G. lamblia*. Infections correlate with poor hygienic conditions, poor water quality control, and overcrowding. Disease may be superimposed on coeliac disease or hypogammaglobulinaemia. Infection may be asymptomatic.

Distinguishing features
• Incubation is 2–3 weeks
• Transmission is through contaminated water or faecal–oral route

---

Box 7.4 Differential diagnosis of malabsorption from abroad

Infective
G. lamblia
HIV enteropathy
AIDS and associated conditions (p. 393)
Cryptosporidium spp.
Strongyloides stercoralis
Small intestinal tuberculosis
Visceral leishmaniasis
Clonorchis sinensis cirrhosis
Filariasis
Tropical sprue
Non-infective
Hypolactasia
Lymphoma (immunoproliferative small intestinal disease)
Calcific chronic pancreatitis
Idiopathic

- Travel abroad is not necessary to acquire infection, although it is more prevalent outside Britain or North America, and in male homosexuals
- Persistent diarrhoea and weight loss after an acute attack of 'gastroenteritis' is characteristic and may continue for months
- The diagnosis should be suspected when a patient first presents with diarrhoea after travelling

Investigations
- Stool examination for cysts or trophozoites detects only about 60% and stool ELISA is therefore preferred (92% sensitivity and 98% specificity)
- Jejunal aspiration (Table 7.1, p. 207; Table 7.3, p. 217) is the most reliable method but rarely required
- Measure immunoglobulins if *G. lamblia* is acquired in the UK or USA or if there is recurrent infection
- Treatment (see below) may be given before a jejunal biopsy if stool examination is negative, but only if the patient is going to be followed up and biopsy performed if there is an incomplete response

Management
- Metronidazole 750–800 mg three times daily for 3 days
- Mepacrine (quinacrine) 100 mg three times daily for 1 week is an alternative for the rare problem of resistant giardiasis, but specialist advice should be sought. Reinfection or an underlying disease is a more common cause of persistent symptoms after treatment

Bacterial overgrowth
Bacterial contamination of the small intestine results in diarrhoea or typical features of malabsorption. An underlying cause (Table 7.4) is almost always present. Bacteria

Table 7.4 Clinical conditions associated with bacterial overgrowth of the small intestine

Site	Associated clinical condition
Gastric hypochlorhydria or achlorhydria	Gastric atrophy
	Vagotomy
	PPI therapy
	Old age
Small intestinal stagnation	
Anatomical	Duodenal-jejunal diverticulosis
	Obstruction (stricture, adhesion, tumour)
	Surgical blind loop
Motor	Pseudo-obstruction
	Scleroderma
	Diabetic autonomic neuropathy
	Absent or disordered migrating motor complex
Abnormal communication between distal and proximal gastrointestinal tract	Ileocaecal resection
	Fistulae
Miscellaneous	Cirrhosis
	Pancreatitis
	Immunodeficiency syndromes

(anaerobes, *E. coli* and *Klebsiella* spp.) deconjugate bile salts, metabolise B_{12} and carbohydrate, but folate and fat-soluble vitamins are not malabsorbed. Normal jejunal juice contains $< 10^4$ Gram-positive organisms.

Distinguishing features
- Diarrhoea or malabsorption in patients with abnormal small bowel structure or motility, decreased gastric acid secretion or when immunocompromised
- May occur in elderly patients without small intestinal pathology
- Onset of diarrhoea in patients with otherwise stable chronic disease (diabetes, systemic sclerosis, Crohn's disease)
- Malabsorption with a low B_{12} and normal (or elevated) folate

Investigation
- Small bowel radiology is the first investigation when the diagnosis is suspected, to look for jejunal diverticulosis or strictures (Fig. 7.3, p. 215)
- Jejunal aspiration is the gold standard and is convenient if a biopsy is being performed to exclude other causes of malabsorption (after normal small bowel radiology), but air insufflation may destroy anaerobes. The normal concentration in healthy jejunum is $< 10^4$ cfu/mL; $> 10^6$ cfu/mL, suggests bacterial overgrowth
- Hydrogen breath test after lactulose is non-invasive but the low sensitivity and specificity limit its use. Breath hydrogen > 20 ppm in < 2 h indicates bacterial overgrowth (p. 427)

Management
- Consider if surgery will correct an underlying anatomic problem contributing to bacterial overgrowth; it rarely will
- Metronidazole 500 mg twice daily or ciprofloxacin 500 mg twice daily for 1 week is often effective
- Tetracycline 250 mg four times daily together with metronidazole 400 mg three times daily for 2 weeks is appropriate if there is no response
- Augmentin/Clavulin (amoxicillin and clavulanate potassium) 875 mg twice daily is effective in suppressing both the aerobic and anaerobic flora
- Replacement vitamin B_{12} (1000 μg intramuscularly once daily for 5 days)
- Retreat without investigation when symptoms relapse
- Cyclical antibiotics (for the first week of every month, rotating through the antibiotics above) are often necessary, because surgical correction of the cause is rarely possible

Bile acid malabsorption
- Bile acids in the colon cause watery postprandial diarrhoea by inhibiting absorption and promoting secretion of water and electrolytes and may occasionally lead to steatorrhoea
- Commonly due to Crohn's disease, ileal resection, cholecystectomy or post-infectious diarrhoea. Primary (or idiopathic) bile acid malabsorption (BAM) is underdiagnosed and should be considered in patients with unexplained diarrhoea
- Diagnosis is by ^{75}Se-HCAT test (synthetic radiolabelled analogue of taurocholic acid). $< 15\%$ retention at 7 days strongly suggests BAM. In the absence of diagnos-

tic tests a therapeutic trial of cholestyramine may be used; a response is typically seen within 3 days
- Treatment with cholestyramine (4–20 g daily) is usually well tolerated, because it controls the diarrhoea

Disaccharidase deficiency

Hypolactasia
- Hypolactasia is a common autosomal recessive small intestinal enzyme deficiency. Alactasia is rare and presents in neonates
- Primary hypolactasia results from a physiological decline in activity of the lactase-phlorizin hydrolase (LPH) after weaning. The age of LPH decline varies in different races (age 1–2 in Thais, but 10–20 in Finns). In some races, including UK and US white Caucasoids, LPH activity persists throughout life. Polymorphisms in the LPH gene have been used to track population migration
- Secondary hypolactasia may follow any cause of mucosal damage (viral gastroenteritis, coeliac disease, giardiasis, Crohn's disease) and resolves once the disease is treated. Cow's milk protein intolerance in children may cause villous atrophy, but not in adults
- Symptoms are similar to those of IBS and include osmotic diarrhoea and excessive flatulence from fermentation of undigested lactose. The colon adapts to absorb excess intestinal fluid, so diarrhoea is variable
- The presence or absence of hypolactasia correlates poorly with symptoms. Many patients with lactose intolerance can drink milk without symptoms, and milk intolerance commonly occurs in the absence of hypolactasia, leading many to question the value of detecting hypolactasia
- Diagnosis is confirmed by a lactose-hydrogen breath test: a rise of > 20 ppm. $H_2 > 2$ h after ingestion of 50 g of lactose is abnormal, but a negative result does not exclude the diagnosis. This amount of lactose is equivalent to that found in four glasses of milk. More physiologic doses of lactose, such as 12.5 and 25 g, have been advocated with correspondingly lower rise in breath hydrogen (10 ppm) considered to be abnormal. A low lactose diet should be considered if clinical suspicion is high
- Avoiding milk is generally all that is required (p. 390). Yoghurt, cheese and butter contain less lactose and can be included in moderate amounts

Other deficiencies
- Sucrase—isomaltase deficiency is a rare disorder of childhood
- Trehalase deficiency results in mushroom intolerance

Adverse reactions to food

Terminology
It is important to distinguish between food allergy, food intolerance and food aversion.
- *Food allergy* is immunological (IgE-mediated type I hypersensitivity) (also now recognised as non-IgE mediated) and uncommon (1.5% adults, or 6–8% children). Reactions are most prevalent in infants and children < 5 years. Associated atopy (eczema, hay fever, asthma) and drug allergy are clues to diagnosis. Foods responsible for $> 90\%$ of significant food allergy are shown in Table 7.5. Labial or pharyn-

Table 7.5 Foods responsible for most food allergy

Infants	Children	Adults
Cow's milk	Cow's milk	Peanut
Soy	Egg	Tree nut
	Peanut	Fish
	Soy	Shellfish
	Wheat	
	Tree nut (walnut, hazel, etc.)	
	Fish	
	Shellfish	

geal oedema, urticaria, wheeze or anaphylaxis occur rapidly and the relationship is usually readily recognised

- *Food intolerance* refers to non-immunologically mediated adverse reactions to food, which resolve following dietary elimination and are reproduced by food challenge. The mechanism for a small number of such reactions is understood. These include the effects of pharmacologically active foodstuffs (e.g. tyramine in cheese, caffeine in coffee), host factors (e.g. hypolactasia), or fermentation of resistant starches (or insoluble fibre) to cause bloating, flatulence or diarrhoea. For the majority with food intolerance, however, the mechanism is unclear
- *Food aversion* or fads are psychological and not a reproducible cause of symptoms on blind testing
- Very few patients who believe food to be the cause of their symptoms have true food allergy. Some will have food intolerance/sensitivities for reasons that cannot be defined scientifically at this stage. Psychological aversion to certain foods is the most common reason for symptoms

Investigations

- Encourage patients to document the relationship between exposure to the specific food and symptoms with a food diary (e.g. diet on one page, symptoms opposite). Dietetic support helps
- Tests for IgE antibody to specific foods include skin prick tests (through glycerinated food extracts), and *in vitro* radioallergosorbent tests (RASTs). These may be useful adjuncts in specialist settings. Although the false-positive rate is high, a negative test may be helpful in ruling out an IgE-mediated reaction, as the negative predictive value is high
- Intradermal skin tests with food extracts, provocation/neutralisation tests, applied kinesiology and IgG_4 antibody tests are of *no* value
- Confirmation of food intolerance is determined by resolution of symptoms through elimination and recurrence after oral challenge. An exclusion diet of low allergenicity with planned reintroduction of common food allergens (dairy products, eggs, fish, nuts, additives and colouring agents) should be supervised by a dietician
- Invasive investigation to exclude other causes of symptoms (small bowel radiology or jejunal biopsy) is only indicated if clinical suspicion of an organic cause is very strong

Management

- Dietetic support from a qualified, interested and experienced dietitian (not a 'nutritionist', who may have no qualifications) is the single most useful factor
- Sweeping generalisations by doctors to 'exclude wheat' or 'dairy products' are often unhelpful (since wheat starch intolerance depends on the processing) and may be harmful (inappropriate reduction in calcium intake)
- Patients with true food allergy should be encouraged to wear a Medic Alert bracelet and carry injectable adrenaline
- Specific foods should be avoided after being identified through a thorough process of dietary exclusion and reintroduction. Foods to which there has been intolerance can often be gradually reintroduced after a few months. Both dose-response and threshold effects occur
- Mebeverine 135–270 mg three times daily may help abdominal pain, or codeine phosphate 15–30 mg as needed can be prescribed for diarrhoea

Short bowel syndrome

General

- Short bowel syndrome occurs when < 1 m of functioning small intestine remains. In adults this is usually related to multiple or massive resection due to Crohn's disease, vascular catastrophe, volvulus, trauma, or tumour resection
- Functional short bowel syndrome is characterised by severe malabsorption in the presence of a normal length bowel. This may occur in severe intestinal dysmotility ('pseudo–obstruction'), refractory coeliac disease, or radiation enteropathy
- The result is diarrhoea, hypomagnesaemia and malnutrition, due to loss of fluid, electrolytes, fat, bile acids, B_{12} or other nutrients. In the acute phase, loss of fluid and electrolytes are most important. Patients with a stoma loss > 1.5 L/day rarely manage without intravenous fluids and magnesium
- Adaptation occurs over 2 years. Factors determining clinical outcome include the presence of the colon, ileocaecal valve, length and health of remaining bowel, age and comorbidity
- The colon is crucially important for absorbing fluid and electrolytes. Gastric emptying is slower in patients who retain their distal ileum and/or colon due to the action of peptide YY, glucagon-like peptide I and neurotensin, released from L cells in the distal ileum and colon
- Preservation of the ileocaecal valve, some terminal ileum and some jejunum have the greatest effect on subsequent symptoms: some patients with 30 cm total (18 cm jejunum, 12 cm terminal ileum) will survive as long as the colon is retained. Patients with < 100 cm bowel and a stoma will almost all need daily parenteral fluids and electrolyte supplements
- Net absorption of electrolytes from the jejunum only occurs when luminal sodium concentration is 90 mmol/L or more. Since almost all oral fluids contain little sodium, the more the patient drinks the more intestinal secretion is provoked and the greater the stomal loss. The same may be true for hyperosmolar nutritional supplements, including elemental feeds
- Gastric acid hypersecretion in short bowel syndrome may contribute up to 1500 mL/day

Symptoms and signs
- Weight loss, electrolyte imbalance and high stomal output (> 1500 mL/day) or diarrhoea, despite a good appetite, indicate intestinal failure
- Other causes of ileostomy dysfunction should be considered (p. 280)
- The condition is best anticipated and surgeons encouraged to measure the length of remaining small intestine at surgery
- Chronic vitamin and trace element deficiency develop insidiously. Unexplained skin rashes or non-specific symptoms (malaise, weakness, paraesthesiae) are highly suggestive

Management
- Management of the chronic phase is shown in Table 7.6
- High sodium fluids in place of ordinary drinks are essential if the residual small intestine is to absorb fluid and electrolytes. Most patients can be encouraged to eat normally. The dietary fat/carbohydrate balance makes no difference to patients without a colon, although patients with a colon absorb more when the diet is high in carbohydrate
- *Wrong advice* to 'drink plenty of (hypotonic) fluids' and (hyperosmolar) nutritional supplements is commonly given
- The *key to management* is a modification of the WHO rehydration solution: commercial preparations contain too little (only 60 mmol/L) sodium. The hospital pharmacy can formulate: glucose powder 20 g (110 mmol), sodium chloride 3.5 g (60 mmol) and sodium bicarbonate 2.5 g (30 mmol), made up to 1 L of tap water
- Chilling these drinks, using a straw or replacing the bicarbonate by sodium citrate (2.9 g, 30 mmol) all help palatability
- The patient should drink 750–1000 mL/day of this solution, whilst *restricting* intake of other fluids to 500–750 mL/day
- Oral rehydration solutions are commonly called '*isotonic drinks*'. Commercial isotonic drinks are marketed for use in sports and are *inappropriate to use unless* salt is added (1/2 teaspoon/500 mL)

Additional therapy
- Give a PPI to reduce gastric secretion
- Octreotide 100 µg subcutaneously three times daily may reduce intestinal secretions and stoma output, but should be reserved for when other measures fail
- Very high doses of loperamide (up to 60 mg/day) and/or codeine phosphate (up to 480 mg/day) may also help
- Magnesium deficiency is common. Intravenous magnesium 10–12 mmol/day rapidly restores serum magnesium, followed by oral magnesium 12–24 mmol/day as magnesium glycerophosphate (500 mg twice daily) or heavy magnesium oxide (320 mg two to three times daily) or magnesium glucoheptonate (15–30 mL, which is equivalent to 1500–3000 mg three times daily) as tolerated and according to availability
- Non-total parenteral nutrition is an important concept if nutrition or electrolyte balance cannot be maintained with oral intake alone. Most patients can eat and absorb some or most, but not all, of their daily requirements. A tunnelled central venous line for administering electrolytes, trace elements and vitamins three or four nights a week is a useful option

Table 7.6 Management of chronic short bowel syndrome

Problem	Mechanism	Management
Salt and water depletion	Jejunal absorption [Na] > 90 mmol/L	Drink WHO oral rehydration solution (p. 232)
		Restrict ordinary fluids
Diarrhoea or stomal output > 1.5 L/day	Hyperosmolar luminal contents	Avoid elemental/polymeric drinks
	Gastric secretions (1.5 L/day)	Proton-pump inhibitor
	Bile salts stimulate colonic secretion	Cholestyramine 4–12 g daily (if colon retained)
	Lack of absorptive capacity	Small, frequent meals
	Rapid transit	Opioids (loperamide up to 60 mg/day and/or codeine up to 480 mg/day)
	Secretion > absorption	Octreotide 150–300 µg/day subcutaneously
Malnutrition	Steatorrhoea (calorie wastage)	Low-fat diet, but rarely vital
	Reduced absorptive capacity	Check Mg, folate, Zn, Ca, every 4–12 weeks: give supplements
		Medium-chain triglyceride diet*
		Nontotal home parenteral feed*
	Terminal ileal resection	B$_{12}$ 1 mg injection every 3 months
Gallstones	Bile acid depletion	Cholecystectomy* if symptomatic
	Octreotide (gall bladder stasis)	
Renal stones	Chronic dehydration and chronic salt depletion	Encourage WHO oral rehydration solution
		Restrict ordinary fluids
	Hyperoxaluria	Low-oxalate diet or cholestyramine if colon present, and CaCO$_3$ 7.5 g/day

*When other measures fail.

- Total home parenteral nutrition is necessary in a small proportion: such patients are best referred to a centre used to managing patients with intestinal failure

Specialist procedures in short bowel syndrome

Medical
- Expert nutritional, fluid and electrolyte support are fundamental
- Glucagon-like polypeptide (GLP-2) analogues promote small intestinal mucosal growth and have shown encouraging initial results, but remain experimental

Non-transplant surgery
- The aim is to increase nutrient and fluid absorption by slowing intestinal transit or increasing absorptive area
- Restore continuity of remaining small intestine with colon if possible
- Operations to slow intestinal transit by creating an antiperistaltic segment are of limited value
- Increasing surface area by the longitudinal intestinal lengthening and tailoring (LILT) procedure has been tried in children with severe dysmotility and dilated intestine. Surgery involves isolation of the dual blood supply to the small intestine, followed by longitudinal incision and iso-peristaltic end-to-end anastomosis, effectively doubling the length of the bowel

Intestinal transplantation
- Rarely indicated but should be considered for patients with intestinal failure who cannot be sustained on long-term parenteral nutrition, due to loss of vascular access or liver failure
- World experience of intestinal transplantation is documented by the international transplant registry (www.lhsc.on.ca/itr). At the last update (May 2001) there had been 696 transplants in 651 patients from 55 centres
- Small bowel transplant has been performed as an isolated intestinal transplant (42%), together with a liver transplant (45%) or as part of multivisceral transplant (13%)
- 61% of transplants were for children < 16 years
- Graft (and patient) survival are improving (Table 7.7), but specialist management of long-term TPN has a 90% 5-year survival in the UK
- Major causes of death are sepsis (50%), rejection (10%), technical (7%) and lymphoma (7%)

Table 7.7 1-year survival figures of all intestinal transplants performed since 1999 in large centres (> 10 transplants/year)

	1-year survival	
	Graft	**Patient**
Small intestine only	60%	76%
Small intestine/Liver	60%	63%
Multivisceral	66%	68%

- Post-transplant lymphoproliferative disease is more common (15%) in multivisceral transplants

Other causes of malabsorption

- Post-infective malabsorption may occur after gastroenteritis from any cause—bacterial, viral, toxin (traveller's diarrhoea) or parasitic (*G. lamblia*). Hypolactasia is the usual reason
- Drug-induced causes include:
  - neomycin
  - cholestyramine
  - liquid paraffin and irritant purgative abuse
  - magnesium-based antacids (interfere with iron, antibiotic and antimalarial absorption) and PPI
  - alcohol
- *Lymphangiectasia* may be primary, or secondary to lymphoma, tuberculosis, severe right heart failure or filariasis. Protein leaks into the lumen ('protein-losing enteropathy') causing chylous ascites (p. 150)
- *Whipple's disease* is a rare condition caused by the actinomycete *Tropheryma whippelii*. It usually affects middle-aged men, causing malabsorption, pleuritic pain, migratory arthritis, finger clubbing, pericarditis, pigmentation and occasional neurological features. Diagnosis has traditionally been based upon histology of jejunal biopsies (infiltration of the lamina propria by PAS-positive foamy macrophages). Molecular methods, allowing diagnosis from blood or faeces, have raised the possibility that Whipple's may cause a wider spectrum of disease (e.g. juvenile chronic arthritis, intractable idiopathic thrombocytopaenia) in which small intestinal disease may not be apparent. Treatment with cotrimoxazole (or penicillin, or tetracycline) for a year is effective. Relapse may occur after many years. Patients are best referred to a specialist centre
- *Eosinophilic gastroenteritis* is a rare disorder characterised by an intense eosinophilic infiltrate which is mucosal (type 1), submucosal (type 2) or transmural (type 3). There is usually a peripheral eosinophilia, which suggests the diagnosis once parasitic infections have been excluded. Symptoms are non-specific, with pain, diarrhoea and occasionally frank malabsorption, but type 3 causes ascites with a high eosinophil content. The triad of eosinophilic gastroenteritis, asthma and mononeuritis multiplex comprise the Churg–Strauss syndrome. Rapid response to steroids is usual
- *Metabolic defects*, except hypolactasia, are not acquired by adults. Aminoacidurias (cystinuria, Hartnup disease), chloridorrhoea and acrodermatitis enteropathica (zinc deficiency) occur in children
- *HIV enteropathy* is characterised by diarrhoea and partial villous atrophy without an identifiable cause (p. 364)
- *Starvation* (including anorexia nervosa) may cause partial villous atrophy, defective intestinal immunity and possibly calcific pancreatitis. Susceptibility to enteric infection is increased. Impaired digestion of nutrients influences refeeding (calorie intake should be increased gradually, with replacement of vitamins and minerals). Chronic

illness and post-operative complications are the commonest cause of starvation in adults in UK and the USA (Section 12.1)

- *Small intestinal lymphoma*, and immunoproliferative small intestinal disease or (α-chain disease is discussed on p. 241
- *Intestinal amyloidosis*, an extremely rare condition usually associated with primary amyloidosis, may cause malabsorption or pseudo-obstruction. Specialist advice after diagnosis by small intestinal biopsy is appropriate

7.3 Diverticulosis

Small intestinal diverticula are asymptomatic, or result in stasis of intestinal contents, bacterial overgrowth and malabsorption (pp. 227 and 214). Perforation, inflammation and haemorrhage are much less common than in colonic diverticula.

Duodenal

- A single diverticulum is usually an incidental finding at ERCP or on a barium meal (about 2%), adjacent to or involving the papilla, and associated with gallstones. They make cannulation of the CBD more difficult at ERCP
- A diverticulum in the duodenal cap rarely follows ulceration
- Treatment is unnecessary unless complications occur. Surgery is appropriate for perforation, haemorrhage or contamination due to stasis, but these are very unusual

Meckel's diverticulum

2% of the population have this embryological remnant located within 100 cm of the ileocaecal valve, but < 5% cause symptoms, most frequently in males

Haemorrhage

- More common than in other small intestinal diverticula, because 20% have heterotopic gastric or pancreatic tissue that can become inflamed
- Occult gastrointestinal bleeding may occur, especially in the young (p. 20)

Diverticulitis and perforation

Cannot be distinguished clinically from appendicitis. Immediate management is similar (p. 237), but the surgeon must look carefully for a Meckel's diverticulum if the appendix is normal.

Other

Bacterial overgrowth, intussusception, herniation (Littre's) and malignant transformation are all very unusual.

Diagnosis and treatment

A ^{99m}Tc isotope scan, which detects heterotopic gastric mucosa, should be carried out before a small bowel enema to avoid interference with the scintigraphic counter. Pretreatment with pentagastrin or acid suppression reduces the false-negative rate. Surgical resection is the treatment of choice.

Small intestinal diverticulosis
- Jejunal diverticula are usually multiple, on the mesenteric margin
- Diarrhoea due to bacterial overgrowth is the commonest presentation (p. 226), but most are asymptomatic
- Small bowel radiology is diagnostic (Fig. 7.3, p. 215)
- Maintenance antibiotics (p. 228), or repeat courses when symptoms recur are indicated once bacterial overgrowth has occurred
- Angiography is necessary for obscure gastrointestinal bleeding in a patient with multiple diverticula, prior to surgery, but such patients are best referred to a specialist centre

7.4 Appendicitis

Appendicitis is usually due to obstruction and invasion by *E. coli* with anaerobes. Crohn's disease, *Y. enterocolitica*, tuberculosis, carcinoid tumour, or *Enterobius vermicularis* infestation are other rare causes.

Clinical features
- Occurs at any age, but most commonly diagnosed in the young. Mortality is 25% when age > 70 years
- The *three cardinal symptoms and signs* most predictive of acute appendicitis are migration of pain from the periumbilical region to the right lower quadrant, tenderness in the right lower quadrant and rigidity (95% accuracy in the presence of all three)
- Abdominal rigidity may be absent when the appendix is retrocaecal or pelvic, and in obese or elderly patients
- The iliopsoas test (with the patient in the left lateral position, pain is produced on extension of the right hip) is highly specific (although sensitivity is poor) and may be useful if the appendix is retrocaecal
- Rectal examination is essential in all cases of abdominal pain
- The pain is higher and more lateral in pregnancy, with a higher incidence of peritonitis
- Subacute obstruction or diarrhoea may occur in the elderly
- An appendix mass may be confused with a caecal carcinoma, Crohn's disease, tuberculosis, or an ovarian tumour
- Clues to the differential diagnosis (Table 1.4, p. 22) include:
  - recent sore throat (mesenteric adenitis)
  - previous episode (Crohn's disease)
  - anaemia (Crohn's disease, caecal carcinoma)
  - weight loss (Crohn's disease, caecal carcinoma)
  - dyspepsia (cholecystitis, perforated ulcer)
  - arthralgia (*Y. enterocolitica*, Crohn's disease)
  - vaginal discharge (salpingitis)
  - midmenstrual cycle (ruptured follicular cyst)
  - frequency (urinary tract infection)
  - preserved appetite (non-specific, or gynaecological)
- Asian origin (ileocaecal tuberculosis)

Management
- β-HCG (human chorionic gonadotropin) to exclude uterine or ectopic pregnancy
- Dipstix urine for nitrites to exclude a urinary tract infection
- In the presence of the three cardinal clinical features (above), surgery is indicated, as diagnostic accuracy will not be improved by imaging. Metronidazole 1 g suppository should be given 1 h before and 8 h after operation
- Metronidazole 1 g suppository, oral clear fluids and observation for 8 h is reasonable if peritonism is absent and the diagnosis uncertain. Imaging by ultrasound or spiral CT should be carried out. These have a sensitivity of 75–95% and a specificity of 85–100% and help exclude other diagnoses (see above). Spiral CT is superior to ultrasound and should be used as the first choice except in women who might be pregnant
- A normal appendix is found in up to 30%. Mesenteric adenitis, *Y. enterocolitica* ileitis, Crohn's disease, Meckel's diverticulitis, tubo-ovarian and non-specific causes (p. 41) should then be considered

Conservative management
- Indicated for an appendix mass, or when the risk of operation is too great—such as in a ship at sea
- Intravenous fluids, metronidazole 500 mg, ampicillin 500 mg and gentamicin 80 mg are given 8-hourly
- 30 mL water can be allowed every hour
- Careful charts of pulse and temperature, as well as regular examination, determine progress
- Surgery must be performed if peritonitis develops

Appendix mass and abscess
- A tender right iliac fossa mass may be palpable after 5 days of untreated appendicitis. Pain and pyrexia resolve with bed rest
- Interval appendicectomy is indicated after 3 months. Small bowel radiology to exclude Crohn's disease is necessary before operation, if the history is atypical in any way
- An appendix abscess is distinguished by a swinging pyrexia and point tenderness on rectal examination. Spiral CT or ultrasound will identify the site and surgical drainage is indicated forthwith

'Grumbling appendix'
- Recurrent right iliac fossa pain has often been attributed to a 'grumbling appendix'. The diagnosis is doubtful
- Repeated attacks of appendicitis may occur, but the patient is well in between
- Chronic pain with evidence of organic disease (weight loss, elevated ESR) is usually due to Crohn's disease at any age, caecal carcinoma in the elderly or, rarely, lymphoma or tuberculosis
- Pain without signs or abnormal investigations is likely to be due to IBS (p. 335), but a small bowel enema is still warranted if pain persists, to exclude more unusual causes

7.5 Small intestinal tumours

Polyps

Single

Isolated small intestinal polyps are rare and suggest malignancy (Table 7.8), although they may be benign. Secondaries from melanoma or lung should be considered. Symptoms are unusual, but bleeding or intussusception can occur. Surgical resection is indicated to establish the nature of a polyp if one is detected by small bowel radiology, but localisation at operation is difficult without peroperative endoscopy.

Polyposis

Multiple polyps are more common (Table 7.5) than single polyps. They are usually lymphoid (nodular lymphoid hyperplasia, in the ileum or rectum of children, or associated with hypogammaglobulinaemia), non-neoplastic hamartomas (Peutz–Jeghers syndrome, associated with buccal or labial pigmentation and intussusception, p. 300) and rarely adenomatous (Cronkhite–Canada syndrome, associated with alopecia and nail dystrophy, p. 297).

Associated features are usually sufficient for diagnosis, although jejunal biopsy or laparotomy may be necessary to exclude lymphoma.

Carcinoid

See also Chapter 4 (p. 128) for general comments on neuroendocrine tumours. 45% of carcinoid tumours arise in the appendix, 30% in the small intestine and 20% in the rectum. Metastases must occur before the carcinoid syndrome develops, in 2% of carcinoid tumours. 5-HT (or serotonin) accounts for only some of the effects; kinins, prostaglandins and other vasoactive substances may also be secreted.

Carcinoid syndrome
- Flushing and cyanosis, often provoked by alcohol or food
- Tears, excess nasal secretion
- Diarrhoea, may be episodic
- Hepatomegaly
- Bronchoconstriction
- Cardiac involvement, fibrosis, tricuspid or pulmonary incompetence
- Cutaneous infiltration, often on the lower limbs that become indurated

Table 7.8 Causes of small intestinal polyps

Single	Multiple
Adenocarcinoma	Nodular lymphoid hyperplasia
Carcinoid	Peutz–Jeghers syndrome (hamartomas)
Secondary deposit	Lymphomatous polyposis
Benign adenoma	Multifocal adenocarcinoma
Lipoma	Endometriosis
Leiomyoma	Cronkhite–Canada syndrome (adenomas)

Diagnosis and treatment

- Clinically silent tumours are often diagnosed incidentally at appendicectomy. Intussusception may occur with ileal tumours
- 24 h urinary 5-hydroxyindoleacetic acid (5-HIAA) excretion > 0.3 mmol/24 h. Borderline tests should be repeated after excluding foods rich in 5-HT (walnuts, bananas, avocados)
- Chest X-ray, liver ultrasound, small bowel radiology and echocardiography are necessary to establish the extent of disease. An isotope octreotide scan is useful for detecting metastases if the tumour expresses octreotide receptors, but is expensive and not widely available (Fig. 7.6)
- Surgical resection of the primary tumour is curative if the tumour is < 2 cm and has not metastasised. Resection will also decrease systemic effects in metastatic disease
- Octreotide (a synthetic analogue of somatostatin) is the treatment of choice and is generally well tolerated, although it increases the risk of gallstones. Octreotide, starting at 50 µg subcutaneously twice daily, should be given and a specialist referral made. The longer acting analogue (Sandostatin LAR) is generally substituted, because it need only be given every 4 weeks

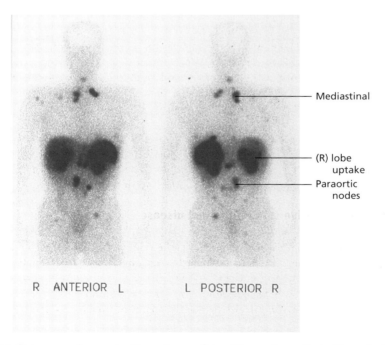

R   ANTERIOR L   L   POSTERIOR R

Mediastinal

(R) lobe uptake

Paraortic nodes

Fig. 7.6 Octreoscan for carcinoid syndrome. Octreotide scan in a patient with carcinoid syndrome. Massive uptake in both lobes an the liver, with mediastinal and para-aortic nodes. Radio-labelled octreotide (Octreoscan) is a good way of detecting functioning, metastatic, or recurrent neuroendocrine tumours.

Outpatient checks
- Ask about flushing, diarrhoea and breathlessness
- Palpate for hepatomegaly and record the BP
- Record peak flow rate
- Measure 24 h urinary 5-HIAA and perform a CT scan annually to monitor progress in patients who have had the carcinoid syndrome, but not in other patients unless symptoms develop

Lymphoma

Intestinal lymphoma is rare, but, after the stomach (p. 99 and classification, is the most common extranodal origin of lymphoma. Mediterranean lymphoma (immunoproliferative small intestinal disease) is discussed below.

Features
- May be associated with coeliac disease (< 5%, usually > 50 years and following dietary non-compliance, p. 223). These are usually T-cell lymphomas, as opposed to the more common B-cell lymphomas
- Present with obstruction (70%), haemorrhage (50%) or perforation
- Weight loss, non-specific symptoms or failure to respond to gluten withdrawal in coeliac disease are characteristic. A mass may be palpable

Management
- Diagnosis is established by CT scan and small bowel radiology, followed by laparotomy. Lesions may be annular, ulcerating, multiple or occasionally diffuse, or missed by contrast radiology. Lymphoma may occur anywhere in the bowel
- Staging is performed by thoracoabdominal CT scan, bone marrow and frozen-section biopsies at laparotomy
- Resection of annular lesions is often possible, but lymphoma in coeliac disease has a bad prognosis
- Post-operative chemotherapy is usually indicated and should be discussed with an oncologist
- Annual follow-up after treatment should include abdominal examination for a mass, blood count, ESR and small bowel radiology if intestinal symptoms recur

Immunoproliferative small intestinal disease
- Immunoproliferative small intestinal disease is seen in Mediterranean Arabs and Jews, Iranians, Pakistanis, Taiwanese or South African black people. It is important to recognise in Europe or the USA, because the early stage can be cured by antibiotics
- Chronic antigenic stimulation from bacterial flora leads to the proliferation of IgA-producing cells in the small intestine. The immunosuppression that accompanies malnutrition may play a permissive role. Subsequently malignant transformation occurs
- A dense, continuous infiltration confined to the mucosa and submucosa of the entire small bowel is characteristic
- Diarrhoea, malabsorption, finger clubbing, fever and weight loss in a young Middle Eastern adult are characteristic

> **Box 7.5 Causes of small intestinal strictures**
>
> Crohn's disease
> Adenocarcinoma
> Lymphoma
> Tuberculosis
> Vasculitis
> Secondary deposit
> NSAIDs
> Radiation
> Surgical anastomosis
> *Y. enterocolitica*

- In 70% of patients an α-heavy chain paraprotein is found on electrophoresis of serum or intestinal fluid. Hypogammaglobulinaemia is common

Staging by laparotomy is recommended to identify stage 0 disease (prelymphomatous), in which sustained remission can be achieved with a prolonged course of tetracycline (500 mg four times daily for > 6 months). Treatment of more advanced disease is with chemotherapy.

Carcinoma

- Small intestinal carcinoma is rare and usually of unknown cause
- It is occasionally associated with coeliac disease, Crohn's disease, familial adenomatous polyposis, Gardner's syndrome and Cronkhite–Canada syndrome (p. 297)
- Obstruction or chronic blood loss are the usual presenting features. Other causes of a small intestinal stricture are shown in Box 7.5
- Laparotomy is necessary, after small bowel radiology, for histological diagnosis and resection. Duodenal carcinomas are treated by pancreaticoduodenectomy (Whipple's procedure)

8 Inflammatory Bowel Disease

8.1 Crohn's disease

Crohn's disease is characterised by chronic transmural granulomatous inflammation, with a tendency to form fistulae or strictures. It predominantly affects the ileocaecal region, but may affect any part of the gastrointestinal tract, often in discontinuity. The cause remains unknown.

General information
A few facts are helpful when explaining the disease to the patient:
- First recognised in 1932, but described earlier (1913, Dalziel)
- Affects 70–100 : 100 000 population, but epidemiologic studies have found prevalence in excess of 200 : 100 000 population in some areas
- 4–11 : 100 000 new cases per year in northern Europe, USA and Australia, but appears uncommon in other areas of the world. Incidence in southern Europe is increasing
- Incidence has doubled since 1950, and increased until 1990, but appears stable in northern Europe. It does not differ markedly between race, sex or social class in Europe, although more common among Jews in the USA
- Presents at any age, but usually 15–40 years. The site of disease and pattern of onset are unrelated to age
- 15% have a relative with Crohn's disease or ulcerative colitis; children of an affected parent have an 80–90% chance of not being affected. Affected parents are older at diagnosis than their affected children (may indicate genetic anticipation) and pattern of disease within families is similar. Twins (44% of monozygotic pairs) often have Crohn's disease together
- Intensive efforts to identify genes predisposing to IBD in the past decade have identified mutations in the NOD2/CARD15 gene on Chr 16 that account for about 40% of small intestinal (but not colonic) Crohn's disease. Two genes recently (2004) reported to be associated with Crohn's disease are OCTN1 & 2 (cationic transporter genes on Chr 5, the IBD 5 locus, possibly associated with perianal disease) and DLG5 on Chr 10 (coding for an epithelial structural protein), but these need to be confirmed by independent studies. Other confirmed linkages to chromosome areas (but not yet specific genes) include loci on Chr 6p (IBD 3 locus), 14q (IBD 4 locus) and 3p. The field is complex, rapidly evolving and only beginning to be associated with clinical patterns of disease
- Twice as common in smokers as non-smokers; stopping smoking reduces risk of relapse, need for immunosuppression and surgery. Probably not associated with oral contraceptive use
- Infective agents, mucins and altered cell-mediated immunity, diet (high refined sugar) and anti-inflammatory drugs are postulated causes, but none explain disease discontinuity. Associations with measles virus infection, vaccine and *M. paratuber-*

culosis have not been confirmed. Microvascular changes are probably secondary to inflammation
- At least half the patients have periods of remission lasting 5 years

Clinical features

It is clinically useful to classify Crohn's disease according to the site, extent and pattern of disease, since this influences medical management, likelihood of surgery and prognosis. This has been formalised in the 'Vienna classification', largely for research purposes (Table 8.1). The site of disease influences the presentation. Exacerbations of existing disease produce similar features that may be due to active inflammation, infection or other complication. Although one pattern of disease tends to predominate in an individual, patterns are not mutually exclusive.

All sites and patterns
- Three symptoms occur in most patients: diarrhoea, abdominal pain and weight loss
- Acute abdominal pain may be confused initially with appendicitis or yersinia ileitis (Table 1.4, p. 272), but a careful history usually detects previous episodes that have not been recognised
- Fever, malaise, anorexia and lassitude are usual in active disease
- Weight loss alone, without diarrhoea or pain, may be the presenting feature in extensive inflammatory small bowel disease and may be confused with anorexia nervosa in adolescents

Small bowel disease
- Aphthous ulcers are common with active disease, but true oropharyngeal Crohn's ulcers are rare
- Duodenal ulcers that are postbulbar, difficult to heal or associated with a high ESR may be due to Crohn's disease, although they are exceptionally rare
- Colicky abdominal pain without systemic illness or local tenderness suggests a fibrotic stricture
- Abdominal pain may also be due to biliary colic or renal calculi
- Malnutrition is usually due to anorexia
- Malabsorption is rare except in extensive small intestinal disease, or after resection
- An abdominal mass is frequently palpable in small intestinal disease, often in the right iliac fossa, but can be anywhere

Colonic disease (Crohn's colitis)
- Severe diarrhoea is more common than in small intestinal disease

Table 8.1 Vienna classification of Crohn's disease (Gassche *et al. Inflamm Bowel Dis 2000*; **6:** *8*)

Age at diagnosis	Site of disease (prevalence)	Disease behaviour
A1: < 40 years	L1: terminal ileum (29%)	B1: non-stricturing, non-penetrating
A2: ≥ 40 years	L2: colon (30%)	B2: stricturing
	L3: ileum and colon (33%)	B3: penetrating

- The rectum is usually spared, although perianal disease is common and can be very difficult to treat (p. 265)
- Extraintestinal manifestations (Table 8.2) are more common than in small intestinal disease
- Rectal bleeding is uncommon compared to ulcerative colitis, but profuse haemorrhage is a very rare complication. Bleeding may indicate a colonic carcinoma in chronic Crohn's colitis, but this is rare
- Toxic dilatation is also much less common than in ulcerative colitis, but may be the presenting feature (p. 39)

Perianal disease
- Associated with ileocolonic disease, less common in isolated small bowel disease
- Recurrent abscesses, fistulae and violaceous fleshy skin tags, with or without ulceration, are characteristic. Appearance is often disproportionately severe compared to symptoms: pain and systemic illness are infrequent except with an abscess
- Anal or rectal stenosis may cause constipation and spurious diarrhoea

Extent of disease
- Extensive (> 100 cm) colonic or small bowel disease is associated with more profound weight loss and poor nutrition
- > 100 cm distal ileum must be diseased or resected before B_{12} malabsorption occurs
- Localised disease tends to follow a fibrostenotic or fistulating course, rather than an inflammatory pattern

Pattern of disease
- Fibrostenotic disease is commonly ileocaecal or small bowel, causing localised strictures and obstructive symptoms

Table 8.2 Extraintestinal manifestations of Crohn's disease

	Common (5–20%)	Unusual (< 5%)

Related to activity	Aphthous ulcers
	Erythema nodosum
	Finger clubbing
	Ocular
	   conjunctivitis
	   episcleritis
	   iritis
	Arthritis (large joint)
	Osteoporosis
		Pyoderma gangrenosum

Unrelated to activity	Gallstones	Liver disease fatty liver primary sclerosing cholangitis
	Sacroiliitis	Ankylosing spondylitis
	Arthralgia (small joint)	Renal stones ureteric stricture right hydronephrosis nephropathy (oxalate) amyloid
	Nutritional deficiency	Osteomalacia Sweet's syndrome Systemic amyloidosis

- Inflammatory disease is more commonly colonic, causing profuse diarrhoea, pronounced weight loss and marked elevation in inflammatory markers (CRP, ESR)
- Perineal Crohn's disease is the most common form of fistulising disease. Other manifestations of fistulising disease pattern are enterocutaneous fistulae with or without pelvic and abdominal abscesses when there is small bowel or colonic disease

Extraintestinal manifestations

Occur in about 15%, but up to 30% in colonic disease. Some are markers of active disease and respond to treatment, others are unrelated to disease activity (Table 8.2, p. 247). Differences from ulcerative colitis are discussed in Table 8.9 (p. 268).

- Sacroiliitis is unrelated to HLA–B27, unlike ankylosing spondylitis
- Fatty liver and abnormal liver function tests are common in sick patients and non-specific
- Renal calculi are more commonly due to chronic dehydration and salt depletion than hyperoxaluria
- Nutritional deficiencies may account for obscure symptoms (p. 371), including weakness (vitamin D, potassium, magnesium), lassitude (iron, B_{12}, folate), rashes (niacin, zinc) or altered taste (zinc), but only occur in very extensive disease or after major resection

Investigations

Diagnosis depends on clinical and radiological and endoscopic and histological features. There is no specific diagnostic test. All patients should be completely investigated to establish the site, extent and pattern of disease, even if the diagnosis is confirmed on a single test (e.g. finding granulomas on rectal biopsy).

Establishing the diagnosis

Sigmoidoscopy and rectal biopsy

Necessary even when the mucosa is macroscopically normal (up to 20% have microscopic granulomas).

Small bowel radiology (See p. 423)

Performed first if diarrhoea, pain and weight loss are the presenting features. Colonoscopy should subsequently be arranged to exclude Crohn's colitis (Fig. 8.1, Table 8.3).

Colonoscopy

Colonoscopy is preferable to a barium enema if there is diarrhoea or visible rectal bleeding, since aphthoid ulcers are more readily detected and multiple biopsies can be taken. Complete small bowel radiology is then advisable, even if the terminal ileum has been demonstrated by reflux of barium, to exclude more proximal disease.

Blood tests

- Anaemia is common, usually due to iron deficiency rather than B_{12} or folate deficiency

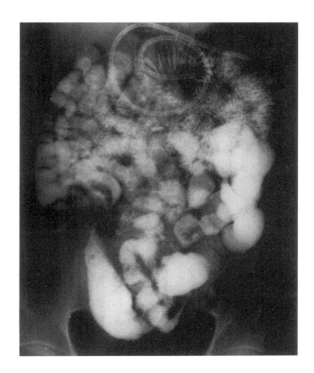

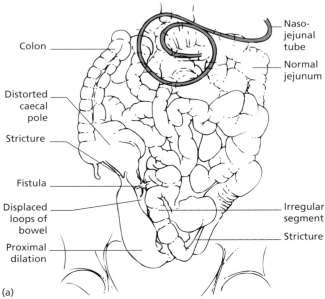

Colon

Naso-
jejunal
tube

Normal
jejunum

Distorted
caecal
pole

Stricture

Fistula

Displaced
loops of
bowel

Irregular
segment

Stricture

Proximal
dilation

(a)

Fig. 8.1 Radiological appearance of Crohn's disease. (a) Small bowel enema in distal ileal Crohn's disease, showing dilatation of the ileum proximal to a stricture, displaced loops of bowel due to a mass, a distorted caecum and a fistula. *(Continued)*

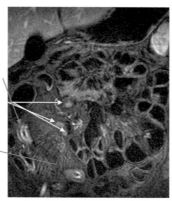

3d FLASH in a patient with Crohn's disease, 1 min after Gd-DTPA IV Injection
Note layered enhancement of an involved ileal loop and enhancing mesenteric lymph nodes

Mesenteric hypervascularity

(b)   Courtesy: N. Gourtsoyiannis, MD, University of Crete

Fig. 8.1 *(continued)* (b) MR enteroclysis, showing layered enhancement, mesenteric hypervascularity and lymph nodes, consistent with active disease.

Table 8.3 Summary of radiological features of Crohn's disease

General	Structural	Mucosal
Rectal sparing	Strictures	Aphthoid ulcers
Discontinuity ('skip lesions')	Fistula	Rose-thorn ulcers
	Asymmetrical disease	Linear ulcers
	Dilatation	Thickened valvulae
	Pseudodiverticula	Cobblestoning
	Caecal distortion	Pseudopolyps
	Mass effect	

- CRP is the most sensitive inflammatory marker, but an elevated ESR or platelet count and a low albumin in a patient with recurrent abdominal pain and weight loss is usually due to Crohn's disease
- Antibodies to *Y. enterocolitica* are indicated when terminal ileal disease is diagnosed at laparotomy for suspected appendicitis

Stool
- Examination for pathogens and *Cl. difficile* toxin assay if diarrhoea is severe
- Laparotomy is occasionally necessary to distinguish Crohn's disease from other causes of a small bowel stricture (Box 7.5, p. 242), including malignancy. Resection will also be therapeutic

Assessing activity

Once the diagnosis has been made it is necessary to establish whether symptoms are due to active disease or complications. Assessment of disease activity is often difficult, because symptoms such as diarrhoea or abdominal pain may be due to conditions other than active disease (Table 8.6, p. 258). A combination of clinical, blood and imaging tests is needed, as no one test is sufficient.

Clinical
- Anorexia, malaise, fever, tachycardia and weight loss indicate active disease
- Severe disease may be present without all these features and superimposed infection can mimic any of them

Blood tests
Low serum albumin or anaemia, a high ESR, CRP, plasma viscosity or platelet count all indicate active disease.

Radiology
Ulcers (aphthous, rose-thorn or linear), fistulae or disease at a new site found on small or large bowel radiology suggest activity.

Endoscopy and other techniques
- Visible ulcers or histological evidence of acute inflammation on biopsies are specific indicators of activity, although these do not correlate well with symptoms and the site of active disease (small intestine) may be inaccessible
- Ultrasound of the abdomen is valuable in experienced hands. It can demonstrate thickened bowel loops, an inflammatory mass or an abscess
- ^{111}I-labelled leucocyte scanning helps differentiate active disease from a fibrotic stricture and may locate an abscess, but may not be available locally
- Crohn's disease activity index or the Harvey–Bradshaw index are useful for clinical trials, but of less value when assessing individual patients

Investigation of recurrent symptoms

Recurrent symptoms may have to be investigated as above, to detect active disease or disease at a new site, but the reasons for reinvestigation must be clearly formulated. They should be relevant to subsequent therapeutic strategies, rather than documenting the current extent of disease for its own sake. Crohn's disease is a chronic condition and patients will have numerous investigations over the years.

Contrast radiology should be limited to symptoms of subacute intestinal obstruction that do not resolve rapidly with treatment, or investigation of complications (fistulae), when surgery may be indicated. Endoscopy is appropriate for colonic or upper gastrointestinal symptoms.

If symptoms do not follow the previous pattern of disease, arrange:
- MSU—for ureteric or renal involvement
- Plain abdominal X-ray—for subacute obstruction or stones
- Ultrasound—for gallstones, nephrolithiasis or hydronephrosis
- White cell scan—if the CRP is normal despite recurrent symptoms, to assess disease activity

Differential diagnosis

As much care must be taken to avoid inappropriately labelling a patient as having Crohn's disease, as not to overlook the diagnosis in the first place. Features are diverse and the clinical alternatives are many, but only a few cause real difficulty (Table 8.4). Do not forget that other disease can also develop after a diagnosis of Crohn's disease has been made.

Table 8.4 Differential diagnosis of Crohn's disease: site of disease

Site	Condition	Differentiating features
Duodenal	Tuberculosis	Biopsy persistent ulcers, chest X-ray
	Sarcoidosis	Chest X-ray, serum ACE, Kveim test
	Zollinger–Ellison syndrome	Diarrhoea common. Serum gastrin
Jejunoileal	Appendicitis, mass or abscess	Abrupt onset. No anaemia
	Laparotomy	
	Tuberculosis	Asian/African patients, Mantoux test
		Laparotomy
	Lymphoma	Smooth stricture(s). Laparotomy
	Adenocarcinoma	Single or multiple strictures (p. 241)
	Other tumours	Ovarian, carcinoid, metastases
	Y. enterocolitica	Acute ileitis. Yersinia antibodies
	Behçet's disease	Aphthous ileal and orogenital ulcers
	Coeliac disease	Ulcerative jejunitis may occur (p. 389)
	NSAID stricture	Ingestion of slow-release NSAID, with no systemic illness
Colonic	Ulcerative colitis	Table 8.12, p. 272
	Indeterminate colitis	p. 282
	Ischaemic colitis	Table 9.5, p. 310
	Carcinoma	Shouldered stricture(s). Biopsy
	Infective colitis	Stool samples, biopsy
	Amoebic colitis	Hot stool, biopsy (p. 359)
	Schistosomiasis	Japan/Middle Eastern patients Cyst excretion, biopsy
	Radiation	History of pelvic malignancy, biopsy
	Solitary rectal ulcer	Constipation, anterior position, biopsy, no systemic illness (p. 296)

ACE, angiotensin-converting enzyme.

Weight loss as the sole symptom
- May be inappropriately attributed to anorexia nervosa in an adolescent. Anaemia, a high ESR or platelet count strongly suggest Crohn's disease
- In older patients, gastrointestinal malignancy (pancreas, gastric carcinoma or lymphoma) must be considered. Gastroscopy and ultrasound are also indicated
- Diabetes can cause weight loss and recurrent perianal sepsis

Abdominal pain
- Symptoms resembling IBS (p. 337) with weight loss or anaemia are indications for further investigation
- Gallstones or renal calculi may coexist with Crohn's disease

Diarrhoea
- Ulcerative colitis, indeterminate colitis (p. 282), pseudomembranous, infective or ischaemic colitis (Box 9.2, p. 323) are usually distinguished by biopsy and stool culture, which must be repeated in cases of doubt
- Isolated diarrhoea that remains undiagnosed after colonic investigation is an indication for small bowel radiology, then distal duodenal biopsy and ultrasound of the pancreas (Fig. 7.1, p. 211)

Right iliac fossa mass
- Caecal carcinoma is more common than Crohn's in the elderly
- Appendix abscess and ileocaecal tuberculosis occur at any age. Tuberculosis, amoeboma or actinomycosis should be considered in Asian, African or South American patients. Ultrasound and serology help, but laparotomy may be necessary. The surgeon needs as much information as possible before operating

Rectal and perianal ulceration
Carcinoma, lymphogranuloma venereum, syphilis, Behçet's disease, HIV infection, *Herpes simplex*, cytomegalovirus and tuberculosis are less common causes than Crohn's disease. Biopsy and serology are usually diagnostic.

Disease at other sites
Radiology resolves most of the dilemmas, but other conditions occasionally mimic the radiological appearances of Crohn's disease (Table 8.3, p. 250).

Management principles

General
- A consistent approach, attention to nutrition, medical treatment of active disease and surgical management of complications are the principles of management
- Close liaison between medical and surgical teams is essential for optimal management of functional and structural problems
- Crohn's disease is only treated if there are symptoms: treat the patient, not the X-ray

Approach
- Explain that although the cause is unknown, inflammation and infection can be treated effectively. General information (p. 440) is often helpful for the patient
- Availability to deal with recurrent problems is reassuring. The patient should have a telephone number to call either the medical secretary for an appointment or an experienced nurse
- Patients should be seen and followed up by an experienced gastroenterologist, who can avoid unnecessary investigations and provide continuity of care
- Cautious optimism is advisable, but reasonable expectations should be discussed with the patient
- Patients often benefit from contact with national patient organisations and their local groups. The National Association for Colitis and Crohn's (NACC), the Crohn's and Colitis Foundation of America (CCFA) and the Crohn's and Colitis Foundation of Canada (CCFC) have useful websites (Appendix 1, p. 437)

Nutrition
Most patients can eat anything. Patients should avoid foods that upset them and try to eat a balanced diet. A special diet is occasionally needed (Table 8.5). Many patients find that avoiding vegetables and other foods high in fibre mitigate abdominal pain during an acute episode, especially if there is small intestinal disease. Patients usually find

Table 8.5 Indications for special diets in Crohn's disease

Situation	Diet
Small intestinal stricture	Low-residue diet (p. 391)
Persistent diarrhoea without active disease	Reduce resistant starches and try a lactose-free diet (p. 390), but see also Table 8.7 (p. 264)
Malnourishment during active disease perioperatively	Enteral supplements Parenteral nutrition, central or peripheral (p. 380)
jejunoileostomy	Isotonic drinks for excess fluid loss (p. 232)
short (< 100 cm) bowel	Enteral or parenteral nutrition (pp. 376 and 380)
Steatorrhoea	Low-fat diet (p. 391)
Active disease unresponsive to steroids	Liquid diet, but see also p. 257 for 6 weeks
Specific deficiencies	Iron, folate, B$_{12}$, fat-soluble vitamins, calcium, zinc, p. 393

it helpful to see a dietitian at diagnosis, who can ensure that calcium or iron intake are not inappropriately restricted

- Good nutrition is especially important in children and adolescents, to ensure adequate growth
- A liquid diet for 6 weeks is beneficial for active disease, but less effective than steroids. Polymeric feeds are as effective and more palatable than elemental feeds and offer an alternative treatment for active disease, especially for extensive small bowel disease, or if consequences of steroids and surgery are to be best avoided (children, multiple operations). About 60% respond to 6 weeks' elemental or polymeric feeding. An experienced dietitian is essential to maintain compliance (p. 377).
- Adequate nutritional supplementation (as sip-feeds, nocturnal nasogastric tube feeding or parenteral nutrition) improves growth velocity in children and helps maintain remission in children
- Parenteral feeding is only indicated when there is gut failure, due to obstruction, high output fistulae or massive resection

Medical management

The drugs of major importance for inducing remission are steroids (systemic and controlled release), aminosalicylates and new biological agents. Immunomodulators (azathioprine or mercaptopurine and methotrexate) are largely used for modifying the pattern of disease. New biological agents such as infliximab are changing the medical approach, but have not yet shown that they can reduce surgical resection or change long-term disease outcome. Benefit (numbers needed to treat, NNT) has to be weighed against side-effects (number needed to harm, NNH). The threshold for using steroids or infliximab differs between Europe and the USA. In Europe, infliximab is generally reserved for active disease refractory to steroids or immunomodulators, while in the USA infliximab is often used in place of steroids if active disease does not respond to aminosalicylates.

Principles of medical management

- Confirm disease activity. Basic investigations for any acute episode include a full blood count, ESR or CRP, albumin, electrolytes and stool sample for pathogens, including *Cl. difficile* toxin. A plain abdominal X-ray is indicated in severe attacks to look for large or small bowel dilation and contrast radiology is advisable before surgical intervention

- Assess severity (can be difficult to assess). All symptoms should be taken seriously. The differentiation between severe and mild attacks is not as clear as in ulcerative colitis (p. 268)
- Consider the location (controlled-release steroids are more effective for ileal than colonic disease) and pattern of disease (≥ 2 relapses a year is an indication for azathioprine/mercaptopurine)
- Discuss treatment options with the patient and consider patients' views
- Agree a strategy for inducing remission (with aminosalicylates, steroids, new biological agents or nutritional therapy) and modifying the pattern of disease (with azathioprine/mercaptopurine or methotrexate)

Severe attacks

- Patients look ill, with severe symptoms, vomiting, fever > 38°C, tachycardia > 90 b.p.m. or laboratory evidence (albumin < 35 g/dL, high ESR, leucocytosis) of inflammation or infection. These features are indications for admission to hospital
- Intravenous fluids and replacement of electrolytes (especially K) are important. The patient may be dehydrated
- Intravenous hydrocortisone 100 mg three to four times daily should be started. Infliximab may be appropriate (p. 256), but specialist advice should be taken before it is given
- Metronidazole 400–500 mg two to three times daily and ciprofloxacin 500 mg twice daily, orally if possible, because it is often impossible to distinguish infection (from an abscess) from inflammation until imaging is performed
- Arrange investigations to confirm active disease and exclude complications. If abdominal pain predominates, arrange abdominal ultrasound or CT scan. If diarrhoea predominates, arrange flexible sigmoidoscopy. If perianal disease is present, arrange pelvic MRI
- Blood transfusion may be needed to bring the haemoglobin up to 10 g/dL
- Fluids are allowed by mouth, but no food. It is uncertain whether avoiding food is of specific value, but patients are often anorexic and symptoms may be exacerbated by food
- If treated with steroids, intravenous hydrocortisone and fluids are best continued for 5 days, then feeding restarted, with oral prednisolone 40 mg/day
- Response should be monitored by symptoms (bowel frequency, pain, anorexia), examination (abdominal tenderness, fever, tachycardia) and blood tests (alternate day full blood count, CRP, albumin, electrolytes)
- Deterioration during intravenous treatment suggests a complication, or disease that is not going to respond to medical treatment, and is usually an indication for infliximab (p. 256) or surgery (p. 265). Deterioration once feeding is restarted has similar implications
- Further investigations can be arranged when the patient is stable
- Once appetite returns and abdominal tenderness resolves, the patient can be discharged, with an outpatient appointment in 2–4 weeks' time. The weight on discharge should be recorded
- Steroid-tapering regimens vary widely from physician to physician and no regimen has been proven to be superior to any other. One commonly used regimen is to reduce prednisolone from 40 mg/day over 2 weeks, then continue at 20 mg for 1 month,

before decreasing by 5 mg/day every 1–2 weeks. It has been the experience of most gastroenterologists that more rapid reduction can provoke early relapse, but the aim must always be to stop steroids during remission
- Alternatives to steroids and maintenance therapy are discussed below

Mild attacks
- Patients are symptomatic and uncomfortable, often with abdominal tenderness and an elevated ESR or CRP. Vomiting, fever or a low albumin usually indicate a severe attack (p. 255)
- Outpatient treatment is reasonable
- Decisive treatment with steroids (European approach) may be preferred by the patient (NNT 2). Start with prednisolone 40 mg daily for 1 week, then 30 mg daily for 1 week, then 20 mg/day for 1 month. A low-residue diet is advisable if colicky pain is prominent. Prednisolone is then withdrawn by 5 mg/day every 1 week (more rapid withdrawal may lead to early relapse). Budesonide CIR (9 mg daily for 6 weeks, then 6 mg/day for 4 weeks before stopping) is an alternative for those with ileo–ascending colonic disease, but this is slightly less effective than prednisolone (NNT 3)
- Initial treatment with high-dose aminosalicylates (US approach, e.g. Pentasa 4 g daily) or antibiotics (metronidazole 0.75–1.5 g daily) is an alternative for those concerned about steroid side-effects, but is less effective than corticosteroids (NNT 6–21)
- Response should be regularly assessed in outpatients (every 2–4 weeks). Symptoms, examination and blood tests (full blood count, CRP, albumin) are the guide

Maintenance therapy
- All patients should be encouraged and supported to stop smoking (reduces risk of relapse two- to fourfold)
- No maintenance therapy is an option for those with mild disease and infrequent (≤ 1 year) relapse
- Mesalazine 2–4 g/day appears to halve the risk of relapse if started within 3 months of steroid-induced remission or surgery (especially for isolated small bowel resection). Lower doses do not work
- Steroids have no effect on maintaining remission but budesonide 6 mg/day may delay the time to relapse in patients who have had remission induced by budesonide 9 mg/day. However, outcome at 1 year does not seem to be improved by maintenance doses of budesonide.
- Azathioprine 2.0–2.5 mg/kg/day halves the risk of relapse and is indicated when relapse occurs during or within 6 weeks of steroid withdrawal, if two or more courses of steroids are needed in 1 year, after treatment with infliximab, or after a second or subsequent surgical resection (p. 280). Treatment should continue for at least 4–5 years if tolerated

Infliximab
- Infliximab (5 mg/kg infusion over 2 h) is effective in 70% with active Crohn's disease
- For perianal disease, it is customary to give infliximab (5 mg/kg) infusions at 0, 2 and 6 weeks
- National guidelines may govern its use. In the UK, NICE guidelines limit its use to patients with severe active Crohn's disease (Harvey–Bradshaw index ≥ 8, Crohn's

disease activity index > 300), refractory to, or intolerant of, steroids and immuno-suppression, for whom surgery is inappropriate. Criteria are less exacting in the USA and some European countries, when active disease in spite of aminosalicylates or antibiotics are acceptable indications

- Before using infliximab, infection (local abscess, including perineal), previous cancer, tuberculosis (history and chest X-ray, but Mantoux test often unhelpful), cardiac failure (deaths reported) and tight intestinal strictures (obstruction may be exacerbated through rapid healing) must be excluded
- Side-effects, affecting up to 25%, include infusion reactions, arthralgia, lupus-type syndrome and sepsis. Antibodies to infliximab (human antichimeric antibody, HACA) increase the risk of side-effects from subsequent infusions, but are not sufficiently predictable to justify their routine measurement
- The patient should know that infliximab is a novel therapy. The long-term effects remain to be determined, but initial concern that it may predispose to lymphoma appears to be unfounded. Nevertheless, 1% of 500 patients receiving infliximab at the Mayo clinic died from causes (usually sepsis) directly attributable to infliximab
- Infliximab has a modest effect on the pattern of disease if responders have repeat infusions at double dose (10 mg/kg) every 8 weeks (39% remission at 1 year, compared to 24% given 5 mg/kg every 8 weeks and 17% given placebo)
- Azathioprine/mercaptopurine or methotrexate should be started or continued after infliximab infusion, and common European practice is to repeat infliximab infusions when symptoms of active disease recur (on-demand or intermittent treatment). In other regions the use of regular maintenance retreatment (i.e. every 8 weeks) is common

Other alternatives to steroids
- Surgery should always be considered for steroid-resistant disease, including stricturoplasty for small bowel strictures, split ileostomy for colonic or perianal Crohn's disease and resection when necessary (p. 265)
- It often helps to discuss the following options with patients:
  - Mesalazine 4 g/day (less effective than steroids)
  - Metronidazole 200–500 mg three times daily (for perianal disease, or when infection coexists with active disease)
  - Budesonide-CIR (for ileocaecal or ascending colonic Crohn's disease, above)
  - Azathioprine (2.0–2.5 mg/kg/day) or mercaptopurine (1.0–1.5 mg/kg/day) (useful steroid-sparing agent, but ineffective alone for active disease and takes from 1 to 4 months to have a clinically apparent effect)
  - Methotrexate 15–25 mg oral or intramuscular/subcutaneous once weekly (effective in 40% with active, steroid-resistant disease when surgery needs to be avoided). Orally administered methotrexate, although sometimes used, has not been shown to be as effective as parenteral methotrexate.
  - Liquid (polymeric or elemental) diet for 6 weeks (used alone or as an adjunct to steroids for extensive small intestinal, perianal or steroid-resistant disease). Palatability is poor and needs expert dietetic support to be tolerated (pp. 254 and 377). Administration by a nasogastric/nasoenteral or percutaneous gastrostomy tube is an option where palatability is an issue
  - Ciclosporin has not been shown to work in controlled trials

- Other new biologicals (such as natalizumab, an α4 integrin antagonist, or CDP 870, a pegylated anti-TNF monoclonal antibody) are on the threshold of practice

Outpatient review in Crohn's disease
Routine follow-up of patients (every 3–6 months) aims to detect early recurrence or complications and to monitor long-term therapy.

Documentation
Needed for each patient and most helpfully recorded on a special card at the front of the notes:
- Date of onset of symptoms
- Site and extent of disease
- Presence or absence of positive histology
- Date of last small bowel/colonic examination
- Chronology of operations and complications

At each review
- Ask about present symptoms and extraintestinal manifestations
- Consider causes of diarrhoea or abdominal pain other than active Crohn's disease (Table 8.6)
- Record weight and abdominal signs
- Check full blood count and liver function every 6 months, even if asymptomatic, to detect subclinical nutritional deficiency or other complications such as sclerosing cholangitis. Full blood count every 4–8 weeks is necessary during azathioprine/mercaptopurine therapy
- Explain the importance of early review if symptoms recur

Indications for surgery
70–80% of patients have an operation at some stage. The decision to operate depends on the degree of disability caused by the symptoms.

Major indications
- Symptomatic disease despite medical therapy
- Intestinal obstruction (subacute or acute) from strictures
- Local complications:

Table 8.6 Causes of abdominal pain in Crohn's disease

Inflammatory markers present	Inflammatory markers absent
Active Crohn's small intestinal colonic	Stricture small intestinal colonic
Abscess	Biliary colic
Pyelonephritis	Renal colic
Cholecystitis	Adhesions
Drug-induced pancreatitis (azathioprine, mesalazine, steroids)	Steroid-induced peptic ulcers
	Other disease—ovarian, pelvic

- fistulae
- abscess
- perforation

Principles

- Limited resection of the most diseased area by an experienced surgeon
- Avoid bypass surgery: recurrence is common. End-to-end anastomosis is preferable
- Nutritional support prior to surgery for complex (especially fistulising) Crohn's disease is essential. Surgery is better delayed, if possible, in malnourished patients (BMI < 18 kg/m²), by some months so that parenteral feeding (or enteral feeding if not obstructed and no fistulae) can improve nutritional status. This reduces the risk of major postoperative complications
- Postoperative mesalazine 3 g daily after the first (small bowel) resection reduces the risk of relapse by approximately one-third and should be started before the patient leaves hospital. After a second or extensive (> 1 m) resection, or surgery for fistulating disease, azathioprine/mercaptopurine is more appropriate

Special situations

- Strictureplasty is preferable for small intestinal strictures, since it avoids resection and anastomosis and minimises loss of bowel
- Limited resection (rather than a right hemicolectomy) is appropriate for ascending colonic or terminal ileal disease
- Localised transverse or distal colonic disease with a stricture or fistula may first be resected, but the relapse rate is high and more extensive disease that needs surgery is best treated by proctocolectomy, which has a lower relapse rate
- Ileorectal anastomosis may avoid a permanent ileostomy if the rectum is spared, but the relapse rate is higher than with a proctocolectomy. Ileoanal pouch formation is considered absolutely contraindicated by most surgeons because of the risk of postoperative sepsis or fistulae
- Split ileostomy and hydrocortisone 100 mg in 100 mL instilled into the distal limb daily may heal resistant colonic or perianal disease. Continuity can be restored after 12–24 months and a permanent ileostomy avoided in about half of patients
- Local surgery should be avoided for perianal ulcers, skin tags or haemorrhoids, because symptoms are usually few and recurrence common. Single, simple fistula may be amenable to fistulotomy but surgical management of perianal fistula is usually limited to placement of draining setons or diversion procedures

Complications

Small intestinal obstruction

Diagnostic investigations
Plain abdominal X-ray, markers of activity and small bowel radiology.
- Usually due to active disease, but may be caused by bolus obstruction at a fibrotic stricture
- Chronic symptoms with few signs of active disease suggests a fibrotic stricture
- Radiographic intestinal diameter correlates poorly with symptoms

Toxic dilatation (See p. 39)

Diagnostic investigations

Temperature > 38°C, colonic diameter ≥ 6.0 cm on plain X-ray (Fig. 1.5, p. 36) repeated daily, stool culture for pathogens and *Cl. difficile* toxin and blood cultures.

• Much less common than in ulcerative colitis

Abdominal, pelvic or ischiorectal abscess

Diagnostic investigations

Temperature chart, white cell count, ultrasound and culture of pus after aspiration. MRI (Fig. 8.2) effectively demonstrates the location and any fistulous connections of pelvic abscesses, but may not be locally available.

[111]In-labelled leucocyte scanning is sometimes helpful if an abscess is suspected and cannot be detected by other methods.

• Radiological or surgical drainage of the abscess is necessary before antibiotics can be effective (intravenous cefuroxime 750 mg and metronidazole 500 mg three times daily until apyrexial, then oral equivalent for 1 week). Steroids are also indicated (oral for ischiorectal, intravenous for abdominal abscesses) to suppress active Crohn's disease, but infliximab should be avoided until sepsis has resolved

Fistulae

Diagnostic investigations

Contrast radiology, preferably when disease is quiescent, MRI is best for perianal fistulae if available, but surgical examination under anaesthetic by an experienced surgeon is the traditional alternative.

• Infliximab (5 mg/kg infusions at 0, 2 and 6 weeks) followed by azathioprine/mercaptopurine should be considered for all fistulae, but only if local sepsis has been excluded by imaging and drained if present. Healing (drying up of fistulae) is often temporary and the optimum combination of infliximab and surgery remains to be defined. Specialist advice should be taken
• Perianal fistulae produce a discharge and may interfere with anal sphincter function (faecal soiling) or produce a stricture (palpable on rectal examination). Treatment is only indicated for symptoms (p. 265). MRI defines the complexity of fistulous tracks in relation to the levator muscles
• Enterovesical or vaginal fistulae (causing pneumaturia or faecal vaginal discharge) usually connect with the terminal ileum. Small bowel radiology is indicated before surgery. Rectovaginal fistulae can heal spontaneously
• Enterocutaneous fistulae often follow surgery. Antibiotics, steroids and nutritional support allow a minority to heal spontaneously, but surgical resection of the fistulous track and connecting bowel is usually needed. The anatomy must be clearly defined by sinograms, small and large bowel radiology before surgery. Infliximab should be used with caution, because it may convert local sepsis into life-threatening septicaemia

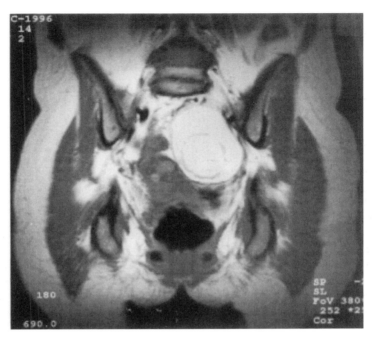

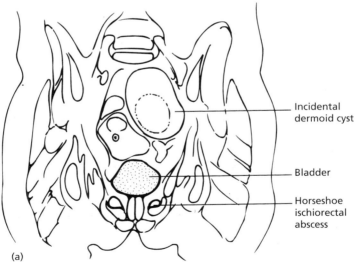

(a)

Fig. 8.2 Pelvic MRI scan of complex perineal abscess. (a) Coronal section. *(Continued)*

- Enterocolic or enteroenteric fistulae cause profound weight loss, often, but not always, with diarrhoea. Metronidazole (400–500 mg three times daily) may help diarrhoea temporarily, and nutritional support should be given for several months, before considering surgery

261

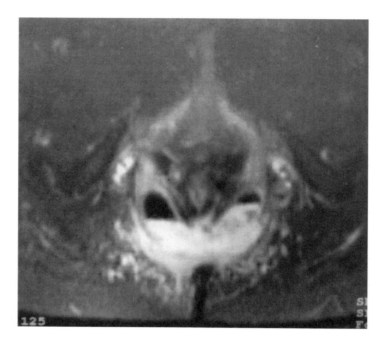

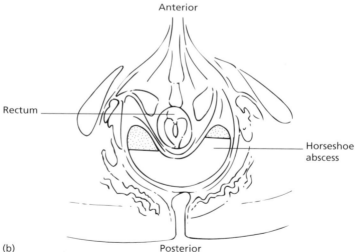

Fig. 8.2 *(continued)* (b) Pelvic MRI showing enlarged sagittal section of horseshoe abscess in (a).

Short bowel syndrome

- Resection to < 100–150 cm leads to short bowel syndrome, especially if there is persistent small intestinal disease or if the colon has been removed
- The cause is rarely serial resection of recurrent Crohn's disease. It is most commonly due to massive resection after complications from an initial operation

- Surgeons should measure the length of bowel from the ligament of Treitz at the time of laparotomy for resection in any patient with Crohn's disease
- Management is discussed on p. 232

Perforation

Diagnostic investigations
Plain abdominal and erect chest X-rays
- Rarely presents acutely because an abscess cavity often forms, although features may be suppressed by steroids
- Surgery is indicated if perforation is detected

Massive rectal bleeding

Diagnostic investigations
Clinical evidence, full blood count, prothrombin time and urgent mesenteric angiography if blood loss > 4 units in < 24 h
- Rare in colonic disease (1%) and very rare in terminal ileal disease
- Transfusion alone is usually sufficient. Colonoscopy is indicated after the bleeding stops
- Surgery for persistent bleeding (> 8 unit transfusion) should be preceded by angiography

Carcinoma

Diagnostic investigations
Colonoscopy, biopsy.
- Occurs in < 5% of patients with colonic disease, related to the extent and duration (> 10 years) of Crohn's colitis. Diagnosis is often too late for curative colectomy
- New symptoms, such as rectal bleeding without signs of active disease, are an indication for colonoscopy
- The risk of small intestinal carcinoma is increased, but remains very rare (2 : 373 patients followed up for > 10 years)

Extraintestinal complications (See Table 8.2, p. 247)

Management problems
Recurrent symptoms are not always due to active disease. When inflammation or infection is present, the ESR, CRP and platelet count are usually elevated and the albumin low ('inflammatory markers').

Persistent abdominal pain (See Table 8.6, p. 258)
- Urine examination is always necessary, to look for haematuria (calculi), proteinuria (infection or inflammation) and for culture
- A plain abdominal film may show fluid levels, dilated bowel, loops separated by a mass or calcified calculi

- Ultrasound of a mass, to look for an abscess cavity, inflammatory mass, thickened bowel loops or calculi, is advisable before repeat small bowel radiology, because it is less invasive. When intestinal gas obscures views, CT scanning is necessary

Persistent diarrhoea (See Table 8.7)
- Dietary modification to reduce ingestion of resistant starches (some types of wheat starch), insoluble fibre or sorbitol (in fizzy drinks) often helps. Dietetic advice should be sought
- Small bowel bacterial overgrowth is characterised by explosive, malodorous diarrhoea without pain. Such symptoms justify empirical treatment with metronidazole 200–500 mg three times daily (or ciprofloxacin 500 mg twice daily, or tetracycline 250 mg four times daily if not tolerated) for 1 week. Lactulose hydrogen breath test is diagnostic (p. 427), except after ileocolonic resection or enteroenteric fistula, but rapid clinical response to antibiotics is characteristic. Cyclical antibiotics (first week of each month) is a pragmatic approach to recurrent symptoms
- Avoiding milk helps patients with hypolactasia, but calcium supplements are then necessary
- Diarrhoea due to distal ileal disease or resection responds to cholestyramine 4–12 g daily
- Active Crohn's colitis may be extensive or an enteroenteric fistula unsuspected. Imaging should be reviewed and colonoscopy or small bowel enema arranged if necessary
- Symptomatic control with codeine phosphate (up to 90 mg/day) or loperamide (up to 12 mg/day) is appropriate if other measures fail

Rapid relapse upon steroid withdrawal
Patients who relapse when steroids are reduced below 10 mg, or within 6 weeks of complete withdrawal (p. 256), are best treated by:
- Azathioprine 2–2.5 mg/kg/day (usually 100–150 mg/day) or mercaptopurine 1.0–1.5 mg/kg/day
- Either increase prednisolone to 30 mg/day to induce remission again and then reduce by 5 mg every 2 weeks, or consider infliximab (above). Budesonide-CIR 3–9 mg daily is appropriate in place of prednisolone for ileal or ascending colonic disease if steroids cannot be withdrawn and surgery considered for persistent symptoms
- Continue azathioprine after steroids are withdrawn for up to 5 years or more
- A full blood count 2–4 weeks after starting treatment and then every 1–2 months, or during any acute infection, is advisable to detect neutropenia (< 3%). Measuring thiopurine methyl transferase (TPMT) activity or genotype may predict the likelihood of neutropenia in some patients. While some advocate this before starting treat-

Table 8.7 Causes of persistent diarrhoea in Crohn's disease

Inflammatory markers present	Inflammatory markers absent
Active Crohn's disease	Small intestinal bacterial overgrowth
	Hypolactasia
	Bile-salt malabsorption after ileal resection
	Short bowel after resection
	Irritable bowel syndrome
	Other disease (coeliac, chronic pancreatitis)

ment, it cannot be stipulated because most cases of neutropenia occur after several months and are not closely related to TPMT activity

- Concomitant treatment with allopurinol or co-trimoxazole should be avoided because toxicity is enhanced
- Patients intolerant of azathioprine may be tried on mercaptopurine unless pancreatitis or hepatitis has occurred. Methotrexate 25 mg once a week, with folic acid 5 mg 2 days before dosing, is an appropriate alternative

Perianal disease
- Treatment is only necessary for symptoms, which are frequently mild compared to the appearance
- Resolution may be independent of disease activity elsewhere
- Metronidazole 200–500 mg three times daily is indicated for mild, symptomatic disease
- Fistulisation is an indication for MR scanning, and if the fistula is transphincteric (Fig. 9.8, p. 326), then examination under anaesthetic to insert a drainage seton should be carried out. Infliximab is then often appropriate (above), followed by azathioprine
- Steroids are often ineffective unless there is active disease elsewhere
- Complicated fistulae that fail to respond to intensive medical treatment usually respond well to defunctioning of the colon or rectum (split ileostomy or colostomy), but are best treated at a specialist centre

Ileostomy dysfunction (See p. 280)

Crohn's disease in pregnancy (See also p. 398)
- Advise patients to avoid conception until disease is inactive. There is then little risk to the pregnancy or the course of Crohn's disease
- Active disease during pregnancy is treated with nutritional support, steroids or aminosalicylates in the normal way (p. 279), because the risks of active disease are greater than any drug side-effects
- Immunomodulation with azathioprine/mercaptopurine is best continued during pregnancy if remission has been difficult to achieve or if prevention of recurrent relapse has only been achieved with azathioprine
- Delivery by caesarean section is advisable if there is active perianal disease or previous anorectal surgery for fistulae

Crohn's disease in adolescence
- Retardation of growth and puberty, as well as loss of schooling, are additional problems, although the course of disease and treatment principles are the same as in adults
- Nutritional assessment and support are essential. Height and weight must be recorded on a centile chart at each visit. Falling below centile lines for height or weight is an indication for blood tests to assess activity and nutritional status (full blood count, folate, B_{12}, iron studies, calcium). Nutritional supplements (enteric sip feeds, p. 376) are usually tolerated, but if not, continuous or nocturnal enteral feeding are alternatives
- Active disease may be treated as in adults, with prednisolone (starting at 1 mg/kg daily) or infliximab. However, many paediatric gastroenterologists use nutritional

therapy in place of steroids as first-line therapy. Surgical resection of the most diseased area should be considered if the response is slow

Prognosis

It is currently impossible to predict the course of Crohn's disease in an individual patient. Relapses tend to follow the previous pattern of disease (fibrostenotic, fistulating, inflammatory). Up to 80% concordance of disease distribution or pattern has been reported in family members affected by Crohn's. Most patients have a good prognosis, although morbidity may be considerable for short periods.

Risk of relapse

- Crohn's disease cannot be cured
- 1 year after diagnosis, about 50% have no symptoms, 25% have low activity and 25% high disease activity in any given year
- Working capacity is normal in 75%. After 5–10 years, 15% are not working due to the disease
- Patients with jejunoileal disease relapse more commonly than those with Crohn's colitis

Need for surgery

- 60% have an intestinal resection within 10 years of the onset of symptoms and 80% after 20 years
- Half the operations are emergencies
- After 15 years, one-third have had no operation, one-third have had a single operation and one-third have had two or more operations
- The need for surgery is more common (80% at 5 years) in those presenting with ileocaecal disease compared to those with Crohn's colitis or disease at other locations (40%)
- About 10% with colonic disease have a permanent ileostomy after 10 years

Recurrence after surgery

- 30% relapse within 5 years and 50% within 10 years, but only half of these need further surgery
- Recurrence is less common in colonic disease and the elderly, but more common in children

Mortality

- In population-based studies, overall mortality is no different from that of the general population
- Patients with extensive (> 100 cm) small intestinal disease, proximal (gastroduodenal or jejunal) disease, or those aged 20–29 years at diagnosis, however, have a higher mortality in the first 5 years after diagnosis (relative risk three- to sixfold)

8.2 Ulcerative colitis

Ulcerative colitis is an inflammatory disorder of the colonic mucosa characterised by relapses and remissions. The cause remains unknown.

General information

A few facts are helpful when explaining the disease to patients:

- Affects 90–170 : 100 000 population (more common than Crohn's), but studies from primary care on hospital-diagnosed cases report a higher prevalence (up to 268 : 100 000)
- 7–22 : 100 000 new cases per year, with no apparent increase in incidence recently. Sex and social class are not associated, although it is uncommon outside Western societies. Asian immigrants to Western countries have a much higher incidence than those in the countries of origin
- Most patients present at age 15–30 years, but 10% present over the age of 60 years. Proctitis is more common than total colitis, especially in the elderly
- 15% have a member of the family with ulcerative colitis or Crohn's, but the genetic influence is less strong than Crohn's disease
- HLA genes are more strongly linked to ulcerative colitis than to Crohn's. The genotype may be related to the pattern of disease (HLA-DR1 *103 is 5–11 times more common in patients who have a colectomy than those who do not)
- Three times as common in ex-smokers, or non-smokers
- Seasonal variation occurs, with presentation in the winter (1.48-fold increased risk in December) being twice as common as in early summer (0.76-fold risk in May, relative to annual mean)
- Appendicectomy reduces the risk by 70%, independently of smoking, for reasons that are unclear
- The cause is unknown, but deficient immunoregulation, NSAIDs, cell-wall deficient bacteria and diet (low fibre, milk) have been implicated. Stress may exacerbate existing symptoms, but not cause the disease
- The pattern is usually intermittent. Chronic continuous symptoms with varying severity are less common. Single attacks with no recurrence probably represent infection rather than ulcerative colitis

Clinical features

General

- Bloody diarrhoea is the hallmark, usually with mucus
- Onset is usually gradual but can be abrupt, and there may sometimes be a previous history of episodic diarrhoea. Infection may trigger an abrupt onset or toxic dilatation
- Bowel frequency is broadly related to the severity of disease
- Abdominal cramps causing discomfort is common, but severe persistent pain suggests a complication or different diagnosis
- Systemic features (anorexia, malaise, fever) are common during an acute attack, except in ulcerative proctitis
- Signs (tachycardia, fever, abdominal tenderness or distension) are important when assessing severity (Table 8.8)
- Other features that help distinguish severe attacks are systemic upset (anorexia, malaise, weight loss), tender colon (often notable by its absence), leucocytosis and hypoalbuminaemia
- Steroids can mask clinical features of severity
- Young patients with severe disease may appear misleadingly well

Table 8.8 Assessing the severity of ulcerative colitis

Feature	Mild	Moderate	Severe
Motions/day	< 4	4–6	> 6
Rectal bleeding	Small	Moderate	Large amounts
Temperature	Apyrexial	Intermediate	> 37.8°C on 2 days out of 4
Pulse rate	Normal	Intermediate	> 90 b.p.m.
Haemoglobin	> 11 g/dL	Intermediate	< 10.5 g/dL
ESR	< 20 mm/h	Intermediate	> 30 mm/h

Extraintestinal manifestations
- 10–20% are affected, especially those with pancolitis
- Similar to those in Crohn's disease (Table 8.2, p. 247), with some important exceptions (Table 8.9)

Investigations
The aim is to confirm the diagnosis, assess the severity and extent of disease, and to detect complications.

Establish the diagnosis

Sigmoidoscopy and biopsy
- Diffuse mucosal changes in the rectum are invariable during active disease
- Infective colitis and occasionally Crohn's disease or ischaemia can look similar
- Characteristic microscopic features are a chronic inflammatory infiltrate, glandular distortion, goblet-cell depletion, crypt abscesses and villiform pattern of the surface epithelium

Colonoscopy
- Always preferable to a barium enema as the initial investigation of bloody diarrhoea, because it provides better mucosal definition and allows biopsies to be taken

Table 8.9 Distinctions between extraintestinal manifestation of ulcerative colitis and Crohn's disease

Extraintestinal feature	Comment
PSC (p. 200)	Affects 2–3% 80% with PSC have UC, 70% are male Less common in Crohn's disease
Cholangiocarcinoma	Usually complicates PSC, but very rare in Crohn's disease
Skin lesions	Consider drug-induced lesions, such as sulphasalazine, especially in UC
Large joint arthritis	Possibly becoming less common in UC due to maintenance sulphasalazine
All extraintestinal manifestations	Relieved by proctocolectomy in UC, except ankylosing spondylitis and hepatobiliary disease, but not in Crohn's disease

PSC, primary sclerosing cholangitis.
UC, ulcerative cholitis.

- In the acute stages a flexible sigmoidoscopy is more appropriate than full colonoscopy, which can be dangerous (perforation); bowel preparation is often not necessary but, if required, the procedure can be performed 30–60 min after a phosphate enema

Stool examination
Always necessary to exclude pathogens (*E. coli* 0157, *Shigella* spp., *Campylobacter* spp., *Cl. difficile* toxin, *Salmonella* spp., *Entamoeba histolytica* after foreign travel, or CMV in immunocompromised).

Establish the severity
- Clinical and radiological criteria (Table 8.8, p. 268; Table 8.10)
- Sigmoidoscopy (Table 8.11), but mucosal changes may have been ameliorated by rectal steroids
- Blood tests
  - anaemia (Hb < 10.5 g/dL) and an ESR > 30 mm/h indicate severe disease. If the ESR is normal, a CRP > 30 mg/L has the same significance
  - leucocytosis, hypoalbuminaemia and hypokalaemia are common in severe disease

Establish the extent of disease
- In a population-based study of 1161 patients, distribution of disease at diagnosis was proctitis (48%), distal or left-sided (33%) or total (19%)
- Proctitis means that the upper limit of inflammation can be seen on rigid sigmoidoscopy (usually < 15 cm from anal verge)
- Distribution of faecal shadows on a plain abdominal X-ray during an acute attack is a useful guide to the extent of disease: faecal shadows are absent from bowel with active mucosal inflammation. It can be misleading, however, in those with proximal constipation
- Colonoscopy and serial biopsy is the best way of establishing the extent. Biopsies frequently show microscopic inflammation proximal to the limit of macroscopic inflammation, but the implications of microscopic changes are not clear. Prognostic factors (for carcinoma, or risk from a severe attack) are based on the extent of macroscopic disease
- The risk of proximal extension of distal disease is about 15% at 5 years and 30% 10 years after diagnosis

Table 8.10 Summary of radiological features of ulcerative colitis (approximate order of severity)

Acute	Chronic
Normal (proctitis)	Increased retrorectal space
Granular mucosa	Granular mucosa
Absent faecal shadows*	Loss of haustra
Punctate ulcers	Tubular colon
Collar-stud ulcers	Pseudopolyps
Mucosal islands*	Backwash ileitis (pancolitis)
Toxic dilatation (≥ 6.0 cm)*	Carcinoma

*Visible on plain abdominal X-ray.

Table 8.11 Sigmoidoscopic appearances in ulcerative colitis

Mild	Moderate	Severe
Diffuse erythema	Granular mucosa	Intense inflammation
Loss of vascular pattern	Petechial haemorrhages	Purulent exudate
Contact bleeding	Spontaneous bleeding	Discrete ulcers

Investigation of relapse

- Sigmoidoscopy and biopsy are necessary to assess the severity (Table 8.11), in association with the clinical features
- Stool for culture and *Cl. difficile* toxin assay must be taken
- Full blood count, ESR or CRP, electrolytes and albumin should be measured. The CRP may be elevated when the ESR is normal
- A plain abdominal X-ray is necessary in severe disease to look for signs of toxic dilatation or mucosal islands (Fig. 1.6, p. 41). When a moderate relapse is slow to settle, proximal constipation may be visible (p. 279)
- Repeat colonoscopy is unnecessary unless the extent of the disease is thought to have changed (such as after a severe attack in a patient with previous proctitis)

Outpatient follow-up in remission

- Duration, extent and pattern of disease should always be documented
- Sigmoidoscopy is only necessary if a relapse occurs
- Rectal biopsy is recommended at every sigmoidoscopy, because it provides an independent record of the macroscopic appearance, consolidates the diagnosis and, rarely, detects dysplasia
- Colonoscopy to reassess the extent of disease is generally appropriate 8–10 years after onset of symptoms. Surveillance colonoscopy and multiple biopsies for dysplasia surveillance is indicated for extensive or total colitis beginning 8–10 years after onset of symptoms and for left-sided colitis after 15–20 years. Surveillance biopsies are not necessary for patients with proctitis (discussed in Fig. 8.3). However, the pros and cons of surveillance strategies should be discussed with the patient (p. 277)
- Annual full blood count and liver function tests are recommended. Macrocytosis can be due to sulphasalazine or azathioprine therapy, but other causes (alcohol, B_{12} or folate deficiency, myxoedema or haemolysis) should not be overlooked
- A mildly elevated AST is an indication for complete abstinence from alcohol for 4–8 weeks before repeating the test. Drug-induced liver damage should be considered (p. 140) and if the AST continues to rise, all drugs should be stopped if possible. A liver biopsy is indicated if > twofold elevation persists for 3 months
- Persistent (> 3 months), or > threefold elevation in ALP, are indications for ultrasound to exclude gallstones, before ERCP to look for primary sclerosing cholangitis

Differential diagnosis

There are many causes of bloody diarrhoea, but only a few cause diffuse rectal changes visible on sigmoidoscopy. The main problems are differentiating ulcerative colitis from infective or Crohn's colitis (Table 8.12).

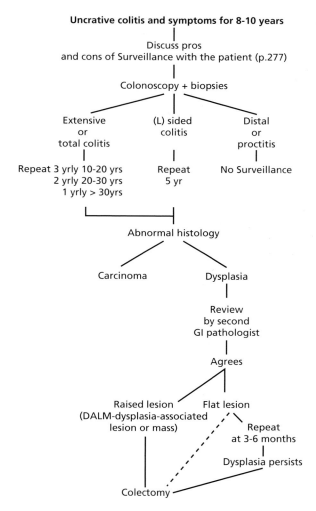

Fig. 8.3 Surveillance colonoscopy in ulcerative colitis.

Infective colitis

- Identification of *E. coli* 0157, *Campylobacter* spp., *Cl. difficile*, *Salmonella* spp., *Shigella* spp. or *E. histolytica* in the stool do not exclude ulcerative colitis
- Infective colitis causes macroscopic and microscopic inflammation, but unlike ulcerative colitis, does not usually distort microscopic glandular architecture
- Repeat sigmoidoscopy and biopsy after the acute episode has settled is always advisable if doubt exists. The patient can be reassured if the second biopsy is normal (acute self-limited colitis), but follow-up is necessary if inflammation persists
- Colitis caused by CMV, herpes simplex or other opportunistic pathogens can be a feature of AIDS (p. 356), but may complicate ulcerative colitis if the patient is immunosuppressed

Table 8.12 Differentiation of ulcerative from Crohn's colitis

	Ulcerative colitis	Crohn's colitis
Clinical		
Bloody diarrhoea	90–100%	50%
Abdominal mass	Very rare	Common
Perianal disease	Very uncommon	30–50%
Sigmoidoscopy		
Rectal sparing	Never	50%
Histology		
Distribution	Mucosal	Transmural
Cellular infiltrate	Polymorphs	Lymphocytes
Crypts	Distorted	Normal
Goblet cell depletion	Common when active	Absent
Granuloma	Absent	Diagnostic
Radiology		
Distribution	Continuous	Discontinuous
Symmetry	Symmetrical	Asymmetrical
Mucosa	Shallow ulcers	Deep ulcers
Strictures	Very rare	Common
Fistulae	Never	Common

Crohn's colitis

A definitive diagnosis is not initially possible in 10–15% (see indeterminate colitis, p. 282) and some turn out to have Crohn's colitis on long-term follow-up. This is one reason for repeat rectal biopsies (p. 294).

In distinguishing ulcerative from Crohn's colitis, the clinical *and* endoscopic *and* histological *and* radiological features should all be considered, rather than depending on a single investigation such as rectal biopsy or barium enema for diagnosis.

Other possibilities

- Drug-induced colitis—NSAIDs may cause colitis identical to ulcerative colitis. Increased apoptotic bodies, eosinophils and limited glandular distortion suggest the diagnosis on biopsy. Colitis may or may not resolve on steroid-withdrawal. COX-2 inhibitors, mycophenolate and other drugs may also cause colitis
- Ischaemic colitis—clinical features can be identical. Rectal sparing, 'thumb-printing' on plain abdominal X-ray and a flexible sigmoidoscopy establish the diagnosis (Fig. 9.6, p. 319)
- Radiation colitis—history of pelvic or abdominal node irradiation, with mucosal telangiectasia
- Microscopic colitis—no bleeding and macroscopically normal mucosa (p. 302)
- Pseudomembranous colitis (p. 283)
- Diverticular-colitis, polyps and colorectal carcinoma are readily distinguished as the cause of bloody diarrhoea, by colonoscopy, as long as a rectal biopsy is taken in addition to areas of inflamed colon
- Minimal change colitis—ulcerative colitis with little or no colonoscopic abnormality
- IBS may coexist with ulcerative colitis (p. 345)

Management

The principles of management are:
- Prompt treatment of acute attacks
- Maintenance therapy to reduce the relapse rate
- Selection of patients for colectomy
- Detection of colorectal carcinoma
- Patient education is essential to ensure early presentation during relapse. Treatment of an acute attack involving any site other than proctitis depends on the severity (Table 8.13). The term 'fulminant attack' is best avoided, because treatment is no different from that for a severe attack. Proctitis is a special case because systemic complications are uncommon.

Mild attacks

General
- Prompt and decisive treatment brings rapid relief to the patient and reduces the risk of complications
- The European approach is to use systemic steroids at an early stage, although in the USA the tendency is to use high-dose oral and topical mesalazine. Response (improvement) on mesalazine 4 g/daily is 70%, but remission is only achieved in 30% after 6 weeks, compared to 80% after 2 weeks on steroids
- Whilst it is reasonable to give a trial of local treatment (such as mesalazine suppositories or enemas) alone in the very early stages (bleeding for < 2 weeks), far too many patients are expected to suffer continuing symptoms from inadequate treatment with oral aminosalicylates and enemas for prolonged periods

Recommended treatment
- 2-week trial of topical mesalazine (1 g suppository, foam or liquid enema) and double the dose of oral mesalazine to ≥ 4 g daily
- If not improving within 2 weeks, start oral prednisolone 20 mg daily for 1 month, then reduce by 5 mg/week
- Failure to improve after 2 weeks is an indication for treatment as a moderate attack. Deterioration is an indication for admission

Table 8.13 Treatment of active ulcerative colitis after topical mesalazine for up to 2 weeks

Drug	Mild	Moderate	Severe
Prednisolone	20 mg/day 1 month 15 mg/day 1 week 10 mg/day 1 week 5 mg/day 1 week	40 mg/day 1 week 30 mg/day 1 week Then as for mild attacks	Admit for i.v. steroids Telephone gastroenterologist

Aminosalicylates	or mesalazine 4 g/day
	or balsalazide
	    6.75 g/day
	or olsalazine 3 g/day
		Continue unchanged	None until oral therapy
			    restarted

Enemas	Mesalazine 1 g once daily whilst bleeding		

Moderate attacks

- Prednisolone 40 mg daily for 1 week, then 30 mg/day for 1 week, then 20 mg/day for 1 month, before decreasing by 5 mg/day
- Mesalazine enemas at night (or steroid enemas if mesalazine not tolerated)
- Continue oral aminosalicylates at previous dose
- Admission is not essential unless symptoms fail to improve within 2 weeks, although for some patients (especially the elderly), bed rest and enemas in hospital are more comfortable

Severe attacks

- Immediate admission is necessary when clinical features of a severe attack are present (Table 8.8, p. 268). Surgical colleagues should be informed. A severe attack may occur without colonic dilatation ('toxic dilatation'), although this may subsequently develop
- A plain abdominal X-ray and blood tests (full blood count, CRP, electrolytes, magnesium, cholesterol and group & save) are taken on the way to the ward. Daily abdominal X-rays are appropriate until fever, abdominal tenderness or tachycardia resolve, to detect mucosal islands, dilatation (Fig. 1.6, p. 41) or perforation
- Intravenous hydrocortisone 100 mg three to four times daily or methylprednisolone 15–20 mg three times daily is given for 5 days
- Rectal steroids should also be given once to twice daily as tolerated. Hydrocortisone 100 mg in 100 mL 0.9% saline, dripped into the rectum through a soft catheter via an intravenous giving set, is often more comfortable for the patient than commercial enemas
- Stool frequency and appearance should be carefully documented by nursing staff, as well as pulse and temperature every 6 h, because these provide objective measurements for clinical decisions
- Sips of fluid only by mouth; although the benefit of withdrawing food does not affect the colitis, patients are usually anorexic and the response to reintroduction of food may help determine the need for colectomy (p. 275). Parenteral nutrition is only needed for malnourished patients
- Intravenous fluids are needed to correct dehydration and maintain serum potassium at 4.0–4.5 mmol/L
- Blood transfusion is advisable if Hb < 10 g/dL. Serum should be grouped and saved for possible surgery
- Daily (or twice daily in very sick patients) re-examination is essential, looking for a rise in pulse or temperature, increasing abdominal girth or tenderness
- After 3 days' treatment, simple prognostic factors (stool frequency and CRP) should be assessed (p. 275). If the CRP on day 3 is > 45 mg/L, discuss contingency plans for surgery (stomatherapist, surgical review) with the patient, consider ciclosporin (below) and continue intravenous hydrocortisone
- Daily full blood count, CRP and electrolytes should be checked until it is clear that the patient is responding to treatment
- Failure to respond after 5–7 days, or deterioration at any stage, is an indication for colectomy. Delay increases the mortality
- 40% are in remission after 5 days, and 30% deteriorate and have a colectomy. Another group (30%) improve, but make an incomplete response. Relapse on reintroducing food and changing to oral steroids usually means that colectomy is required

- For those who improve, oral prednisolone 40 mg/day can be started after 5–7 days and decreased after 1 week to 30 mg/day for 1 week, then to 20 mg/day for 1 month. It can then be decreased by 5 mg/week unless relapse occurs (p. 276)
- Aminosalicylates are poorly tolerated in severely ill patients and should be stopped. They can be reintroduced as oral steroids are tapered
- Antibiotics, including metronidazole or ciprofloxacin, offer no benefit in controlled trials. However, for first attacks of < 4 weeks' duration, metronidazole and ciprofloxacin as well as steroids are sensible to cover both infective and ulcerative colitis
- Ciclosporin (2 mg/kg daily infusion over 6 h, then 5–8 mg/kg/day orally) may help avoid surgery when severe colitis fails to respond to intravenous steroids. Specialist supervision is appropriate. About 60–70% respond, but there is a risk of morbidity (and mortality) from further delaying surgery, opportunistic infections or renal impairment. The risk of seizures is higher in hypomagnaesemia (Mg < 0.5 mmol/L) or hypocholesterolaemia (< 3.0 mmol/L). Ciclosporin should only be used if there is a prospect of maintaining medical remission with azathioprine/mercaptopurine, because most patients relapse when cyclosporin is withdrawn. It works rapidly (within 2–5 days) and if effective, then oral ciclosporin is continued for around 3 months. Azathioprine can be started in the last month of treatment as steroids are withdrawn and prophylaxis for pneumocystis is unnecessary.

Indications for emergency surgery
- Toxic dilatation (p. 39)
- Perforation
- Massive haemorrhage
- Failure of a severe attack to respond to intravenous steroids within 5 days. The decision and timing is always difficult, and should be made jointly by a senior physician and surgeon. Whilst some prefer to continue steroids for longer periods, the operative morbidity (and mortality) increases if surgery is inappropriately delayed
- A prospective study has provided a simple clinical guide to the need for surgery in severe colitis without colonic dilatation. If, after 3 days' intravenous treatment the stool frequency is > 8/day, or if the frequency is 3–8/day together with a CRP > 45 mg/L, then there is an 85% chance that colectomy will be needed on that admission
- Mucosal islands on a plain abdominal X-ray, a sustained fever > 38°C and stool frequency > 8/day after 24 h treatment, predict a high probability that colectomy will be needed
- Patients with a severe attack who make an incomplete response to intravenous steroids after 5 days, but then deteriorate when food is reintroduced usually need surgery. 40% of incomplete responders (stool frequency > 3/day, or visible blood in the stools after 1 week of intensive treatment) come to colectomy within a few months of admission

Proctitis
- Topical mesalazine (e.g. Pentasa suppository 1 g at night) and oral aminosalicylates (mesalazine 2–4 g, balsalazide 6.75 g or olsalazine 1.5–3 g daily) are often sufficient, but proctitis can be very refractory, even to oral steroids

- Mesalazine enemas are more effective than steroid enemas, but less well tolerated. The combination (steroid enema in the morning, mesalazine at night) may be better than either alone and is useful for refractory disease
- Patients usually find foam enemas or suppositories easier to retain than liquid enemas. It is a matter of personal choice, although suppositories are useful for very localised disease
- Failure to control symptoms within 2–4 weeks is an indication for prednisolone (above)
- Refractory proctitis is discussed on p. 279

Maintenance treatment
- All 5-ASA compounds (sulfasalazine, mesalazine, olsalazine, balsalazide) reduce the relapse rate by about fourfold, from 80 to 20% at 1 year. Compliance is probably more important than the individual drug and measures to improve compliance (twice daily dosing, calendar packs) help
- Maintenance treatment should be continued for life, because the benefit is sustained and it may reduce the risk of malignancy
- Sulfasalazine 1 g twice daily is still a drug of first choice, because it is cheap (25% of the cost of other salicylates), may be more effective than mesalazine and it is tolerated by 80%. However, concern about serious, but very rare reactions (Stevens–Johnson syndrome) means that some gastroenterologists advocate Asacol, Pentasa, balsalazide or olsalazine from the start
- Nausea or abdominal discomfort occurs in 10–20% taking sulphasalazine 2 g/day, but idiosyncratic side-effects (rash, leucopenia) are rare. Reversible oligospermia is frequent, so potential fathers should be started on olsalazine or mesalazine
- Mesalazine (Asacol 400 mg or Pentasa 500 mg three times daily), olsalazine (500 mg twice daily), or balsalazide 1.25 g twice daily are indicated for sulfasalazine intolerance
- Higher doses of olsalazine (2 g/day) are more effective at maintaining remission in proctitis after a relapse. Diarrhoea can be provoked by olsalazine, but is ameliorated by taking tablets with food
- Nephrotoxicity may occur with any aminosalicylate and may even be an extraintestinal manifestation of ulcerative colitis. Monitoring renal function at clinic visits (or every 6–12 months) is a sensible precaution although of unproven value
- Steroids have no effect on relapse rate and should be tapered and stopped once remission occurs
- Patients often benefit from contact with the NACC, CCFA, CCFC or similar patient-based organisations, even if symptoms are mild (Appendix 1, p. 437).

Detection of colonic carcinoma

Risk
- The risk of cancer increases with the extent and duration of disease. It is probably reduced by maintenance therapy with aminosalicylates, which should encourage compliance in those with extensive disease
- It is more prevalent in patients whose symptoms run a chronic continuous course, those not having specialist follow-up, or those with a family history of colorectal cancer

- An active medical and surgical approach to treatment as outlined above also found no increase in the risk of colorectal cancer among 1161 patients with ulcerative colitis treated in Copenhagen

Surveillance
- Surveillance colonoscopy is accepted practice for patients with extensive colitis of more than 10 years' duration, but its value remains debated. Once symptomatic and interval cancers that present between planned colonoscopies are excluded, > 100 colonoscopies have to be performed to detect the occasional case of dysplasia or early cancer. Colonoscopy carries a definable risk of perforation and > 50 biopsies are needed for > 90% chance of detecting dysplasia. Since many colonoscopists take < 20 biopsies, there may be a 30% chance of missing dysplasia if present. However, many patients with pancolitis like the reassurance that surveillance colonoscopy affords
- The decision about surveillance is best discussed with individual patients after discussing the pros and cons and current evaluation of risk, taking into account the patient's own preference
- Proctitis does not justify surveillance but, in many centres, surveillance is undertaken after 15–20 years in patients with left-sided disease extending beyond the rectum
- Patients with PSC appear to represent a subgroup at higher risk of cancer who should have more frequent (perhaps annual) colonoscopy
- If a surveillance programme is part of the unit's policy, a register and recall system for patients with total colitis is essential
- Current advice is that all patients have a colonoscopy to reassess extent of disease after 8–10 years and then to perform colonoscopy in those with extensive colitis every third year in the second decade of disease, every second year in the third decade and annually thereafter (Fig. 8.3, p. 271; Table 9.5, p. 310)
- The alternative is to offer long-term outpatient follow-up for those with extensive colitis and promptly investigate by colonoscopy any new or persistent symptoms

Indications for surgery
Colectomy is the only cure for ulcerative colitis, although it does not affect some of the extraintestinal manifestations (Table 8.9, p. 268). Colectomy with a temporary ileostomy and later ileoanal pouch construction is now the operation of choice, but proctocolectomy and permanent ileostomy retains a definite place.

Indications for elective surgery
Disease is usually extensive, but colectomy is occasionally needed for distal colitis. The patient should see a stomatherapist and may want to talk to an ileostomist of the same gender and similar age before surgery. Indications are:
- Continuous symptoms (often with general ill health and anaemia) despite treatment or significant medication-related side-effects or toxicities
- Frequent relapses unresponsive to medical treatment that materially affect the patient's life
- High-grade dysplasia, or frank malignancy

Indications for emergency surgery (See p. 275)

Type of operation
- Colectomy and later formation of an ileoanal pouch ('restorative proctocolectomy', J or S pouches) is popular because there is no permanent ileostomy. Good results (continence and five or fewer bowel actions/day) are obtained in 80–90% in experienced hands, but 5% need revision to a permanent ileostomy
- Proctocolectomy with a permanent ileostomy remains the standard procedure for older patients or those with poor continence during acute attacks. Mortality is < 2%, but ileostomy dysfunction occurs in about 15% (Table 8.14)
- For emergency surgery in patients who may subsequently have an ileoanal pouch, subtotal colectomy is appropriate, leaving the rectal remnant in place
- Segmental resection or ileorectal anastomosis cannot be justified in ulcerative colitis, because disease starts distally or will recur in the colonic remnant. A potential exception is in highly selected cases when there is relative rectal sparing *and* when both pelvic dissection (with the small risk of reduced fertility or impotence) *and* a stoma need to be avoided. Continuing symptoms are likely. Patients must recognise that it is only a potential surgical bridge until a family is completed and not a long-term solution

Complications

Toxic dilatation
Clinical features of severe disease with mucosal islands and a colonic diameter of > 6 cm on plain X-ray are diagnostic (Fig. 1.6, p. 41).

Perforation
- Diagnosed by free gas on plain X-ray, usually complicating toxic dilatation when surgery has been delayed too long, or colonoscopy during a severe attack
- Common signs (pain and peritonism) are often few and masked by steroids
- Colectomy after fluid, blood and electrolyte replacement is vital

Massive haemorrhage
- Diagnosis is not difficult except at presentation, when the mucosal pattern may be obscured by blood

Table 8.14 Complications of ileostomies

Early	Late
Ischaemia	Dysfunction (fluid loss > 1500 mL/day)
Wound infection	Small bowel obstruction
Small bowel obstruction	Parastomal herniation
Delayed perineal healing	Stenosis
	Retraction
	Local dermatitis
	Psychosexual/social
	Gallstones
	Renal calculi

- Coagulation should be checked and corrected with FFP if the prothrombin time is > 20 s
- As the underlying disease is likely to recur, colectomy is usually indicated if bleeding has not stopped after transfusing 4 units

Carcinoma (See p. 276)

Management problems

Refractory distal colitis or proctitis
- Distal colitis is resistant to treatment in about 25%, but surgery is better avoided for limited disease. The therapeutic options below also apply to patients who relapse rapidly after a course of steroids, or who appear to be dependent on steroids
- Consider whether poor compliance is contributing and explore the reasons
- Confirm continuing disease activity by sigmoidoscopy and biopsy
- Take a plain abdominal radiograph and treat proximal constipation by sodium pico-sulphate and magnesium citrate (Picolax) 1 sachet orally, magnesium citrate (Citromag 15 g/300 mL, sodium phosphate (Fleet Phospho–Soda) 20 mL with water or polyethylene glycol (Movicol) 2 sachets
- Start mesalazine 1 g suppositories at night, in addition to steroid enemas in the morning. Enemas may bypass the rectum to dwell in the sigmoid colon
- Restart prednisolone 40 mg/day, as for a moderate attack (Table 8.13, p. 273), together with azathioprine 2–2.5 mg/kg/day or mercaptopurine 0.75–1.5 mg/kg/day
- Consider whether IBS is contributing to symptoms (disparity between symptoms and degree of mucosal inflammation). Dietary reduction of resistant starches (p. 340) or milk may help
- Novel therapy with epidermal growth factor enemas may have a role when available, but anecdotal treatment options with lignocaine (lidocaine) 2% gel (10–30 mL twice daily), arsenic suppositories (Acetarsol 250 mg twice daily), bismuth or butyrate enemas have not been substantiated by controlled trials
- Admission for intensive treatment before considering colectomy is appropriate if there is still no response, but patients are best referred to a specialist centre

Osteoporosis
Osteoporosis is common in patients with inflammatory bowel, although the absolute fracture risk is small and role of prophylaxis remains debated. Patients should be encouraged to exercise and have an adequate calcium intake (using supplements if restricting dairy intake). For patients who have been on steroids for more than 3 months in a year, bone mineral density scanning is appropriate and bisphosphonates started (alendronate 70 mg once a week or risedronate 35 mg once a week) if osteoporosis is detected

Pregnancy
- Pregnancy has no consistent effect on colitis
- Maintenance therapy should be continued because long experience with aminosalicylates confirms their safety. Although birth weight may be slightly lower, this may simply reflect disease activity and the risk of relapse is more serious than that of treatment
- Relapse during pregnancy is treated in the standard way

Chronic continuous symptoms

Usually an indication for colectomy if the disease is extensive.

Stomas and pouches

Ileostomists and patients with pouches produce 500–800 mL effluent/day, which is largely fluid and high in sodium and magnesium. Urine volume is decreased to compensate. Ileal adaptation develops over 12 months and volume decreases. Nutrient absorption is normal except when there is coexistent small intestinal disease or terminal ileal resection.

Ileostomy dysfunction

- Ileostomy dysfunction means an overactive ileostomy with an increase in effluent
- Loss of fluid and electrolytes causes lassitude, postural hypotension and dehydration with a classical biochemical picture of hyponatraemia, hyperkalaemia, high urea and hypomagnesaemia
- Partial obstruction (parastomal hernia, adhesions), prestomal ileitis, recurrent disease (in Crohn's), or infection may be the cause, but often no reason is apparent
- Culture of effluent, plain abdominal X-ray and serum electrolytes are necessary. Small bowel radiology, if there is abdominal pain, and urinary and ileal effluent electrolytes guide replacement in severe cases
- Admission and intravenous fluids are indicated if there is clinical evidence of dehydration or postural hypotension
- Prescribe omeprazole 40 mg/day to reduce gastric hypersecretion together with loperamide, up to 20 mg/day once oral intake resumes
- Oral electrolyte solutions (p. 211) are indicated for chronic losses. The amount depends on electrolyte loss, but 2–3 L/day may be needed

Partial ('subacute') small bowel obstruction

- Adhesions, twisted ileal loops, stenosis, recurrent Crohn's disease or parastomal herniation may be the cause
- Ileoscopy with a fibre-optic sigmoidoscope to look for mucosal ulceration is advisable, but may be difficult even in normal ileostomies
- Most settle spontaneously with intravenous fluids, nasogastric suction if there is vomiting and intramuscular pethidine/meperidine 50–100 mg for pain

Stenosis or retraction

- Digital examination of the ileostomy spout will detect stenosis and is advisable at outpatient visits during the first 6 months and if obstruction or bleeding occurs
- Retraction of the spout causes maceration of the skin and difficulties with bag adhesion. Surgical revision is usually necessary

Practical problems

- A specialist nurse (stomatherapist) is invaluable before elective procedures to help plan the site or relieve anxiety and to assist with management after a stoma has been formed
- A badly sited stoma is rapidly recognised by the patient. Revision may be necessary if the stoma substantially interferes with daily activities (including sitting, if at an abdominal crease)

- Odour may be reduced by odour-proof bags or dietary changes (eggs, onions and beans are common culprits)
- Local dermatitis may be due to an allergy to the adhesive, or leaking effluent. Changing the type of appliance and an effective seal are the solutions
- Psychosocial difficulties may be helped through patient support groups (the Ileostomy Association, NACC, CCFA and CCFC, Appendix 1, p. 439), although patients without problems benefit as well

Ileoanal pouches

Indications
- After proctocolectomy for ulcerative colitis or familial adenomatous polyposis and occasionally for other patients with cancer
- Crohn's disease is usually an absolute contraindication, but indeterminate colitis is acceptable if the slightly increased risk of complications is accepted
- Relative contraindications include faecal incontinence during acute attacks, age > 65 years, rectal cancer, during emergency colectomy for severe ulcerative colitis (delay procedure until recovery) and if still planning to conceive (small risk of impotence in men and reduced fertility in women)

Complications
- All the problems of ileostomists may occur with ileoanal pouches
- Pouchitis occurs in 10–20%, causing diarrhoea (occasionally bloody), urgency and an inflamed pouch mucosa. It probably does not occur in pouches for familial adenomatous polyposis. Infection must be excluded and the diagnosis confirmed by pouchoscopy (rigid sigmoidoscopy) and biopsy. Metronidazole 400–500 mg three times daily, ciprofloxacin 500 mg twice daily, or catheter emptying of the pouch should be tried, in that order. Attacks are often isolated, but long-term low-dose metronidazole or ciprofloxacin are potentially effective for chronic pouchitis. VSL3 probiotic therapy (although not widely available) may be used for chronic pouchitis
- Other causes of pouch dysfunction include too small a pouch, incomplete emptying, anastomotic stenosis, cuffitis, or parapouch sepsis. MRI and a pouchogram (isotope or contrast imaging) to assess design and function aid diagnosis
- Local patient groups (such as the Kangaroo Club) provide help and support

Prognosis
- The pattern of relapse and remission 1 year after diagnosis tends to continue for any individual. 90% have intermittent activity and 50% are in remission at any one time. 20% will relapse every year and 10% have continuous symptoms
- Prolonged remission on maintenance therapy occurs, with 50–60% remaining in remission for more than 2 years, but < 5% are symptom-free for 15 years
- Proximal extension in proctitis is rare (< 10%), but occurs in 15–30% with distal or left-sided disease
- The colectomy rate varies with the local approach to refractory disease. Following the approach above, the cumulative colectomy rate in 1161 patients was 24% at 10 years and 32% 25 years after diagnosis

- Distribution of disease affects the likelihood of colectomy. In the study of 1161 patients, 9% with distal, 19% with substantial and 35% with total colitis had a colectomy within 5 years of diagnosis. Thereafter the colectomy rate was 1% per year, whatever the extent
- There appears to be a substantial difference in mortality during a severe attack between those managed in specialist centres (< 1%, including operative mortality) and those managed elsewhere (5%)
- Mortality is otherwise similar to that of the general population
- Up to 12–15% with pancolitis for 20 years develop colonic carcinoma, but some population-based studies have not shown any increased risk (p. 266). The risk of carcinoma in colitis distal to the splenic flexure is no higher than in the general population

8.3 Other types of colitis

General information
If a definitive diagnosis of the type of colitis cannot be made after clinical, endoscopic, histological and radiological examination, this should be stated in the notes. This is an indication for regular follow-up, repeated sigmoidoscopy and biopsy, until a diagnosis is established.

Differentiation between post-infective, ulcerative and diffuse Crohn's colitis is the usual problem (Table 8.12, p. 307). Small bowel radiology is essential if doubt about the diagnosis persists, because typical lesions of Crohn's disease may be asymptomatic.

Indeterminate colitis

Features
- Features of both ulcerative colitis and Crohn's colitis (such as non-bloody diarrhoea with diffuse inflammation on colonoscopy, or bloody diarrhoea with relative rectal sparing and histology suggesting ulcerative colitis, or clinical and endoscopic features of ulcerative colitis, but histology showing submucosal inflammation)
- Distinction between ulcerative colitis and Crohn's colitis is not possible in 10–15%
- Incidence may be 2 : 100 000 and prevalence 27 : 100 000 (giving a total prevalence of inflammatory bowel disease of up to 450 : 100 000 in one study in primary care, or just less than 1 : 200 population)

Treatment
- As for ulcerative colitis
- Careful histological examination of colectomy specimens by an experienced gastrointestinal pathologist prior to ileoanal pouch surgery is necessary in cases of diagnostic doubt. Patients with indeterminate colitis appear to do as well with ileoanal pouch surgery as those with ulcerative colitis, although there is some evidence that a substantial proportion subsequently turn out to have Crohn's colitis

Microscopic colitis

Features
- Watery diarrhoea in the presence of a normal colonoscopy and chronic inflammation in the absence of crypt architectural distortion on mucosal biopsies
- Often female, aged > 60 years, but can occur in much younger patients
- Drugs are implicated as the cause in up to 50% (usually NSAIDs, but also PPIs such as lansoprazole)
- Three types have been defined:
  - lymphocytic colitis, with an increased number of intraepithelial lymphocytes
  - collagenous colitis, with a subepithelial collagen band > 10 μm thick
  - microscopic colitis not-otherwise-specified (NOS), with chronic inflammation but no collagen band or intraepithelial lymphocytes
- Drugs may more commonly cause collagenous colitis, but there are no other clinical differences between the types, and more than one type may occur in the same individual at different times
- Other causes of diarrhoea (Table 7.1, p. 207), including coeliac disease, should be excluded

Treatment
- Stop NSAIDs or PPIs
- Mesalazine 2 g/day is effective in about 50%
- Cholestyramine 4–12 g/day is effective in about half
- Budesonide 9 mg daily is effective in most and is indicated if a prompt response is needed or other trials of treatment fail
- About two-thirds resolve, a quarter improve and the remainder have a relapsing course that needs intermittent or continuous treatment

Diversion colitis

Inflammation in the defunctioned loop of a colostomy, causing a mucous discharge, usually responds to topical steroid enemas. Thought to be due to epithelial short chain fatty acid deficiency and sodium butyrate, enemas may be effective, although these are not commercially available.

Pseudomembranous colitis

Features
- Caused by *Cl. difficile*, usually after prolonged or multiple antibiotics, especially ampicillin or clindamycin
- *Cl. difficile* causes about 4% of acute gastroenteritis in adults and cases in hospitals are increasing exponentially. PPIs predispose to infection
- Pseudomembranous colitis only represents the severe end of the spectrum
- Diagnosed by sigmoidoscopy (punctate, adherent yellow–white plaques on an inflamed rectal mucosa) and detecting *Cl. difficile* toxin in stool. Histology may be diagnostic if a plaque ('summit lesion') is included in the biopsy, but may be difficult

to distinguish from ulcerative colitis or ischaemic colitis (Box 9.1, p. 318). Either condition may coexist

Treatment

- Oral metronidazole 400–500 mg three times daily for 1 week in the first instance
- Relapse may occur (up to 30%) and should be treated with vancomycin 125–250 mg four times daily for 1 week or longer (sometimes several weeks, decreasing the dose gradually)
- Both antibiotics and steroids (p. 273) are advisable if doubt exists about the diagnosis of pseudomembranous or acute ulcerative colitis, followed by colonoscopy once symptoms resolve
- Recurrent infection despite metronidazole and vancomycin is rare and patients are best referred to a specialist centre

Ischaemic colitis (See p. 321)

9 Large Intestine

9.1 Constipation

No single definition of constipation suffices, but most define it by one or more of the following symptoms: the passage of hard stools, infrequent stools (typically < 3/week), the need for straining, a sense of incomplete evacuation, excessive time spent on the toilet, or unsuccessful defecation.

- Constipation affects 2–27% of Western populations, is more common in women, non-whites, children and the elderly. Patients' reporting of constipation depends on early training, preoccupation with the bowel and their expectations (p. 291)
- Risk factors include physical inactivity, low income, limited education, a history of sexual abuse and a history of depression

Classification

Constipation can be classified into three broad categories, although more than one mechanism can contribute in any one individual.

Normal transit ('functional') constipation
- The cause in 60% of patients presenting
- Stool transit and frequency are normal, but patients describe constipation due to hard stools or difficulty with evacuation

Slow transit constipation
- Present in about 15% of patients, typically young women who are otherwise in good health. Onset at puberty is typical
- Characterised by infrequent bowel movements (once a week or fewer), infrequent urge to defecate, bloating and abdominal pain
- The diagnosis is important and should be distinguished from constipation-predominant IBS, because lifelong use of osmotic laxatives is needed, often in large doses
- Barium enema is usually unnecessary, but rarely shows faecal loading in a dilated colon—idiopathic megacolon (p. 296). Patients typically have delayed emptying of the proximal colon and fewer high-amplitude contractions after eating
- Histopathological studies have shown alterations in the number of myenteric plexus neurons and concentration of peptide neurotransmitters

Defaecation disorders
- Present in about 25% of patients
- Recognised by difficulty in initiating evacuation, prolonged and unsuccessful straining, sensation of incomplete evacuation, and often a history of rectal or vaginal digitation to help expel stool

- Most commonly due to dysfunction of the pelvic floor or anal sphincter leading to an inability to coordinate abdominal, recto-anal and pelvic floor muscles during defecation
- Structural abnormalities such as rectal intussusception, rectocele and excessive perineal descent (Descending perineum syndrome, p. 296) are less common causes
- Attempts to avoid pain associated with an anal fissure may contribute to defecation disorders

Causes

- Diet or faulty bowel habit cause the vast majority, but less common, treatable causes should not be overlooked (Table 9.1)
- Dietary causes are common in the elderly or depressed, although tricyclic antidepressants and pseudo-obstruction are additional causes in these groups
- Faecal impaction in the elderly or mentally impaired may cause spurious diarrhoea, urinary retention or exacerbate neurological irritability
- Chronic stimulant laxative use may cause cathartic megacolon, hypokalaemia or melanosis coli
- Neurological disorders may cause constipation due to inactivity or failure of rectal sensation and rectal reflexes. Constipation is a key feature of spinal cord lesions (such as transection, transverse myelitis or cauda equina tumours). Drugs often contribute to constipation in Parkinson's or cerebrovascular disease
- Aganglionosis (due to Hirschsprung's or Chagas' disease) very rarely presents in adults, with constipation and megacolon

Investigation

History
- Determine the frequency, nature and consistency of stool, so as to establish whether the patient really is constipated. Also ask about duration, diet and drugs

Table 9.1 Causes of constipation

Common	Uncommon	Rare
Age	Anorectal disease	Metabolic/endocrine
Diet	Fissure	Hypothyroidism
Inadequate fibre	Stricture	Hypercalcaemia
Immobility	Mucosal prolapse	Hypokalaemia
Pregnancy	Rectocele	Porphyria
Motility disorders	Descending perineum syndrome	Lead poisoning
Irritable bowel syndrome	Intestinal obstruction	Hypopituitarism
Idiopathic slow transit	Carcinoma	Neurological disorders
Drugs	Pseudo-obstruction	Aganglionosis
Opiates	Anorexia nervosa	Hirschsprung's disease
Anticholinergics	Neurological disorders	Chagas' disease
Iron	Cerebral disease	Autonomic neuropathy
Aluminium antacids	Spinal cord lesions	Myopathy

Unusual postures on the toilet, digitation of the rectum or posterior vaginal pressure to facilitate emptying suggest a defecation disorder

Examination
- The perianal area should be examined for scars, fistulae, fissures and external haemorrhoids
- Perineal descent should be examined with the patient bearing down to identify *excessive descent* (below the plane of the ischial tuberosity or > 3.5 cm) indicates laxity of the perineum (usually due to childbirth or many years of excessive straining) and suggests a defecation disorder. *Limited descent* indicates an inability to relax the pelvic floor muscles during defecation, sometimes with prolapse of rectal mucosa
- Rectal examination should determine whether faecal impaction, stricture, or masses are present. The sphincter tone at rest and during voluntary contraction should be noted. Palpation of the posterior rectal wall may identify spasm of the pelvic floor; a defect in the anterior wall is suggestive of a rectocele
- Testing perineal sensation is essential in severe constipation when considering spinal cord pathology

Initial investigations
- The most important investigation is careful clinical examination, including assessment of perineal descent (above and p. 296)
- Blood tests—full blood count, electrolytes, calcium and thyroid function tests will identify most organic causes
- Investigation of the entire colon is indicated in all patients > 50 years, and in younger patients when accompanied by alarm symptoms (e.g. new onset or worsening of constipation, blood in the stools, weight loss, family history of colorectal cancer). Flexible sigmoidoscopy is best performed on patients < 50 years, without alarm symptoms, who do not respond to initial dietary measures

Physiological investigations
- Only necessary in patients with symptoms refractory to both a high-fibre diet and laxatives
- *Colonic transit studies* are indicated when the bowel frequency is less than once a week, but without features of a defaecation disorder. This will help distinguish slow transit from normal transit constipation. Fybogel three sachets/day or psyllium 15–20 g/day is given for 2 weeks (to eliminate dietary causes of slow transit), then 20 oral radio-opaque markers are taken at once. Plain abdominal X-rays at 2 and 5 days normally show > 75% excretion of markers by day 5 (Fig. 9.1). If the markers are retained exclusively in the lower left colon, the patient may have a defecation disorder
- *Balloon expulsion* is a simple test for defaecation disorders but does not define the aetiology. A positive test is defined by the inability to expel a latex balloon filled with 50 mL of water within 2 min. Missing a defaecation disorder consigns a patient to intractable symptoms, but this test is usually limited to specialist centres
- *Anorectal manometry* should be performed if a defecation disorder is suspected. Inappropriate contraction of the anal sphincter at rest and while bearing down is common. Absent anorectal inhibitory reflex suggests Hirschsprung's disease, but is

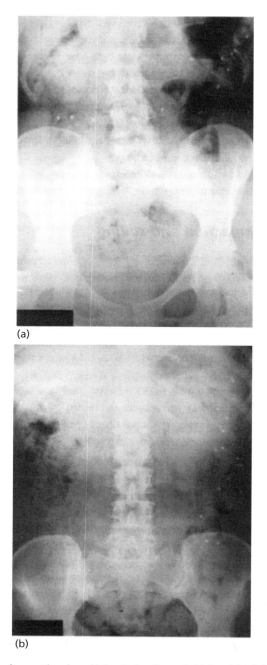

(a)

(b)

Fig. 9.1 Slow transit constipation. Abdominal radiograph (a) 3 and (b) 5 days after ingesting Ed: 20 radio–opaque markers, all of which remain visible, indicating prolonged transit. (*Source*: From Travis SPL. *Shared Care in Gastroenterology*, by permission of Isis Medical Ltd.)

more commonly due to enlargement of the rectum as a result of retained stool. Hyposensitivity to balloon distension suggests a neurological disorder but is more commonly due to increased rectal capacity after prolonged stool retention

- *Defaecography* (defaecating proctogram, Fig 9.2) is appropriate if the results of these investigations are equivocal, or if there is a suspected structural abnormality impeding defaecation. Incomplete emptying of the rectum, reduced change in the anorectal angle (< 15°), reduced perineal descent (< 1 cm), or the presence of a substantial rectocele, enterocele, mucosal prolapse, or intussusception indicates a defaecation disorder (p. 291). Isotope defaecating proctography quantifies the degree of hold-up, but is only available at specialist centres

Other investigations
- *MRI* to exclude a spinal cord or cauda equina lesion if there has been recent onset or progression of symptoms over < 12 months
- *Isotope colonic transit studies* help discriminate between *colonic* and *isolated rectal* slow transit. This is important when considering surgery for intractable cases (below), because ileorectal anastomosis is inappropriate if there is rectal slow transit

Management

General recommendations
- Take a careful and empathetic history. Many patients will have had their symptoms dismissed as 'poor diet', and uncommon causes (such as defaecation disorders) are usually missed because they have not been considered

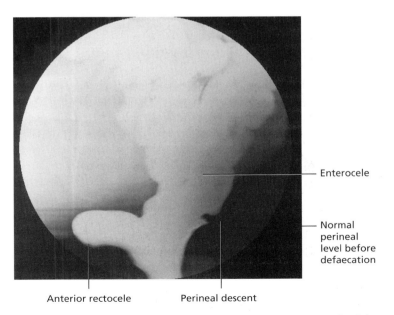

Fig. 9.2 Defaecating proctogram. Defaecation disorder—marked (5 cm) perineal descent, anterior rectocele and sigmoid enterocele.

- Constipation due to colonic, anorectal or systemic disease must be identified and treated appropriately
- The patient's idea of a normal bowel habit should be discussed. Aim for a soft, easily passed motion every 1–2 days
- Re-education is an important part of improving bowel habit:
  - do not ignore the urge to defecate
  - develop a regular time for defecation each day
  - avoid excessive straining—this makes defecation disorders worse
  - avoid prolonged sitting

Diet

- Increased *fibre* intake is the key for patients with normal transit constipation, but is not always well tolerated due to flatulence or bloating. Aim for a gradual increase to 20–25 g/day, either with changes in diet or with fibre supplements. This must be accompanied by adequate fluids (about 1500 mL/day), which the elderly are sometimes reluctant to increase
- *Fibre* (p. 341) is complex. Effects depend on solubility (water-holding capacity, which softens the stool) and fermentability (which produces short-chain fatty acids that accelerate transit, but also generate gas). *Insoluble fibre* (such as wheat bran) increases stool bulk and is least fermentable, but does not trap much water. *Soluble fibre* traps most water, but is most readily fermented. Isphagula (Fybogel) or psyllium (Metamucil, Normacol, Prodiem) is recommended, because it is more soluble than wheat bran and resists fermentation
- 100% wholemeal bread, leguminous vegetable (peas, beans and lentils) and fruit are simple dietary changes (p. 388)
- A tablespoon of bran (added to breakfast cereal, yoghurt or soup) may be necessary, but it should be of the coarse-milled variety
- If bloating or flatulence are prominent, then the intake of soluble fibre (soft fruits) is best reduced
- If constipation alternates with liquid stools, then golden linseed added to yoghurt, soups, or cereals offers a good balance between soluble and insoluble fibre
- Constipation due to slow transit, colonic strictures or spinal cord lesions are usually exacerbated by increased dietary fibre and osmotic laxatives are more useful

Laxatives

Laxatives are indicated to alleviate painful defecation, when straining will exacerbate a condition (such as a hernia), for drug-induced constipation, or before surgery or colonic examination. There are four groups of laxatives and over 60 different preparations, but bran and an osmotic laxative, with only an occasional stimulant, work for most. The diagnosis should be reassessed if two sorts of laxative are ineffective. The ultimate sanction for simple constipation is magnesium sulphate. Any laxative is dangerous in obstruction.

Bulk-forming laxatives

- For functional constipation and painful anorectal conditions, with extra fluid
- Isphagula husk (Fybogel), or sterculia (Normacol) are more palatable than coarse bran (1–2 tbsp/day), but more expensive

Osmotic laxatives
- Poorly absorbed or non-absorbed substances that lead to water secretion into the intestine. Most take several days to start to work
- Indicated when bulk-forming laxatives are ineffective, for proximal constipation in ulcerative colitis or hepatic encephalopathy
- For patients with renal or cardiac insufficiency, osmotic laxatives may cause volume overload due to absorption of sodium; absorption of magnesium and phosphate may lead to hypermagnesemia or hyperphosphatemia particularly in patients with renal insufficiency
- The dose of lactulose (30–100 mL/day) is easy to regulate according to effect. Gas and bloating are common due to bacterial fermentation in the colon
- Sodium picosulphate with magnesium citrate (Picolax 1–2 sachets) works for intractable constipation (p. 294), but has some stimulant action. Smaller doses (Laxoberal 5–20 mL daily, available over the counter in the UK; oral Fleet Phosphosoda (sodium phosphate) or Citromag (magnesium citrate) in North America) can be given regularly to prevent recurrence
- Polyethylene glycol (PEG-3350, Movicol, MiraLax) 1 or more sachets or heaped tbsp daily helps chronic constipation and is the osmotic laxative of choice if lactulose cannot be tolerated. It is not metabolised by colonic bacteria and therefore causes less gas and bloating and has no role in hepatic encephalopathy. It is also effective for faecal impaction (p. 294)

Stimulant laxatives
- Act within hours by increasing intestinal motility and secretions
- For opiate-induced constipation, bowel clearance, neurological disorders or temporary use in stubborn constipation. Long-term use should be avoided because of a perceived risk of causing a 'cathartic colon'
- Colic may be exacerbated
- Anthraquinones (e.g. Senna 2–4 tablets at night) are converted to their active form by colonic bacteria and act the following morning. May cause melanosis coli
- Bisacodyl (e.g. Dulcolax 5–10 mg at bedtime or in the morning) can be used for occasional treatment of severe constipation
- Codanthrusate (1–3 capsules, or 5–15 mL at night) should be given to patients on long-term morphine to prevent constipation, but carries a carcinogenic risk so should otherwise be avoided

Faecal softeners
- Glycerine suppositories or a disposable enema (such as Micralax, or Relaxit or Fleet Enema) are useful for stubborn cases and can be given by a district nurse 2–3 times a week to prevent recurrent faecal impaction
- Docusate sodium is a safe and modestly effective stool softener. It can be given as a 100 mg capsule once or twice daily and provides relief in patients with mild constipation but is generally ineffective in more severe cases; it is also available in a liquid solution of 20 mg/5 mL.
- Liquid paraffin can cause granulomas or lipoid pneumonia, and is not recommended

Management of defaecation disorders

- Initial management includes dietary advice, avoidance of straining at stool, exclusion of serious disease and addressing psychological factors contributing to symptoms
- *Biofeedback* using psychological retraining in conjunction with anorectal electromyography or manometry catheter helps up to two-thirds, but may not be widely available. A good rapport between therapist and patient is central to successful treatment
- Rectal surgery (such as rectopexy) should be considered only for large rectoceles, prolapse or rectal–rectal intussusception, when conservative measures have failed. The functional significance and approach should be discussed between surgeon, radiologist and gastroenterologist, because inappropriate surgery can make symptoms worse
- Psychological distress and anxiety are often prominent, but care should be taken to distinguish between those that are a *result of* an unrecognised defaecation disorder and those *contributing* to symptoms. This is often difficult, but if there is a disparity between severity of symptoms and radiological or manometric abnormality, it is best to avoid surgery
- Preliminary data suggests that injection of botulium toxin into the puborectalis muscle may help those whose pelvic floor does not relax during defaecation. Specialist advice is appropriate
- Topical rectal steroids (e.g. steroid containing suppositories) may relieve bleeding from rectal mucosal prolapse, but are otherwise unhelpful since the condition is not primarily inflammatory. Colonoscopy and repeat biopsies are indicated if rectal biopsies are equivocal, to exclude Crohn's disease and other pathology

Management of slow transit constipation

- The bowel should initially be cleared with Picolax (1–3 sachets), then osmotic laxatives in sufficient doses (lactulose 50–150 mL daily, PEG (e.g. Movicol or MiraLax 1–3 sachets or 1–2 heaped tbsp daily), or Laxoberal 10–20 mL daily). Where Picolax is not available, Dulcolax can be given prior to an osmotic laxative. The patient should adjust the dose according to the stool consistency
- Stimulant laxatives may be needed at times of crisis (no defaecation for > 7 days), but regular use should be avoided, because of the risk of cathartic colon. Bulking agents frequently make abdominal pain worse and recognising this is often greeted with relief by the patient

Intractable constipation

- Many patients with chronic constipation have tried 'all the laxatives'
- First, make a record of the dose, duration and type of all that have been tried; also make note of results and side-effects
- Then work from first principles: retake the history, consider in particular the possibility of a defaecatory disorder, repeat a careful clinical examination including perineal sensation and descent, perform a proctosigmoidoscopy, check that the calcium, thyroid function and other appropriate tests have been performed and then discuss a constipation strategy with the patient

- The best strategy is usually to clear the bowels out with Picolax or Dulcolax (bisacodyl), followed by a regular osmotic laxative in effective (often large) doses to prevent 'silting up' again. Polyethylene glycol (Movicol or MiraLax 1–3 sachets daily or 1–2 heaped tbsp daily) is often best tolerated. An appropriate diet with plenty of fluid is important, but excessive fibre can be counterproductive
- Avoid using two laxatives with the same mode of action and increase the dose of any laxative to a maximum, before changing the type
- Consider the use of novel agents (e.g. tegaserod 6 mg twice daily, a partial $5-HT_4$ agonist)
- Total colectomy and ileorectal anastomosis should be reserved for patients with intractable slow transit constipation. It should *only* be considered if a defaecation disorder or isolated rectal slow transit has been excluded (these patients do badly after surgery because obstructive defaecation persists, or have psychological problems that have not been addressed). Some of these patients may have a more diffuse motility disturbance that also involves the small intestine. In these patients an ileorectal anastomosis may not be effective. Such patients can be identified by means of radio-opaque marker transit studies
- Antegrade colonic evacuation (ACE) procedure is being developed as an alternative to colectomy for patients with slow transit. A button stoma is made in the caecum so that 1 L of water can be instilled daily to act as a lavage. A major advantage is that it can be reversed if unhelpful. Specialist evaluation is appropriate. A loop ileostomy can also be tried. It also has the advantage that it can be reversed if unsuccessful and, if successful, the patient can subsequently undergo a colectomy and end (Brooke's) ileostomy

Faecal impaction and soiling

Faecal impaction is distressing for the patient and may cause stercoral ulceration. Patients usually have neurological disease, or are elderly with multisystem disease. A history of long-standing constipation is followed by anismus, spurious diarrhoea or general irritability in the neurologically impaired. Diagnosis is made by rectal examination revealing a hard mass of stool.

- Polyethylene glycol (Movicol, 8 sachets in 1 L drunk over 6 h) is effective and usually tolerated
- Regular osmotic laxatives (p. 293) or stimulant laxatives in neurological constipation are necessary to prevent recurrence
- In faecal soiling, regular enemas (Micralax, Relaxit, or Fleet Enema three times weekly) will keep the rectum empty and prevent soiling
- Faecal soiling in younger patients is often a feature of psychological distress, which should be explored. It may be a feature of sexual abuse. Biofeedback to relearn early recognition signals of the urge to defecate may help, along with appropriate psychological support

Megacolon

- Megacolon or megarectum in adults is usually idiopathic. A long history of constipation is usual, although it may be intermittent and interspersed with episodes of faecal impaction with spurious diarrhoea. A barium enema is diagnostic. Aganglionosis must be excluded by anorectal manometry (p. 431). Full-thickness rectal biopsy and

silver stain to show the myenteric plexus is only justified if manometry shows inhibition of sphincteric relaxation
- Idiopathic megacolon is treated in the same way as slow transit constipation, but referral to a specialist centre is necessary for manometry and makes subsequent management easier. Laxatives must be continued for life, to avoid episodes of faecal impaction, and this should be made clear to the patient and the general practitioner

Descending perineum syndrome

Women are most commonly affected, sometimes as a sequel to pudendal nerve damage during childbirth. Marked perineal descent (> 3.5 cm) during excessive straining at stool causes a sensation of incomplete evacuation and further straining. This results in rectal mucosal prolapse, ulceration and bleeding. Eventually the stretching of the pelvic floor associated with excessive descent may injure the sacral nerves, reducing rectal sensation resulting in incontinence.

Solitary rectal ulcer

This presents with rectal bleeding and a sensation of incomplete evacuation and must be distinguished from proctitis, Crohn's disease or carcinoma. Patients are often male. Constipation with excessive straining at stool is thought to cause mucosal prolapse with anterior rectal inflammation. Solitary rectal ulcers are sometimes caused by insertion of a finger or foreign body, in a desperate attempt to initiate defaecation by severely constipated patients. Sigmoidoscopy shows a patch of erythema, a single, or sometimes several ulcers. Biopsies are diagnostic and are essential to exclude Crohn's disease, carcinoma or other causes of rectal ulcers (p. 252). Histopathology characteristically shows the muscularis interdigitating into the mucosa, with some fibrosis.

9.2 Colonic polyps

Adenomatous polyps precede colorectal cancer, which can be prevented by the early recognition and treatment of polyps. Not all polyps are premalignant.

Classification

Polyps are mucosal projections into the lumen and may be sessile or pedunculated. There are four types, which cannot be reliably distinguished macroscopically, so polypectomy and histology are always indicated.

Metaplastic
- Commonest type (75% of those in the rectum of adults > 40 years, often multiple, usually sessile, shiny and < 5 mm in diameter)
- No malignant potential

Adenomas
- Adenomas are defined by appearance (pedunculated, sessile or flat) and histology (tubular, villous, tubulovillous, serrated)

296

- Common (50% of colonic polyps in patients > 55 years)
- 25% are multiple
- 30–40% of Western populations will develop an adenoma by age 60, but the lifetime cumulative incidence of colorectal cancer is only 2–3%. Adenomas are diagnosed on average 10 years earlier than colorectal cancer, providing one line of evidence for the adenoma–carcinoma sequence
- Malignant potential in an individual is related to *size* (higher risk with size > 10 mm), *histology* (villous > tubulovillous > tubular, or presence of dysplasia), and *number* of polyps (> 5)
- *Flat* or *depressed* adenomas may progress more rapidly than polypoid adenomas. They account for 10–30% of cancer in Japan but appear to be uncommon in the West
- *Villous* adenomas tend to recur locally after removal
- *Serrated* adenomas have a characteristic 'saw-toothed' histological appearance and have a lower malignant potential

Inflammatory
- Pseudopolyps after severe colitis of any cause
- May have a sessile or cylindrical (finger-like) appearance
- Not neoplastic

Hamartomatous
- Juvenile polyps are developmental malformations, often large, pedunculated and vascular, but usually solitary. Very rarely there are multiple (> 5) polyps–juvenile polyposis (p. 300)
- Peutz–Jeghers syndrome of buccal pigmentation and multiple small intestinal hamartomas also affects the colon in over 50% (p. 300)
- No apparent malignant potential, but occasional foci of dysplasia in solitary polyps increase the risk of small or large bowel cancer in Peutz–Jeghers syndrome and juvenile polyposis
- Cronkhite–Canada syndrome (p. 239) is a rare disorder affecting middle-aged adults, causing diffuse gastrointestinal polyposis (adenomas), malabsorption due to protein-losing enteropathy, nail dystrophy and hyperpigmentation. It is not inherited. Antibiotics may help diarrhoea due to bacterial overgrowth, but there is no specific treatment

Other
- *Nodular lymphoid hyperplasia* in the rectum or terminal ileum is a normal variant in young people and recognised histologically, although radiological features may resemble Crohn's disease or polyposis (p. 242)
- *Pneumatosis coli* (p. 302) can be mistaken for multiple polyps or Crohn's disease by the uninitiated
- Lipomas, leiomyomas or neurofibromas occasionally occur in the colon, but are generally of no significance
- GISTs, including malignant leiomyosarcomas and other rare tumours rarely present as polypoid colonic lesions; GISTs are addressed in Chapter 3 (p. 101)

Clinical features

Most colonic polyps are asymptomatic and detected on barium enema or endoscopy for unrelated gastrointestinal symptoms. Some present with rectal bleeding at any age, but diarrhoea (sometimes with profuse mucus and hypokalaemia) is a rare presentation of a villous adenoma.

Management

- Colonoscopy is currently the gold standard for the detection and removal of polyps although it may miss up to 25% of small polyps. Polyps identified on sigmoidoscopy or barium enema are an indication for total colonoscopy and polypectomy
- All polyps must be examined histologically and the pathologist should say whether polypectomy has been complete
- Suspicious or partially removed polyps can be marked for follow-up or surgical identification by 'tattooing', with 1 mL intramucosal Indian ink
- Complications of polypectomy include immediate (2%) or delayed (2% up to 2 weeks) bleeding. Perforation occurs in 0.06–2.0% of polypectomies
- Polyps recur in 30–40% of patients, so surveillance is appropriate
- The interval from a small polyp to malignancy is measured in years and may be more than a decade. Explanation of the polyp–cancer sequence is important and should reassure patients, who might otherwise think that every examination can be expected to reveal a cancer
- Optimum timing for surveillance remains a matter for debate. Guidelines differ between countries depending on the local factors driving health care. The British Society of Gastroenterology guidelines (2002) are shown in Fig. 9.3). Surveillance is stopped depending on age and comorbidity. It is an individual decision, but at age 75, life expectancy is likely to be less than the average time for new adenomas to become malignant. American guidelines from the US Multisociety Task Force on Colon Cancer (Winawer S *et al.*, *Gastroenterology* 2003) and Canadian guidelines from the Canadian Association of Gastroenterology and the Canadian Digestive Health Foundation (Leddin D *et al.*, *Can J Gastroenterol* 2004) are also available

Inherited polyposis syndromes

The variety of rare, inherited polyposis syndromes is daunting, but the key point is a careful family history and specialist genetic referral if two or more cancers have occurred in first-degree relatives.

Familial adenomatous polyposis

- Characterised by multiple (> 100) adenomatous colonic polyps that invariably progress to colorectal cancer at a mean age of 40, unless colectomy is performed. An attenuated form with fewer polyps is recognised
- The incidence is about 1 : 10 000 live births. Autosomal dominant caused by mutations in the APC (tumour suppressor) gene (detected in 65–95% of families). 30–50% of cases are sporadic due to new mutations

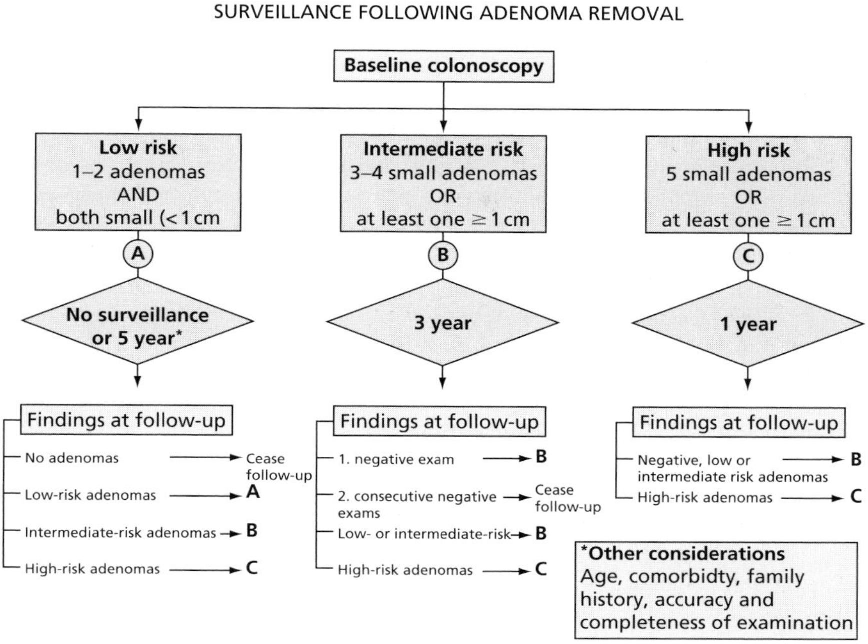

SURVEILLANCE FOLLOWING ADENOMA REMOVAL

```
                          ┌─────────────────────┐
                          │ Baseline colonoscopy │
                          └─────────────────────┘
```

Low risk
1–2 adenomas
AND
both small (< 1 cm

(A)

**No surveillance
or 5 year***

Findings at follow-up
- No adenomas ────────── Cease follow-up
- Low-risk adenomas ────────── **A**
- Intermediate-risk adenomas → **B**
- High-risk adenomas ────────── **C**

Intermediate risk
3–4 small adenomas
OR
at least one ≥ 1 cm

(B)

3 year

Findings at follow-up
1. negative exam ────────── **B**
2. consecutive negative exams ────── Cease follow-up
- Low- or intermediate-risk→ **B**
- High-risk adenomas ────────── **C**

High risk
5 small adenomas
OR
at least one ≥ 1 cm

(C)

1 year

Findings at follow-up
- Negative, low or intermediate risk adenomas ────────── **B**
- High-risk adenomas ────────── **C**

*Other considerations
Age, comorbidty, family history, accuracy and completeness of examination

Fig. 9.3 Surveillance programme for patients with adenomatous polyps. (*Source:* Atkin W, Saunders B. *Gut* 2002; **51(Suppl V):** v7)

- Polyps may occur in childhood, but the increased cancer risk starts in teenagers. Gastric cancer and small intestinal adenocarcinoma are also more common
- Rare variants include Gardner's syndrome (colonic polyposis and osteomas) and Turcot's syndrome (colonic polyposis and medulloblastoma). Other rare associations are congenital hypertrophy of the retinal pigment epithelium (CHRPE), papillary thyroid carcinoma, adrenal carcinoma and large intra–abdominal desmoid tumours

Management

- Early diagnosis is the key to management, usually achieved by meticulous screening of family members (Table 9.5, p. 310). This requires flexible sigmoidoscopy (colonoscopy is generally unnecessary) of all children of the index case, starting at age 12–15, and continuing annually until polyps are detected (indicating the need for colectomy) or until age 40. Endoscopic screening can be replaced by genetic testing in families with a known pathogenic APC mutation. Mutation–positive members and members of families in which no mutation is identified need subsequent endoscopic screening
- Once the diagnosis is made the operation of choice is a proctocolectomy with permanent ileostomy or ileoanal pouch anastomosis. Ileoanal anastomosis should be avoided as it carries a 25% of cancer developing at the anastomosis at 20 years

- The details of all UK patients should be sent to the FAP Registry (St Mark's Hospital, Northwick Park, Harrow, Middlesex)
- Ophthalmological examination to detect congenital hypertrophy of the retinal pigment epithelium (see above), causing multiple areas of pigmentation in the peripheral retina, is appropriate, because this can aid screening of relatives if present
- Long-term follow-up is essential, not only to manage pouch function but also to detect other complications. Ampullary carcinoma is more common and screening by biennial endoscopy (including the use of a side-viewing duodenoscope) is advocated. Chronic abdominal pain may be caused by desmoid tumours, diagnosed by CT scan. Pouchitis (p. 281) is extremely rare in ileoanal pouches for familial adenomatous polyposis, unlike ulcerative colitis

Prognosis
Although colectomy prevents colorectal cancer, mortality is still more than twice the general population owing to the development of desmoid tumours, duodenal or ampullary carcinoma.

Juvenile polyposis
- The syndrome is caused by mutations in at least two genes, SMAD4/DPC4 and BMPR1A/ALK3. The incidence is about 1 : 100 000 live births
- Characterised by multiple hamartomatous polyps (typically 50–200) in the colon, rectum, stomach and small intestine
- The risk of colorectal cancer is 10–40% and gastric cancer 20%
- Endoscopic polypectomy of both upper and lower gastrointestinal tract polyps is the aim of treatment. This decreases the cancer risk and symptoms such as bleeding and diarrhoea
- Colectomy and ileorectal anastomosis is recommended for patients with a very large number of polyps
- Screening of family members is detailed (Table 9.5, p. 310); clinical screening may be replaced by genetic testing in families with a known pathogenic mutation

Peutz–Jeghers polyposis
- Autosomal dominant cancer predisposition syndrome caused by mutations in the LKB1 gene. The incidence is about 1 : 50 000 live births
- Characterised by mucocutaneous melanin pigmentation and hamartomatous polyps, which affect predominantly the small intestine but also the stomach and colon. Excess of non-gastrointestinal cancers include endometrial, ovarian and lung
- Isolated labial freckles in asymptomatic individuals without any family history of malignancy are not due to Peutz–Jeghers, although an occasional cause of gastroenterology referral
- Affected patients require polyp clearance every 2 years by upper gastrointestinal endoscopy and colonoscopy
- Complications from small bowel polyps are common and require intraoperative endoscopy via enterotomies
- Screening of family members is detailed in Table 9.5 (p. 310) but may be replaced by genetic testing in families with a known pathogenic mutation

Hereditary non-polyposis colorectal cancer

- Autosomal dominant cancer syndrome that accounts for 5–8% of colorectal cancer. Associated with germline mutations in mismatch repair genes (MSH2, MLH1, MSH6, PMS1, PMS2). More than 90% of HNPCC demonstrate microsatellite instability (compared to 10% of sporadic colorectal cancers)
- Colon cancer develops predominantly in the right colon at a mean age of 45 without polyposis (although preceded by adenomas). Synchronous or metachronous colonic tumours occur in > 40% of patients
- Other tumours include endometrial, stomach, ovary, ureter, renal pelvis, bile ducts, kidney, small intestine and brain
- A thorough family history is critical to the identification of affected families. According to the Amsterdam II criteria (less stringent than the former Amsterdam I criteria) all of the following conditions should be fulfilled:

Amsterdam II Criteria for diagnosing HNPCC
1. ≥ Three family members with HNPCC-related cancers of whom one is a first-degree relative of the other two
2. ≥ Two generations with colorectal cancer
3. ≥ One HNPCC-related cancer diagnosed before age 50

Indications for HNPCC genetic testing
1. Colorectal cancer patients in families that meet the Amsterdam II criteria
2. Individuals with two HNPCC-related cancers
3. Individuals with colorectal cancer and a first-degree relative with colorectal cancer and/or HNPCC-related extracolonic cancer and/or adenoma; one of the cancers diagnosed < 50 years and the adenoma diagnosed < 40 years

---

- Some patients who do not meet the above high-risk criteria should be prescreened by testing of biopsy material. Evidence of microsatellite instability (increased in HNPCC) and/or loss of gene expression by immunohistochemistry is an indication to then carry out genetic testing:

Indications for immunohistochemistry of biopsy tissue before HNPCC genetic tests
1. Individuals with colorectal or endometrial cancer < 50 years
2. Individuals with adenomas diagnosed < 40 years

- First-degree relatives should have colonoscopic screening every 2 years beginning at age 25 or 5 years before earliest colorectal cancer in family (Table 9.5, p. 310). Gastroscopy should be offered every 2 years from age 50 or 5 years before earliest gastric cancer in family. Endometrial suction biopsy combined with endovaginal ultrasound should be carried out every 2 years after age 25. Endoscopic screening to detect at-risk individuals may be replaced by genetic testing in families with a known pathogenic mutation. However, endoscopic surveillance is required in all patients with known pathogenic mutations or, in the absence of a mutation, in all patients who have a family history that fulfils the criteria for HNPCC.

Pneumatosis coli (pneumatosis cystoides intestinalis)
- A rare condition with gas-filled submucosal cysts that look like polyps at colonoscopy, but which collapse on needle aspiration. A plain X-ray or barium enema shows multiple radiolucencies along the wall of the bowel, or throughout the abdomen if the small intestine is involved. It may be misdiagnosed as multiple polyps, Crohn's disease, lymphoma or carcinoma if the diagnosis is not recognised at colonoscopy or barium enema. Histology of colonic biopsies is diagnostic. Submucosal spaces and associated giant cells are characteristic.
- There may be no symptoms, but diarrhoea with bleeding, mucus or abdominal pain is common. No cause can usually be found, although it may be associated with emphysema
- Treatment is only necessary for symptoms. 70% inspired oxygen through an oxygen mask and rebreathing apparatus for 5 days usually gives relief for long periods. The improvement in colonoscopic appearance is dramatic. Oxygen should be used with care if the patient has emphysema. Metronidazole has been advocated, but is rarely helpful. Hyperbaric therapy also has its advocates, but is very rarely necessary if atmospheric oxygen is properly administered. Persistent symptoms are often due to coexistent irritable bowel

9.3 Colorectal cancer

Adenocarcinoma of the colon is the commonest malignancy in Britain after lung cancer (lifetime incidence 2–3%, about 20 000 deaths per year in the UK). It is potentially curable and preventable.

Causes
The polyp–dysplasia–cancer sequence is now generally accepted. Adenocarcinomas almost always arise from pre-existing adenomatous polyps except in ulcerative or Crohn's colitis. The proposed sequence from normal mucosa through hyperplastic to adenoma then carcinoma is accompanied by serial mutations, first in the APC gene, then in the *ras* oncogene, followed by inactivation of the p53 tumour suppressor gene, resulting in loss of control of epithelial growth and repair mechanisms. Other mutations are certainly involved.
- Genetic—sporadic colorectal cancer is considered a polygenic disorder susceptible to environmental influences. Although only 1% have familial adenomatous polyposis, acquired mutations in the APC gene occur in up to 80% of all colorectal cancers and at least 50% have mutations in the *ras* oncogene
- Environmental—lack of dietary fibre causing slow transit and excessive fat with increased exposure to toxic bacterial products of digestion may explain the prevalence in Western communities. Colonic cancer is rare in the Far East and Africa, but the incidence is increasing. How dietary factors influence gene mutations is not understood
- Chronic inflammation (ulcerative or Crohn's colitis, p. 276) increases the risk

Clinical features

- Features vary with the site of the tumour. Most colorectal cancers are left-sided, but one-third are proximal to the splenic flexure. Cancers associated with pancolitis are evenly distributed
- Bleeding—less than half have visible rectal bleeding. Fresh blood on the outside of faeces does not exclude a tumour, which may coexist with haemorrhoids. Negative occult blood tests do not exclude a colorectal cancer
- Change in bowel habit—more common in distal tumours. Tenesmus is common in rectal cancer. Any patient with change in bowel habit over the age of 45 years should be referred for investigation
- Abdominal pain is non-specific. It may be due to spasm, partial obstruction in distal lesions or local invasion in caecal tumours
- Anorexia, weight loss or an abdominal mass (especially caecal) are late features, but do not always indicate incurable disease
- Emergency presentation with obstruction (15%, usually at the splenic flexure), perforation (< 5%) or other reason (anaemia, jaundice) occurs in 30%
- Iron-deficiency anaemia (IDA) in middle-aged men or postmenopausal women suggests a caecal neoplasm until proven otherwise (Section 9.7, p. 327)
- Colorectal cancer is an unusual cause of a persistent pyrexia, and is rarely the cause of pyogenic liver abscesses

Investigations

Patients with rectal bleeding, change in bowel habit or IDA (especially in men and post-menopausal women) must always be investigated for colonic cancer. Once the diagnosis is established, operability must be assessed.

Initial investigations

Rigid or flexible sigmoidoscopy

- Any patient with rectal bleeding
- If colon cancer or polyps are discovered, the whole colon should then be examined by colonoscopy or barium enema, because cancers may be multiple in 3%. The term 'synchronous' describes more than one tumour at one time and 'metachronous' a second tumour after resection of the first

Blood tests

- Anaemia may be the only feature of caecal tumours. ESR is often normal
- Raised ALP may be due to hepatic or bony metastases. Elevated γ-GT or AST indicates hepatic origin

Colonoscopy

- Appropriate initial colonic investigation for patients with rectal bleeding, change in bowel habit, polyp(s) seen on sigmoidoscopy, or those with a strong family history of colorectal cancer
- Detects polyps or cancer that has been missed at barium enema in 20–30% with rectal bleeding

- Provides a histological diagnosis, which is desirable before surgery, but not essential if radiological appearances are typical

Barium enema
- Radiological features of cancer are strictures with shouldering ('apple core'), or irregular filling defect in the bowel wall (Fig. 9.5, p. 314)
- Colonoscopy is necessary if a barium enema is normal or views were poor in a patient with persistent rectal bleeding
- Barium enema may be the preferred initial investigation of choice for patients with a change in bowel habit in areas where the waiting list for colonoscopy is excessive

CT Colonography
- The sensitivity of this technique is improving and may be reaching levels comparable to colonoscopy. It offers the advantage that sedation is not usually required. Adequate bowel preparation is required for optimal visualisation and diagnostic accuracy. Findings usually require colonoscopic confirmation and treatment of resectable polypoid lesions. Rectal air insufflation (pneumocolonography) may enhance resolution, but the most important factor seems to be the imaging software in the helical CT scanner
- A CT colon (different to CT colonography, see p. 425) does not require bowel preparation other than oral gastrograffin and is appropriate for elderly (age > 80 years) or frail patients who would tolerate barium enema or colonoscopy badly

Staging investigations
The purpose of staging is to define the extent of tumour spread and aid decision-making before and after surgery. The TNM (Tumour, Node, Metastasis, Table 9.2) classification is internationally accepted, but some surgeons and pathologists still use Dukes' staging (Table 9.3). This is further complicated by the overall staging of the Cleveland Clinic (I–IV, Table 9.3).

Table 9.2 TNM Staging of colorectal cancer

Stage	Description
T: Primary tumour	Tx: Cannot be assessed
	To: No evidence of tumour
	T1, T2, T3, T4: Different depths of invasion
N: Lymph nodes	Nx: Cannot be assessed
	No: No nodes
	N1: Positive nodes
M: Distant metastasis	Mx: Cannot be assessed
	Mo: No metastasis
	M1: Metastasis
R: Resection margin	Rx: Cannot be assessed
	Ro: No involvement
	R1: Involved

Cancers are defined by the combination of features for each patient (e.g. T3, N1, M0), to which may be added the results of resection (R).

Table 9.3 Dukes' and Cleveland Clinic staging and prognosis in colorectal cancer

Stage	Description for patients	5-year survival (%)
Dukes' A (T1–2, N0, M0) Stage I (Cleveland Clinic)	Tumour limited to the bowel wall. It has spread beyond the innermost lining of the colon to involve the inside wall of the colon, but has not spread to the outer wall of the colon or outside the colon.	95–100
Dukes' B (T3–4, N0, M0) Stage II (Cleveland Clinic)	Tumour extends through the muscular wall of the colon to the outside surface, but there is no cancer in the lymph nodes	65–75
Dukes' C (T any, N1, M0) Stage III (Cleveland Clinic)	Tumour has spread outside the colon to one or more lymph nodes. Tumours within the colon wall are classified as Dukes' Stage C1, while tumours that have grown through the wall, and have spread, are classified as Dukes' Stage C2.	30–40
Dukes' D (T any, N either, M1) Stage IV (Cleveland Clinic)	Tumour has spread outside the colon to other parts of the body, such as the liver or the lungs. The tumour can be of any size and may or may not include affected lymph nodes	< 1

Imaging

- *Abdominal CT scan*—appropriate for all patients to identify nodal or metastatic spread
- *Pelvic MRI*—appropriate for rectal cancers, because it provides better definition of tumour margins and mesorectal spread than CT scan. This correlates with local recurrence and helps decision-making about preoperative downstaging radiotherapy or chemoradiation
- *Endoanal ultrasound*—for rectal cancers without extramural spread (T1 or T2, stage I, Table 9.3), to identify T1-2 tumours amenable to local excision. Correlation of ultrasound and pathologic T-scores approaches 80–90%

Surgery

Preoperative management

- Staging should be complete and discussed at a multidisciplinary meeting with surgeons, histopathologists, radiologists, medical and radiation oncologists and nurse specialists to decide strategy for any preoperative downstaging chemoradiotherapy (p. 307)
- The site and prospect of a possible stoma should be discussed with the patient with the support of a stomatherapy nurse specialist
- Bowel preparation is needed before elective surgery. Prophylactic antibiotics (intravenous metronidazole 500 mg and cefuroxime 750 mg three times daily, although

regimes vary) should be started on induction and continued for 24 h. Low molecular–weight heparin should be given 2 h before surgery and continued until the patient's discharge

Rectal cancer (below the peritoneal reflection)
- Experienced colorectal or oncologic surgeons produce the best results in terms of survival and local recurrence, making a strong case for subspecialisation in surgery
- *Anterior resection* (rectal excision and total mesorectal excision, TME, with stapled anastomosis and no colostomy) is now possible provided that at least 10 mm of full-thickness rectal wall can be resected distal to the tumour. *Abdominoperineal resection* is now reserved for very low rectal tumours. Consequently preservation of sexual and urinary function is possible in 80–95% of patients
- *Transanal endoscopic microsurgery* (TEM) may be considered by an experienced surgeon for favourable tumours (size < 3 cm, located within 8 cm of the anal verge, staged by endoanal ultrasound as T1-2, N0, involving < 40% of the rectal circumference)

Colon cancer
- The surgical procedure is determined by the cancer location. For caecal and ascending colon cancers a right hemicolectomy and ileo-transverse anastomosis is performed. For transverse colon cancers a transverse colectomy, left or right extended hemicolectomy, or subtotal colectomy with ileo-sigmoid anastomosis may be performed (no comparative data is available to help make the choice between these options). For distal colon cancers a left hemicolectomy or segmental colectomy is performed
- There is no difference between sutured and stapled anastomoses
- Laparoscopic surgery is improving and evidence from a large randomised trial comparing laparoscopic with open surgery suggests that there is no difference in the two techniques with respect to tumour recurrence or survival

Obstructive colorectal cancer
- Obstructive colorectal cancer carries a poor prognosis (< 20% survival at 5 years)
- For obstructive right colonic cancers primary anastomosis is usually feasible
- For obstructive left colonic cancers, options include diversion loop colostomy, Hartmann's procedure (resection of the left colon, closure of the rectal stump and end colostomy), resection and primary anastomosis, or the use of a self-expanding metal stent (SEMS)
- SEMS are transforming management of sick, elderly patients with distal colonic obstruction. SEMS may be used as a bridge to surgery, or as a definitive palliative procedure. Stenting at the time of emergency presentation permits resolution of the obstruction, giving time to resuscitate the patient and perform accurate staging. Patients with potentially curable disease may then be offered surgical resection and primary anastomosis

Adjuvant therapy
Adjuvant therapy may be pre- or postoperative and include chemotherapy, radiotherapy, or both. The sequence and optimal combination is hotly debated. Several ran-

domised controlled trials are in progress and colorectal surgeons should work closely with an oncology colleague. Decisions are made on expert local opinion, but the following is a synthesis of current data.

Rectal cancer

• *Preoperative radiotherapy* is frequently used for patients with stage II or III disease (Table 9.3, p. 305), because this reduces the rate of local recurrence and may improve overall survival by 10%. Radiotherapy may be short course (5 days) or long course (6 weeks). Opponents cite the need for a defunctioning colostomy prior to radiotherapy and debate the benefit

• *Preoperative combined chemotherapy and radiotherapy* should be considered for patients with distal rectal tumours (stage II and III) to downstage tumours and facilitate sphincter-sparing surgery

• *Postoperative chemotherapy* in stage II and III disease is based on 5-fluouracil (5-FU), with an additional agent (irinotecan or oxaliplatin). Local expert advice is appropriate and the threshold for using irinotecan or oxaliplatin is lower in the USA than in Europe

• *Adjuvant chemoradiotherapy after TEM* should be considered for all patients with T2 tumours and those with T1 tumours with high-risk histological features (poorly differentiated, lymphatic, or blood vessel involvement)

• Patients with unresectable disease should be carefully discussed at the multidisciplinary meeting (above) to agree on the best palliation of local symptoms (bleeding, pain, continence). Radiotherapy is useful for controlling pain; laser ablation or argon plasma coagulation for bleeding and poor continence is likely to necessitate defunctioning. The benefit of chemotherapy and all treatment modalities should be discussed with the patient

Colon cancer

• The overall survival benefit from chemotherapy is modest (around 7% absolute benefit), but chemotherapy extends disease-free intervals and delays recurrence. The benefits and side-effects should be carefully discussed between patient and oncologist and a joint decision made. Care should be taken to be realistic rather than over-optimistic, but also not to destroy hope

• Adjuvant therapy with 5-FU and leucovirin should be considered for patients with stage III disease and high-risk patients with stage II disease (e.g. T4 tumours or tumours associated with obstruction or perforation)

• Irinotecan and oxaliplatin are second-line agents (for recurrent disease or intolerance of first-line therapy) in Europe, but are increasingly used as part of first-line combination chemotherapy

• The role of radiotherapy is not well defined but appears limited to patients with cancer invading or adherent to surrounding structures and palliation of pain

Surveillance

• Local protocols vary, but despite complex protocols involving colonoscopy, CT scanning, and carcinoembryonic antigen (CEA) measurements, an overall survival benefit has yet to be demonstrated

• Surveillance colonoscopy is recommended for patients who have had a curative resection, since this reduces recurrent carcinomas. If preoperative colonic evaluation was incomplete, colonoscopy should be performed within 6 months of resection to look for synchronous tumours. Following this, colonoscopy is appropriate every 3–5 years (see Appendices 1 and 2)

- A CT scan should be performed once during the first 2 years after resection, to detect operable liver metastases. Some advocate ultrasound surveillance every 6–12 months in younger patients to detect liver metastases at a resectable stage
- A detailed family history and screening of relatives at risk of cancer is essential (Tables 9.4 and 9.5, pp. 309, 310)
- CEA measurements are often used as an adjunct to surveillance, but early recognition of recurrence through a rising CEA increases the lead-time without conferring an overall survival benefit
- Resection of isolated (< 3, none > 5 cm) hepatic metastases should be considered at a specialist centre in younger (age < 65) patients, because survival appears to be improved. The age, size and number of metastases considered suitable for resection are increasing

Secondary chemoprevention
A randomised controlled trial of the use of aspirin in patients with previous colorectal cancer has demonstrated a 35% reduction of recurrent adenomas. Further work is required before aspirin can be recommended as secondary chemoprevention. Even if recommended, it will not replace the need for colonoscopic surveillance.
Recurrent or inoperable disease

- Symptoms of obstruction or clinically significant recurrent rectal bleeding must be relieved even when a cure is not possible, because the quality of life (and death) is poor with no intervention
- SEMS provide effective palliation for obstructive colonic lesions. A high rate of stent displacement limits its use in patients with rectal cancers. Local laser therapy, ethanol injection or argon plasma photocoagulation help alleviate bleeding

Prognosis

Histopathological criteria of spread and differentiation are the most useful guide. The TNM and Dukes' classification are most widely used (Tables 9.2 and 9.3, p. 304).

- Well-differentiated tumours have a better prognosis than poorly differentiated tumours at any stage
- Older patients have a higher operative mortality. Young patients may have more aggressive tumours, but this is disputed
- Women have a better prognosis than men
- Duration of symptoms is inversely related to prognosis, except in obstruction, when survival is halved, or perforation, when 5-year survival is < 10%

Screening for colorectal cancer

Screening aims to detect cancer at a treatable stage. The target groups and method of screening remain controversial, but there is good evidence that screening for colorectal cancer in the general population over the age of 50 would be at least as cost-effective as mammography screening for breast cancer.

Table 9.4 Summary of recommendations for non-familial colorectal cancer screening and surveillance in high-risk groups

Disease groups	Screening procedure	Time of initial screen	Screening procedure and interval
Colorectal cancer			
Colonic adenomas	Consultation + LFTs + colonoscopy	Colonoscopy within 6 months of resection only if colon evaluation preoperatively incomplete	Liver scan within 2 years postoperative Colonoscopy 5-yearly until age 70
Low risk			
1–2 adenomas, both < 1 cm	Colonoscopy	No surveillance, or repeat at 5 years	Cease follow-up after negative colonoscopy
Intermediate risk			
3–4 adenomas, or at least one adenoma > 1 cm	Colonoscopy	3 years	Every 3 years until two consecutive negative colonoscopies, then no further surveillance
High risk			
≥ 5 adenomas or ≥ 3 at least 1 cm	Colonoscopy	1 year	Annual colonoscopy until out of high-risk group, then interval colonoscopy as per intermediate risk group
Large sessile adenomas removed piecemeal	Colonoscopy or Flexi Sig (depending on polyp location)	3-monthly until no residual polyp; consider surgery	
Ulcerative colitis or Crohn's colitis	Colonoscopy + biopsy every 10 cm	Pancolitis 8 years, left-sided colitis 15 years from onset of symptoms	Colonoscopy 3-yearly in second decade, 2-yearly in third decade and annually thereafter; four biopsies every 10 cm
IBD and PSC +/– liver transplant	Colonoscopy	At diagnosis of PSC	Annual colonoscopy with four biopsies every 10 cm
Uretero-sigmoidostomy	Flexi Sig	10 years after surgery	Flexi Sig annually
Acromegaly	Colonoscopy	At age 40	Colonoscopy 5-yearly

Table 9.5 Summary of recommendations for familial colorectal cancer screening and surveillance in high-risk groups

Family groups	Lifetime risk of death from colorectal cancer	Screening procedure	Age at initial screen	Screening procedure and interval
Familial adenomatous polyposis	1 : 2.5	Genetic testing + Flexi Sig + OGD	Puberty	Flexi Sig 12 monthly. Colectomy if +ve
Juvenile polyposis or Peutz-Jeghers	1 : 3	Genetic testing + colonoscopy + OGD	Puberty	Flexi Sig 12 monthly. Colectomy if +ve
At-risk hereditary non-polyposis colorectal cancer (according to Amsterdam criteria) > two first-degree relatives MMR carriers	1 : 2	Colonoscopy +/− OGD	Aged 25 or 5 years before earliest colorectal cancer in family. Gastroscopy at age 50 or 5 years before earliest gastric cancer in family	2 yearly colonoscopy and gastroscopy
Two first-degree relatives with colorectal cancer	1 : 6	Colonoscopy	At first consultation or at age 35–40 years, whichever is the later	If initial colonoscopy clear, then repeat at age 55 years
One first-degree relative < 45 years with colorectal cancer	1 : 10	Colonoscopy	At first consultation or at age 35–40 years, whichever is the later	If initial colonoscopy clear, then repeat at age 55 years

Source: Cairns S, Schofield J. *Gut* 2002; **51**(Suppl V): v28)

General population

Screening asymptomatic individuals at standard risk of colorectal cancer aims to detect polyps that are premalignant, or cancer at a curable stage. The present options are faecal occult blood testing (FOBT) or flexible sigmoidoscopy although many specialists, particularly in the USA, advocate the use of colonoscopic screening in the general average-risk population.

Faecal occult blood testing

- Haemoccult is a guaiac-based home-test kit that requires collection of two samples from each of three consecutive stools, which are smeared onto cards and mailed to a processing laboratory. If any of the six cards is positive, the test should be repeated after dietary exclusion of red meat for 5 days, and if still positive, colonoscopy is recommended because up to 50% will have a colorectal cancer or large adenoma ($\geq$ 1 cm)
- Haemoccult screening is the only test shown in a randomised controlled trial to reduce mortality from colorectal cancer (annual frequency—33% reduction; biennial frequency—20% reduction). Unlike the alternative (flexible-sigmoidoscopy screening) it has no effect on the incidence of colorectal cancer. Pilot projects are taking place in Australia (www.health.gov.au/pubhlth/strateg/cancer/bowel/index.html) and the UK (www.cancerscreening.nhs/colorectal/pilot-evaluation.html)
- The problems are low take-up rate (54–75%), poor sensitivity (30–50% for cancer and < 20% for adenomas), false-positive results due to components of the diet (red meat, aspirin, horseradish), bias towards motivated patients (potentially at higher risk) and possible earlier detection of less aggressive tumours (lead-time bias)
- Immunochemical tests (used routinely in Japan) for haemoglobin or other blood components are more sensitive but less specific
- Faecal analyses for tumour DNA markers (k-ras, APC, p53 and BAT26) are being developed. Further studies are required to determine their sensitivity and specificity for screening, but are unlikely to alter the incidence of colorectal cancer or overcome the problem of acceptability

Flexible sigmoidoscopy

Flexible sigmoidoscopy every 3–5 years from the age of 50 is now recommended in the USA, but a single examination at age 55–60 years may be as effective. This would identify most polyp-formers allow more intensive surveillance and reduce the incidence of cancer by removing the polyps. Three randomised trials are underway and will provide additional useful information to help guide practice.

Other techniques

- Colonoscopy screening at 10-year intervals has been endorsed in the USA despite the additional procedural risks and lack of evidence that it reduces proximal colorectal cancer. A pilot study is awaited
- CT and MRI colonography is being investigated as a tool to screen out people without neoplasia to minimise the number of unnecessary colonoscopies. Oral contrast consumed on the day before screening may obviate the need for bowel preparation

High-risk groups

The British Society of Gastroenterology has issued endoscopic screening guidelines (2002) for high-risk individuals. These include previous colorectal cancer (p. 302), inherited polyposis syndromes (p. 300), ulcerative colitis or Crohn's colitis (Chapter 8, p. 266) and acromegaly (Chapter 13, p. 402). These are detailed in Tables 9.4 and 9.5. Faecal occult blood screening in these high-risk groups is not worthwhile, because it has a low negative predictive value.

9.4 Colonic diverticular disease

The prevalence of colonic diverticula increases with age. In developed countries diverticula are present in 50% of the population aged > 50 years but 90% of patients are asymptomatic, Although rare in developing countries, the prevalence is rising, coincident with increasing Westernisation likely as a result in changes in dietary intake patterns.
- The overall prevalence of diverticula is equal in men and women. However, under age 40 symptomatic disease may be more common in men (sex ratio 3.25 : 1)
- 'Colonic diverticulosis' is a more appropriate term than 'diverticular disease' to describe the presence of uncomplicated diverticula. This avoids the connotations of the word 'disease', which may worry patients unnecessarily
- The natural history of colonic diverticulosis is shown in Fig. 9.4. In about 10% of patients diverticulosis may become complicated by bleeding, inflammation (diverticulitis), perforation or abscess formation

Asymptomatic diverticulosis

Diverticula are frequently an incidental finding on barium enema. In developed countries the sigmoid colon is affected in 95% of patients and is the exclusive site in up to

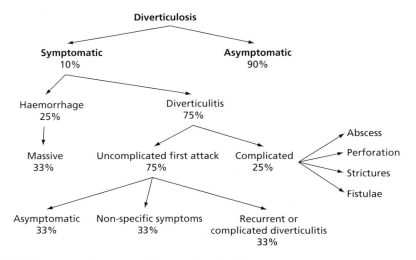

Fig. 9.4 The natural history of colonic diverticulosis.

50% of these cases. Right-sided colonic diverticula are more common in people <40 years and in Asian populations.

Symptomatic uncomplicated diverticulosis

Symptoms

It remains debatable whether uncomplicated diverticula can cause any symptoms. It is likely that colonic symptoms in the elderly are due to IBS and coexistent diverticulosis, but colorectal cancer must always be considered (Fig. 9.5).

Common symptoms
- Colicky left iliac fossa pain relieved by defaecation, lasting for weeks or months. Pain is sometimes central or in the right iliac fossa, and persistent
- Constipation (which is thought to promote formation of diverticula), with pellet-like stools, often covered in mucus
- Bloating and flatulence
- Rectal bleeding, recently altered bowel habit, right-sided or upper abdominal pain, diarrhoea or tenesmus must not be attributed to diverticulosis without investigation

Diagnosis
- Characteristic symptoms, normal blood tests (full blood count, ESR) and diverticula on barium enema or CT scan are sufficient for diagnosis
- Rigid sigmoidoscopy should always be performed before a barium enema, because the rectum can be more closely examined. A biopsy should always be taken, because histology may show disease (Crohn's, or microscopic colitis) even when the rectal mucosa looks normal
- Colonoscopy is only indicated when a barium enema shows distortion of the bowel wall in association with diverticula, but should be performed by an experienced colonoscopist because of the risk of perforation. Carcinoma, Crohn's disease, ischaemia, or a pericolic abscess from diverticulitis may be impossible to distinguish radiologically from muscle hypertrophy or stricture and, in those instances, colonoscopic evaluation is required

Management
- Increasing dietary fibre (p. 388) relieves pain if constipation is present, but existing diverticula do not regress
- Antispasmodic agents (dicyclomine 10–20 mg, hyoscine 10–20 mg, mebeverine 135–270 mg, or two peppermint oil capsules three times daily) may help pain
- Stimulant laxatives should be avoided for treating constipation because these may increase colonic pressure and provoke pain. Osmotic laxatives (p. 293) are preferable

Complicated diverticulosis

Diverticulosis may be complicated by mucosal inflammation (diverticular colitis), subserosal inflammation (diverticulitis), abscess formation, perforation, bleeding, or obstruction. Altogether these complications are responsible for > 40% of all emergency admissions to hospital with large bowel pathology.

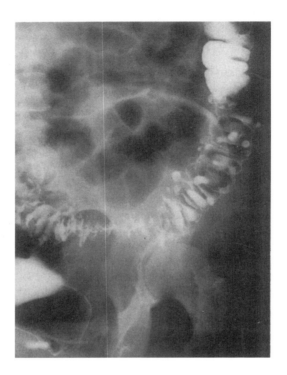

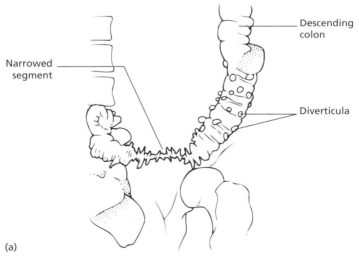

(a)

Fig. 9.5 Colorectal cancer. (a) Barium enema showing a typical annular carcinoma in the mid-sigmoid. *(Continued)*

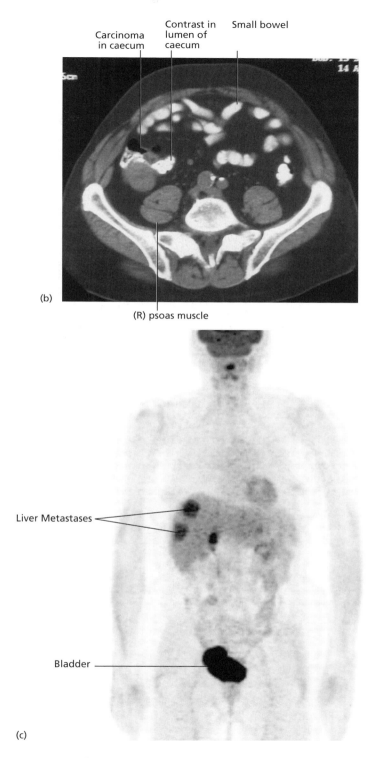

(b)

Carcinoma in caecum

Contrast in lumen of caecum

Small bowel

(R) psoas muscle

Liver Metastases

Bladder

(c)

Fig. 9.5 *(continued)* (b) CT colonography showing a caecal carcinoma. (c&d) PET scan showing colorectal metastases in (c) coronal

315

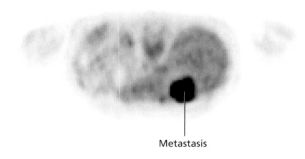

Metastasis

Fig. 9.5 *(continued)* (d) cross-sectional plane.

Diverticular colitis

Sigmoid mucosal inflammation may be seen in up to 25% of patients with diverticulosis. Clinically and histologically it may mimic inflammatory bowel disease presenting with diarrhoea and the passage of blood and mucus. Caution is required before labelling someone as having ulcerative or Crohn's colitis on a background of diverticular disease. The discriminating test is a rectal biopsy. If this shows chronic inflammation, then this *excludes* diverticular colitis since diverticula are never rectal.

Diverticulitis

- Diverticulitis is recognised by pain, fever, leucocytosis and an elevated ESR. Urinary symptoms may result from a sympathetic cystitis but colovesical fistulae with urinary tract infections can occur (see below). Right-sided diverticulitis may mimic appendicitis. Prior symptoms are often absent
- CT scanning is the most appropriate investigation if there is diagnostic doubt, but patients are often treated without diagnostic confirmation if attacks are recurrent
- Pericolic abscess is suggested when a mass is palpable. It may present with obstruction
- Colonoscopy is contraindicated in the acute stage, but may be done when symptoms settle if diverticulitis cannot be distinguished from a carcinoma or Crohn's disease on CT scan
- Management of mild cases of diverticulitis is usually with oral antibiotics (metronidazole 400–500 mg three times daily plus cephradine 500 mg four times daily or ciprofloxacin 500 mg twice daily), but severe cases or diverticulitis in the elderly, the immunosuppressed or those without adequate social support need admission to hospital. In hospital, up to 90% will settle with conservative medical management (intravenous fluids, intravenous antibiotics and analgesia). A CT scan is indicated if a mass is palpable, to exclude an abscess. Surgery is necessary for abscesses, perforation or fistulae. Subsequent treatment with bulking agents and osmotic laxatives (p. 293) are indicated to treat constipation and reduce recurrence
- Portal pyaemia with liver abscesses is often due to diverticulitis in the elderly, but can also be due to a colorectal cancer or appendicitis
- Following the first admission with diverticulitis, one-third will remain asymptomatic, one-third will experience non-specific abdominal symptoms and one-third will have further attacks. Surgery should be considered after two episodes of diverticulitis if

316

the disease is localised, because the recurrence rate rises to 90%. CT colonography or barium enema should define the distribution of diverticula. There is some evidence that recurrent diverticulitis is more common in patients presenting with a first attack at a young age, and in these patients earlier surgical intervention should be considered

Perforation

- Perforation may present with peritonitis, pelvic, paracolic or subphrenic abscess. Chronic pyrexia, ill health and weight loss may be the only features in the elderly or debilitated. Only 20% have a previous history of diverticular disease
- Mortality following perforation is up to 30%, reflecting comorbidity in elderly population
- Risk of perforation and subsequent mortality is particularly high in immunocompromised patients
- Fistulation (colovesical, colovaginal) occurs in 20% of patients with complicated disease. The risk is lower in women because interposition of the uterus affords some protection

Bleeding

- Accounts for 40% of all cases of lower gastrointestinal haemorrhage. Up to 80% of bleeding diverticula are right-sided
- Risks associated with bleeding include increased age, male gender, use of NSAIDs and anticoagulants
- > 90% will settle with conservative management. FFP should be given if the patient is taking anticoagulants
- Rebleed rate in patients who do not receive definitive therapy is 9% at 1 year, rising to 25% at 4 years. After two episodes of haemorrhage the risk of rebleeding rises to 50%
- IDA is never due to uncomplicated diverticulosis. Carcinoma, ulcerative colitis, Crohn's disease and angiodysplasia must be excluded by colonoscopy, but angiography during active bleeding may be necessary to detect the site of bleeding (p. 21)
- Colonoscopic therapy should be attempted by an experienced colonoscopist for persistent diverticular bleeding

Obstruction

- Recurrent attacks of diverticulitis may lead to the development of a fibrotic stricture and subsequent colonic obstruction. Coexistent carcinoma should be excluded by flexible sigmoidoscopy
- Small bowel obstruction during an episode of diverticulitis is more common and is usually due to involvement of small bowel loops in the inflammatory mass

Indications for surgery

Surgery is only indicated for complications of diverticulosis (Box 9.1). Segmental colectomy for symptomatic diverticulosis is very rarely necessary, and only after medical treatment has been vigorously tried and other causes of symptoms have been excluded.

- Recurrent diverticulitis is unusual, but can be cured by resection and primary anastomosis once the acute episode has settled

---

> **Box 9.1 Indications for surgery in diverticulosis**
>
> Infection
>   recurrent diverticulitis
>   paracolic or pelvic abscess
>   peritonitis
> Perforation
> Fistulae
>   colovesical
>   colovaginal
>   ileocolic
> Obstruction
> Major haemorrhage

- Abscesses are best localised by CT scan and drained percutaneously. Colonic resection is rarely necessary, because perforated diverticula causing an abscess usually seal spontaneously
- Patients with perforated diverticula and peritonitis need adequate rehydration and parenteral antibiotics (e.g. metronidazole 500 mg and cefuroxime 750 mg three times daily) before emergency laparotomy. Resection of the affected colon and a double-barrelled colostomy is probably best, but when it is not possible to mobilise an inflamed mass of sigmoid colon, resection with closure of the rectal stump and a colostomy (Hartmann's procedure) is then necessary. Attention to nutrition in the postoperative period is vital, because such patients are often frail, elderly and debilitated
- Fistulae are treated by sigmoid colectomy and closure of the bladder or vaginal connection
- Obstruction can be managed conservatively if incomplete (p. 54), but total colonic obstruction needs decompression by a transverse colostomy, with later resection of the stricture

Prognosis
Treating uncomplicated, symptomatic diverticulosis with increased dietary fibre appears to reduce the complication rate to around 5%.

9.5 Intestinal ischaemia

Intestinal ischaemia includes small intestinal ischaemia, but this is rare compared to ischaemic colitis. Vascular disease may be acute or chronic, but does not always involve arterial occlusion. Focal ischaemia (due to vasculitis) or venous infarction are rare.

Vascular anatomy
The gut is supplied by the coeliac axis (CA), superior mesenteric artery (SMA) and inferior mesenteric artery (IMA) (Fig. 9.6). The stomach and rectum (supplied by CA and inferior mesenteric vessels) are well protected by oesophageal and internal iliac anas-

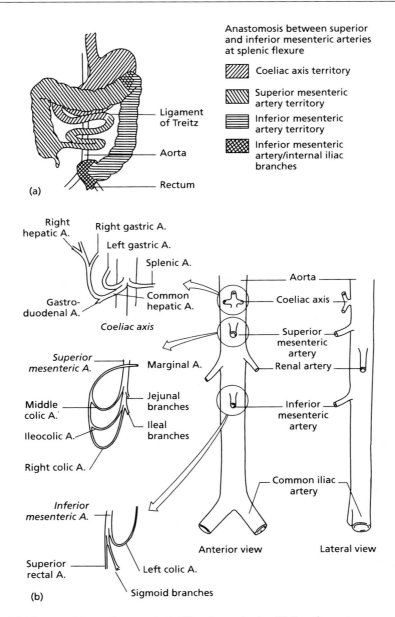

Anastomosis between superior and inferior mesenteric arteries at splenic flexure

- Coeliac axis territory
- Superior mesenteric artery territory
- Inferior mesenteric artery territory
- Inferior mesenteric artery/internal iliac branches

Ligament of Treitz

Aorta

Rectum

(a)

Right hepatic A.

Right gastric A.

Left gastric A.

Splenic A.

Aorta

Gastro-duodenal A.

Common hepatic A.

Coeliac axis

Coeliac axis

Superior mesenteric artery

Superior mesenteric A.

Marginal A.

Renal artery

Jejunal branches

Middle colic A.

Inferior mesenteric artery

Ileal branches

Ileocolic A.

Right colic A.

Inferior mesenteric A.

Common iliac artery

Superior rectal A.

Left colic A.

Anterior view

Lateral view

(b)

Sigmoid branches

Fig. 9.6 **Mesenteric vascular supply.** (a) Vascular territories. (b) Vascular anatomy.

tomoses, respectively. Branches of SMAs and IMAs anastomose through a variable marginal artery, which means that the splenic flexure is at particular risk from ischaemia. Ischaemic colitis is usually microvascular, with no apparent large vessel disease.

Causes

Although there are many causes (Table 9.6), intestinal ischaemia is rare and there are only four clinical syndromes: acute, chronic, or focal intestinal ischaemia, which usually affect the small intestine, and ischaemic colitis.

Acute intestinal ischaemia

See p. 32.

Chronic intestinal ischaemia

Chronic small intestinal ischaemia is rare and no randomised studies on diagnosis and treatment are available.

Clinical features

- Abdominal pain starting within 20–60 min after eating and lasting 1-4 h ('mesenteric angina') in an elderly patient with other cardiovascular disease
- Weight loss, because the patient becomes afraid to eat
- Audible epigastric bruit, but this is often absent and may be normal in thin adults

Management

- The diagnosis should be suspected in an elderly arteriopath when other causes of postprandial pain and weight loss have been excluded

Table 9.6 Causes of intestinal ischaemia

Common	Uncommon	Rare
Atheroma	*Systemic emboli*	*Thrombosis*
stenosis	atrial thrombus	polycythaemia
thrombosis	bacterial endocarditis	sickle cell
embolization	*Non-occlusive infarction*	oral contraceptive
	cardiac failure	antithrombin III deficiency
	septicaemia	factor V Leiden mutation
	trauma	protein C deficiency
	anaphylaxis	antiphospholipid antibodies
		microvascular
		Vasculitis
		rheumatoid arthritis
		polyarteritis nodosa
		systemic lupus
		Takayasu's disease
		Behçet's disease
		Miscellaneous
		aortic dissection
		infiltration by tumour
		iatrogenic (cardiac catheters)
		intestinal volvulus

- *Duplex ultrasound* is an excellent validated screening tool for occlusive disease of the CA and SMA. Chronic intestinal ischaemia is an unlikely diagnosis if the SMA is widely patent
- *Multiplane three vessel angiography* remains the gold standard and should be performed if intervention is planned. Unlike ultrasound, it reveals nothing about arterial flow.
- *CT scan with three-dimensional reconstruction* of the abdominal arteries can provide excellent images of the large to medium-sized vessels without the need for arterial puncture; it is useful when screening for atherosclerotic disease or fibromuscular hyperplasia
- *Magnetic resonance angiography* and tonometry may provide information on the functional deficiency of the splanchnic circulation. It is appropriate if the technical ability to perform duplex ultrasound is not available, or if duplex scanning is negative and the diagnosis still suspected
- Treatment is difficult. Small, frequent meals are advisable
- Angioplasty or arterial reconstructive surgery has been shown to give long-term symptom relief in most patients suitable for surgery, but risks are high since most patients have extensive vascular disease and other comorbidity

Focal intestinal ischaemia

Trauma, radiation, vasculitis or drugs (enteric-coated potassium, slow-release anti-inflammatory drugs) may cause focal ischaemic damage. These cause a small intestinal stricture that presents as subacute obstruction: bleeding or perforation rarely occurs. Diagnosis is made by small bowel enema or enteroscopy (where available) since it may be overlooked on barium follow-through. Management is surgical, to exclude other causes (Box 7.5, p. 242) and to relieve the obstruction.

Strangulated herniae also cause focal ischaemia, but present acutely. The exception is a Richter's hernia (ischaemia of part of the herniated bowel, which subsequently returns to the abdominal cavity), because initial symptoms may resolve temporarily.

Ischaemic colitis

Ischaemic colitis can be acute, chronic or focal, but is classified separately because it is more common and presents differently from small intestinal ischaemia.

Clinical features

- Patients are usually elderly arteriopaths with a history of myocardial infarction, atrial fibrillation, peripheral vascular disease or hypertension (Table 9.6, p. 320). There may be a documented history of a hypotensive episode resulting in low splanchnic blood flow. Colonic ischaemia is a recognised complication of aortic aneurysm repair (< 5%)
- Abdominal pain is usual but not invariable, unlike small intestinal ischaemia
- Diarrhoea may precede rectal bleeding, or vice versa. The onset of either is usually sudden. Bleeding rarely requires transfusion
- Toxic dilatation occurs rarely
- Symptoms may occur for days or weeks before presentation, although patients with colonic gangrene present within hours and cannot be distinguished clinically from those with acute small intestinal ischaemia

Diagnosis

- A plain abdominal X-ray is important to rule out other diagnoses but may show an abnormal segment, usually at the splenic flexure, with mucosal oedema ('thumbprinting', Fig. 9.7)
- Limited flexible sigmoidoscopy after a phosphate enema, performed by an experienced colonoscopist is safe and the best diagnostic investigation provided there is no evidence of peritonism. It should be performed within 3 days of the onset of symptoms
- Biopsies show ulceration and a polymorphonuclear infiltrate. Haemosiderin-laden macrophages are characteristic, but may not be present (particularly in the early phases of the event)

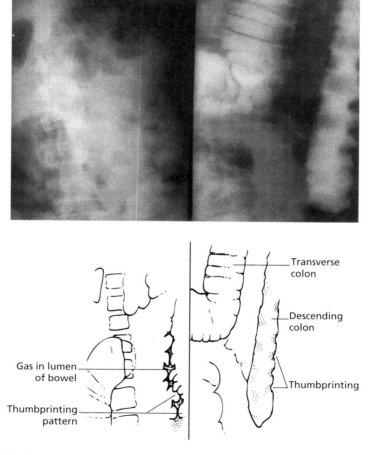

Fig. 9.7 Radiological appearance of ischaemic colitis. Radiographs in acute ischaemic colitis. In the plain film (left) gas outlines smooth indentations of the mucosa in the descending colon: thumbprinting. This is shown on barium enema (right).

- CT is also helpful in ruling out other diagnoses and may provide additional evidence of segmental bowel wall thickening
- Some centres advocate measuring serum D-lactate to aid diagnosis. It is produced by colonic bacteria and is not metabolised by the liver. It rises early in response to an ischaemic episode due to increased intestinal permeability
- A common dilemma is to distinguish ischaemic colitis from acute Crohn's colitis (Box 9.2). It is normally possible to exclude ulcerative colitis, because the rectum is not inflamed, but occasionally the rectal mucosa can look congested
- Colour-flow Doppler ultrasound scanning may differentiate ischaemia from inflammatory disease with high specificity (but low sensitivity). Absence of arterial flow may predict poor outcome

Management
- A conservative approach is appropriate for the majority of patients who will have non-transmural disease. Intravenous fluids to maintain intravascular volume and splanchnic perfusion and transfusion to maintain the haemoglobin at 10 g/dL are indicated, until bleeding, pain and diarrhoea improve. Early nutritional support (by enteral route if possible, but parenteral if there is an ileus) is crucial, because patients are often elderly and relatively malnourished before admission
- Most recover completely within 2 weeks and recurrence is surprisingly rare. Follow-up colonoscopy is unnecessary if symptoms resolve. About 10% subsequently develop a colonic stricture, which may be treated by colonoscopic dilatation or local resection

---

Box 9.2 Features favouring a diagnosis of ischaemic colitis

History
Age > 60 years
Vascular disease (angina, hypertension, previous myocardial infarction, claudication)
Diabetes
Onset with sudden pain, then bleeding

Signs
No abdominal mass
No perianal or extraintestinal features of Crohn's radiology
Single affected segment
Often localised around the splenic flexure
Thumbprinting (mucosal oedema, distinguished from mucosal islands by being larger)
Symmetrical stricture

Endoscopy
Variable appearance, from mild reddening, local ulceration to gangrene

Histology
Minimal changes
Intramucosal haemmorrhage
Fibrosis
Haemosiderin (uncommon)

- Deterioration is an indication for blood cultures, intravenous antibiotics and plain abdominal X-ray. Hypotension at presentation, coexisting diabetes and prolonged ileus predict need for surgical intervention. Toxic dilatation (diameter > 5.5 cm) may rarely occur and is an indication for colectomy

9.6 Anorectal conditions

Haemorrhoids
Haemorrhoids are dilatations of the normal rectal submucosal venous plexus, which develop due to straining at stool. They are often associated with redundant mucosa or perianal skin. The traditional classifications into internal or external, first-, second- or third-degree haemorrhoids are better replaced by descriptive terms (such as bleeding, temporarily, or permanently prolapsed, thrombosed).

Bleeding
- Bright red blood often spurts round the lavatory after defecation, or smears the outside of the stool. This type of bleeding does not exclude a rectal carcinoma or proctitis
- Anaemia should never be attributed to haemorrhoidal bleeding without investigation

Haemorrhoidal prolapse
- Prolapse is recognised by the patient, but has to be distinguished on rectal examination from a polyp, rectal prolapse, anal cancer, or skin tag of Crohn's disease
- Permanent prolapse often causes discomfort from venous engorgement, or mucous discharge and pruritus. Pain does not occur without a fissure, thrombosis or infection

Thrombosis
- Rapid onset; severe perianal pain may take several days to resolve
- Severe pain from a thrombosed haemorrhoid may justify direct admission to hospital
- Anal carcinoma must be considered in the differential diagnosis of a painful, thrombosed haemorrhoid of long duration (several weeks)
- A perianal haematoma is due to thrombosis of a venous saccule

Management
- A serious cause of rectal bleeding must be excluded by sigmoidoscopy, and colonoscopy or a flexible sigmoidoscopy with a barium enema if aged > 40 years
- A high-fibre diet is safe and inexpensive (p. 388) and may reduce bleeding and pain on defecation
- Persistent hard stools suggest that dietary fibre intake remains insufficient (possibly due to poor tolerance) and can be temporarily relieved by lactulose 30–100 mL/day, Movicol 1–2 sachets daily or MiraLax 1–2 heaped tbsp daily
- Topical preparations reduce burning and itching (but exert no effect on bleeding) by a local anaesthetic or anti-inflammatory effect (when combined with a steroid preparation), but evidence supporting their efficacy is lacking. Long-term use of topical anaesthetic agents may cause chronic perianal dermatitis. Mesalazine (5-aminosalicylic acid) suppositories were effective in one randomised controlled trial

- Thrombosis can be managed by the use of a local ice pack to relieve oedema, lignocaine (or lidocaine) 1% gel (no more than 3 days) and lactulose 30–100 mL/day. Surgical intervention should be considered after recovery
- Conservative surgical intervention is only indicated for bleeding or persistent symptoms. Rubber band ligation (RBL) and infrared photocoagulation (IRC) are both superior to injection sclerotherapy with > 90% of patients improved or symptom-free following treatment. IRC is less painful than RBL but requires repeat treatment sessions. Both modalities are delivered endoscopically
- Excisional haemorrhoidectomy should only be considered for large, permanently prolapsed haemorrhoids, or following failed RBL/IRC intervention

Fissures and fistulae

Anal fissure
- A linear break in the distal anal mucosa that extends below the dentate line to the anal verge. Often associated with a skin tag (sentinel pile) or anal polyp
- Pain during defaecation or acute constipation is characteristic, often with bleeding; the blood often drips into the toilet bowl water after passage of stool
- Diagnosis is made by inspection of the anal margin when gently parting the buttocks. Rectal examination is painful, but may be possible after applying lignocaine 2% gel perianally and into the anal canal
- Uncomplicated fissures are anterior. If there is a fissure in another position (posterior or particularly lateral), consider Crohn's disease
- Management is directed at relieving constipation (dietary fibre, with lactulose). Nitroglycerine ointment (0.2% twice daily for 6 weeks) or diltiazem ointment are cost-effective first-line therapies with healing rates between 33 and 86%. Patients should be warned of the risk of headache. Botulinum toxin (BoTox 20U injected into the anterior midline of the internal anal sphincter) is an alternative. This may be delivered under endoanal ultrasound. Lateral sphincterotomy should be reserved for patients with relapse or therapeutic failure of these agents

Perianal fistulae
- Perianal fistulae result from chronic infection in an anal gland. Acute infection causes an abscess
- Most are non-specific, but an underlying cause should be suspected for extensive, bilateral (horseshoe) or recurrent fistulae. Crohn's disease and rarely diabetes or tuberculosis should be considered
- Types of fistulae are shown in Fig. 9.8
- The track of the fistula should be identified by MRI (p. 260) whenever fistulae are recurrent or potentially complex as in Crohn's disease
- Surgery aims to lay open the fistulous track to allow healing by gradual granulation. Biopsies must be taken at every opportunity to exclude Crohn's disease. Complex or deep fistulae may need insertion of a seton of monofilament nylon (p. 265) along the track that prevents premature closure. Alternatively, fibrin glue installation may promote closure, although this is unsuitable for patients with Crohn's disease

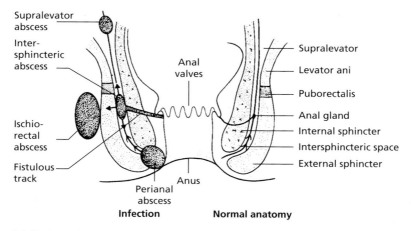

Fig. 9.8 Perianal fistulae and abscesses. Infection starts in the anal glands and may spread vertically, horizontally or circumferentially. An abscess is an acute, localised collection of pus, whilst a fistula, which connects two epithelial surfaces, is the chronic phase of the same disease process.

Pruritus ani

Perianal itching has many causes (Table 9.7). Questions about cleansing, rectal or vaginal discharge, local ointments (for 'piles'), skin disorders, or family members with the condition are relevant.

- Examination must include inspection for skin disease, digital assessment of sphincter tone and proctosigmoidoscopy
- Urine testing for glycosuria, cellophane tape slide from the anus for threadworm/pinworm (*Ent. vermicularis*) and skin scrape for fungi are often helpful. Skin biopsy, high vaginal swab or anorectal manometry (for sphincter dysfunction) are rarely indicated
- Treatment is directed at the cause. Careful washing and drying of the area after defecation is most important. Topical hydrocortisone 1% twice daily for 2 weeks provides symptomatic relief, but reassessment rather than represcription is indicated for persistent symptoms

Table 9.7 Causes of pruritus ani

Common	Uncommon	Rare
Poor hygiene	Rectal discharge (sphincter dysfunction)	Eczema
Haemorrhoids		Lichen sclerosus
Fissure	Fistula	Paget's disease
Threadworm/Pinworm	Fungal infection (diabetes)	Bowen's disease
Skin sensitivity to	Vaginal discharge	
'haemorrhoid' ointment	Spurious diarrhoea	

Proctalgia fugax

Paroxysmal perineal pain lasting a few minutes, often felt deep in the rectum or after defecation and perhaps waking the patient at night, has no known organic cause. Rectal or puborectalis spasm have been suggested as causes.

9.7 Investigation of iron-deficiency anaemia

- In Europe and North America IDA occurs in 2–5% of adult men and post-menopausal women, accounting for 4–13% of referrals to gastroenterology clinics
- The management of IDA is often suboptimal, with many patients being incompletely investigated. IDA in adult men and postmenopausal women requires investigation of the upper gastrointestinal tract, distal duodenal biopsies to exclude coeliac disease, and whole colon. IDA should not be attributed to an uncomplicated peptic ulcer, hiatus hernia, NSAIDs, oesophagitis or haemorrhoids without investigation of the colon
- The cause may not be identified in one-third of patients
- In teenagers suspected of having anorexia nervosa, iron deficiency should provoke a search for Crohn's disease
- Recurrent iron deficiency over a period of years should always raise the suspicion of coeliac disease
- IDA can be expected after partial or total gastrectomy, due to poor chelation and absorption of iron due to a loss of acid, and free iron in exfoliated cells. Investigations are only required in such patients if IDA persists on oral iron, or presents for the first time many years after gastrectomy

Essential investigations

History
A careful history is mandatory. Ask about:
- Evidence of bleeding—menstrual loss in women
- Diet—frequency of meat intake, vegetarian or vegan
- Weight loss—suggests carcinoma, malabsorption
- Diarrhoea—coeliac, Crohn's disease, but by no means universal
- Easy bruising—bleeding diathesis
- Mouth ulcers—coeliac, Crohn's disease
- Drugs—aspirin and NSAIDs
- Family history of haematological disorder

Examination
- Signs of iron deficiency—cheilosis, koilonychia (Table 12.4, p. 372)
- Mouth and lips—for telangiectases (hereditary haemorrhagic telangiectasia usually presents as iron deficiency in adults)
- Abdominal mass—neoplasm, Crohn's disease

- Rectal—for a rectal cancer (although rectal cancer almost never presents with IDA as the sole manifestation)
- Sigmoidoscopy may be omitted if digital rectal exam is negative and there is no history of altered bowel habit or rectal bleeding
- FOBT is of *no benefit* in the investigation of IDA, being insensitive, non-specific and not altering the need for gastrointestinal investigation
- Check urine for haematuria—if positive, perform an intravenous urogram to exclude renal carcinoma

Blood tests
- Full blood count—a hypochromic (MCH < 27 pg), microcytic (MCV < 80 fL) anaemia (Hb < 14 g/dL in men, < 12 g/dL in women) may be due to chronic disease, thalassaemia trait or sideroblastic anaemia, as well as iron deficiency. Microcytosis may be absent in combined iron and folate deficiency. Thrombocytosis indicates inflammation, or acute on chronic bleeding
- Blood film—hypochromic microcytosis and target cells may be seen in the presence of severe IDA; occasional macrocytes (dimorphic film) or Howell–Jolly bodies (hyposplenism) strongly suggest coeliac disease
- Serum ferritin (< 30 pg/L) should always be used to confirm IDA. However, ferritin is an acute-phase reactant and may be raised in patients with IDA who also have coexisting inflammatory disease (Crohn's disease, rheumatoid arthritis), malignancy or hepatic disease. Measurement of iron and total iron-binding capacity is then appropriate: low serum iron (< 10 pmol/L) with a high total iron-binding capacity (> 70 pmol/L) confirms iron deficiency; low iron and low total iron-binding capacity (< 45 pmol/L) suggests chronic disease; normal values suggest a haemoglobinopathy and are an indication for measuring HbA2 (normal < 2%)
- Folate, B_{12}, albumin—if malabsorption suspected
- Endomysial antibody serology to look for coeliac disease is conveniently performed at the first visit, but is strictly unnecessary when an upper gastrointestinal endoscopy and distal duodenal biopsy will be performed
- Upper gastrointestinal endoscopy
- Distal duodenal biopsies should always be taken when any patient with IDA is endoscoped, as 2–3% of patients will have coeliac disease

Colonic imaging
- All patients should undergo examination of the lower gastrointestinal tract as dual pathology occurs in 10–15% of patients
- Colonoscopy is usually the investigation of choice, as it will allow biopsies to be taken, the detection and treatment of angiodysplasia and the removal of polyps. It may be performed immediately after upper gastrointestinal endoscopy, under the same sedation
- Barium enema with sigmoidoscopy is a suitable alternative, especially if the facilities for colonoscopy are limited
- CT colon (different to CT colonography, see p. 425), because it does not require bowel preparation other than oral gastrograffin, is appropriate for elderly (age > 80 years) or frail patients who would poorly tolerate barium enema or colonoscopy

Further investigations for gastrointestinal bleeding of obscure origin

The cause of IDA that has not been diagnosed after the investigations above can present a very difficult problem. Before repeating any of the investigations, it is wise to retake the history and to review the results, to ensure that obvious causes (dietary insufficiency, menstrual loss, coeliac disease) or pitfalls (haemoglobinopathy, renal cell carcinoma) have not been overlooked.

Review results
- Ferritin—iron deficiency confirmed and haemoglobinopathy considered?
- Coagulation—bleeding diathesis excluded, including von Willebrand's disease?
- Endoscopy—by an experienced endoscopist?
- Distal duodenal biopsy—result of histology seen and reviewed?
- Barium enema—complete examination?
- Colonoscopy—good preparation, with views of proximal colon, by an experienced colonoscopist?
- Abdominal ultrasound—any evidence of portal hypertension?

Asymptomatic patients
- Stop iron therapy and repeat the full blood count after 3–6 months
- If anaemia recurs, the next investigation is small bowel radiology, preferably by a small bowel enema to obtain optimal mucosal definition
- In young people (age < 30 years) a Meckel's scan should be performed, although false-negative scans are common
- No further investigations are then required provided the IDA is not transfusion-dependant and there has been no overt blood loss. Regular iron therapy is appropriate, with checks on full blood count every 3–6 months. Follow-up studies have shown this approach to be safe

Symptomatic patients
- This includes those needing repeat transfusions, or in whom there is clear evidence of gastrointestinal blood loss (recurrent melaena, rectal bleeding or positive faecal occult blood)
- The sequence in Fig. 9.9 is recommended, but judgement is needed according to the age and condition of the patient. Whilst catastrophic bleeding (Ch 1, p. 19) is not the province of IDA, it helps to discriminate between the types of obscure gastrointestinal bleeding in the same algorithm
- The most useful investigation is a careful re-evaluation of the notes with repeat endoscopy and colonoscopy by a highly experienced endoscopist. Push enteroscopy and isotope red cell scans are being replaced by wireless capsule enteroscopy (p. 419)
- Capsule enteroscopy is becoming more widely available, but is time-consuming and frequently identifies lesions of doubtful significance. It is indicated if symptomatic iron deficiency recurs and the cause cannot be identified despite good quality endoscopy, distal duodenal biopsy, colonoscopy and small bowel radiology
- On the rare occasions that the source of recurrent bleeding is not detected by other means, elective laparotomy and on-table endoscopy by an experienced endoscopist is

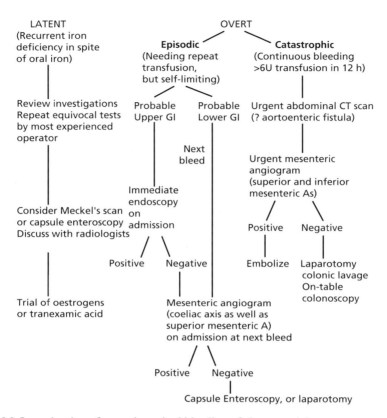

Fig. 9.9 Investigation of gastrointestinal bleeding of obscure origin.

rewarding and potentially therapeutic. The surgeon initially excludes a Meckel's diverticulum, then carefully transilluminates the whole small bowel and colon from the *outside* looking for vascular lesions (room lights are dimmed and a fibre-optic light source is used), *before* feeding the small bowel over a paediatric colonoscope introduced by mouth and then examining the colon

- Mesenteric angiography is usually only performed when there is brisk bleeding (> 1 unit/4 h, Fig 1.3, p. 20), but experienced radiologists can also detect mesenteric arteriovenous malformations or intestinal varices from portal hypertension as an elective procedure. There may also be an inclination to ignore the coeliac axis if upper gastrointestinal endoscopy is normal, but this neglects the possibility of rare hepatic, biliary or pancreatic sources of bleeding. Careful discussion with the radiologist is essential

- Oestrogens (oestradiol 30–50 µg daily) may be effective in reducing recurrent bleeding from angiodysplasia (p. 12). Low doses are ineffective, but higher doses carry a risk of thromboembolism

Iron therapy

- Ferrous sulphate 200 mg or ferrous gluconate 300 mg three times a day is cheap and effective. The haemoglobin should rise by 2 g/dL after 3–4 weeks. A liquid preparation may be tolerated when tablets are not, but in general tolerability reflects the dose. Ascorbic acid may enhance absorption. The use of modified release preparations is unjustified
- Ferrous gluconate or ferrous fumarate may be better tolerated than ferrous sulphate, but all iron preparations may be poorly tolerated by those with intestinal inflammation (such as Crohn's disease). Iron trimaltose delivers less reactive iron and is much better tolerated, but availability is limited
- Oral iron should be continued for 3 months after correction of IDA in order to replenish iron stores
- Parenteral iron should be reserved for patients with intolerance to oral iron, continuing severe blood loss, or malabsorption. Risk of severe anaphylaxis is reduced to < 1% with newer preparations such as iron sucrose (Venofer) and iron dextran III-hydroxide dextran complex (Cosmofer). Nonetheless, a test dose should be given with resuscitation facilities available. The use of Cosmofer is preferred as it can be given as a single total dose infusion (Venofer requires about ten separate visits to receive the total iron dose)

10 Irritable Bowel Syndrome

10.1 Introduction

The term 'irritable bowel syndrome' (IBS) is used to describe a collection of abdominal symptoms for which no organic cause can be found. This does not mean that the symptoms are all psychological. Indeed it seems increasingly likely that IBS encompasses a heterogeneous group of organic bowel disorders, each with characteristic morphological, psychological and physiological changes that are only now being fully appreciated. Classification of these disorders remains limited by current definitions and a lack of sufficiently sensitive diagnostic tests.

- IBS is a common disorder affecting 10–20% of people at any one time. 75% of IBS patients never seek medical advice
- Women have a two- to fourfold increased prevalence of IBS and are more likely to seek health care. IBS is less common in patients > 65 years
- IBS accounts for 2% of consultations in general practice but 30–50% of gastrointestinal outpatient referrals

10.2 Aetiology and potential mechanisms

- Twin studies suggest a *genetic* component to IBS. Whilst this may represent shared genetic susceptibility for psychological disorders, variation in genes controlling inflammation or peristalsis may also be important
- *Enteric infection* may precipitate disease in a subset of patients. Up to 20% of IBS patients date the onset of symptoms to a bout of gastroenteritis (Section 10.5 p. 343)
- *Visceral hypersensitivity* has been demonstrated by ileal and anorectal balloon distension, but is insufficiently sensitive or specific to be used for diagnosis. The location of this hypersensitivity within the brain–gut axis is unclear
- *Altered gastrointestinal motility* and *transit* of food and gas is reported in IBS. Diarrhoea-predominant IBS is characterised by increased propulsive contractions and shorter small bowel and colonic transit times, while constipation-predominant IBS is characterised by decreased propulsive contractions and longer gut transits. > 50% of patients report exacerbation of symptoms after eating, and this can be objectively associated with abnormal gastrointestinal motility
- *Pyschological factors* may either influence health care–seeking behaviour, or sometimes be causal. Up to 50% of IBS patients referred to gastrointestinal clinics have coexisting psychiatric disease including paranoia, anxiety, depression, somatisation or phobias. A history of frequent consultation for minor ailments is common. A history of physical or sexual abuse is said to be 2–3 times more common in IBS patients

- Although objective evidence is lacking, most patients agree that *stress* aggravates IBS. Chronic sustained stress, such as separation or bereavement, is probably more important than acute stressors
- *Food intolerance* (p. 229)
- *Abnormal colonic flora* has been reported in some patients with IBS and is the rationale for treatment with probiotics (p. 343)

10.3 Diagnosis and clinical features

- The diagnosis of IBS is made by validated, consensus clinical criteria, since there is no biological test.

ROME II criteria
Pain or discomfort for 12 weeks of the previous 12 months associated with two of the following three:
1. relief with defaecation
2. onset associated with a change in stool frequency
3. onset associated with a change in stool form (appearance)
- *Although not part of the Rome II criteria, most clinicians include the absence of alarm symptoms (Box 10.1). This increases specificity, but not sensitivity*
- Using these clinical criteria, the diagnosis of IBS can be considered 'safe'. Follow-up studies show that < 2% develop organic disease after a median follow-up of 5 years

Diagnostic confidence may be increased by the following symptoms that are not required for diagnosis:
- Abnormal stool frequency (> 3/day, or < 3/week)
- Abnormal stool form (lumpy/hard or loose/watery)
- Abnormal stool passage (straining, urgency, incomplete evacuation)
- Passage of mucus
- Bloating or abdominal distension
- Fatigue

Box 10.1 Alarm indicators that suggest organic disease is more likely than IBS

Age of onset > 55 years
History < 6 months
Progressive, or very severe, or non-fluctuating daily symptoms
Nocturnal symptoms
Rectal bleeding
Anorexia
Unexplained weight loss
Family history of carcinoma, IBD, coeliac disease
Abnormal physical findings (apart from mild abdominal tenderness)
Mouth ulcers
Anaemia
Fever
Raised inflammatory markers

Less common features not of diagnostic value:
- Nausea
- Dyspareunia
- Pain in the back, thigh or chest
- Malaise after defaecation
- Urinary frequency (irritable bladder)

Gender differences in IBS
- Women are more likely to consult not only for IBS but also for chronic musculoskeletal or abdominal pain
- Constipation, distension, nausea and mucus are more common in women
- A history of hysterectomy is more common in women presenting with IBS than in an age-matched control group without IBS

IBS Subgroups
Clinical subgroups have been suggested. Although controversial, it helps rationalise individual patient management and may reduce clinical heterogeneity in drug trials.

Pain-predominant IBS
- Central, right or left iliac fossa pain, less commonly in several sites. Often poorly localised
- Daily pain for > 6 months is rarely organic in the absence of alarm indicators (Box 10.1)
- Persistent ache, often with sharp exacerbations
- Relieved by defaecation, but sometimes follows defecation
- Worse at times of stress, or during menstruation
- Symptoms frequently but erroneously attributed to diverticulosis (uninflamed diverticula do not produce symptoms)

Diarrhoea-predominant IBS
- Morning frequency, often with urgency
- Usually with pain, but often relieved by defaecation

Constipation-predominant IBS
- Especially women
- Sensation of incomplete evacuation
- Associated with the passage of mucus, but never blood

Alternating-pattern IBS
- Alternating episodes of constipation and diarrhoea
- Often have passage of hard constipated stool in the morning followed by increasingly loose or watery stools through the rest of the day

Overlap with other functional disorders
- Non-ulcer dyspepsia (p. 79)—upper abdominal pain or discomfort
- Food intolerance (p. 229)

- Pelvic pain syndrome—commonly seen by gynaecologists
- Irritable bladder—may indicate a common abnormality of smooth muscle function

Differential diagnosis

IBS is part of the differential diagnosis of many organic disorders and a list is unhelpful. However, common diagnostic pitfalls of treatable disorders can be avoided by thinking of the diagnosis.

Diarrhoea-predominant IBS

Care should be taken before attributing chronic diarrhoea to IBS. Consider:
- Coeliac disease (p. 107). Up to 5% of patients with a diagnosis of IBS have coeliac disease
- Inflammatory bowel disease (especially Crohn's disease)
- Lactose intolerance (p. 228)
- Bile salt malabsorption (p. 429)
- Microscopic colitis (p. 283)

Constipation-predominant IBS

- Pelvic floor dysfunction (p. 288–9)
- Slow transit constipation (p. 287)
- Intestinal pseudo–obstruction (p. 230)
- Obstructive defaecation (pp. 291, 294)

Investigations

The aim is to exclude organic disease by the minimum number of tests.

All patients

- Urine test for protein or blood caused by renal tract disease
- Full blood count, ESR (or CRP, plasma viscosity) and liver enzymes will identify most organic causes of symptoms
- Antiendomysial antibody to exclude coeliac disease (p. 107)
- Proctoscopy, to exclude anterior mucosal prolapse, if there is a sensation of incomplete evacuation after defecation (p. 287)

Diarrhoea-predominant IBS

- Haematinics (ferritin, folate, B_{12})
- Stool culture
- Rectal biopsy (to exclude microscopic colitis)

Indications for flexible sigmoidoscopy or colonoscopy

- Presence of any alarm feature irrespective of age
- *Not* indicated in patients < 50 years in the absence of alarm indicators (Box 10.1, p. 336)
- Patients < 50 years with persistent symptoms refractory to conventional diet or drug management

Further investigations

- *Additional tests should be avoided* unless there are unusual features or markers of organic disease: there is no need to arrange an ultrasound just because the pain is in the right upper quadrant, or an endoscopy just because the pain is epigastric. Gallstones, hiatus hernia or colonic diverticulosis are likely to be incidental to the patient's symptoms
- *Endoscopy* may be justified when the pain is clearly related to meals (dyspepsia), retrosternal (heartburn), or periodic (p. 78). It is essential to obtain distal duodenal biopsies if there is iron or folate deficiency
- *Ultrasound* of the pancreas and biliary tree is appropriate when upper abdominal pain is episodic and the endoscopy is normal. Pelvic ultrasound is indicated for lower abdominal pain related to periods
- *Small bowel radiology* is appropriate when there is weight loss or abdominal pain and diarrhoea, to exclude Crohn's disease
- Diarrhoea without pain is investigated as in Fig. 7.1 (p. 211). Mild symptoms from hypolactasia, coeliac disease or small intestinal bacterial overgrowth may be misattributed to an irritable bowel, especially after an episode of gastroenteritis. Colonoscopic biopsies may show collagenous or lymphocytic colitis (p. 283)
- *Motility tests* (such as transit studies or intestinal manometry) are not diagnostic, probably because IBS represents more than one motility disorder. Many patients have increased sensitivity to rectal balloon distension, but this also occurs in proctitis or other conditions

10.4 Management

General approach

- Taking the history and examining the patient in a careful, sympathetic and thorough manner makes subsequent explanation and reassurance very much easier. A good doctor–patient relationship is associated with a reduced number of return visits
- Make a positive diagnosis based on symptoms and absence of alarm features
- Establish effect of illness and patient's psychosocial resources (e.g. family support)
- Establish existence of coexisting psychiatric disorder or unresolved major loss
- Assess the patients expectations and hidden fears
- Provide firm reassurance, emphasising their symptoms are real and not just 'in their head'
- Provide education and explanation as to the cause of symptoms
- Avoid giving mixed messages, for example, by reassuring the patient and then ordering expensive tests
- If a test needs to be done (e.g. sigmoidoscopy), it helps to explain that the result is expected to be normal. In this way, concern that an inappropriate test has been performed, or the diagnosis missed, is more easily allayed
- Normal results should be stated in a positive and encouraging manner
- Focus on the principle of patient-based responsibility for care

Explanation

Initial

A provisional diagnosis and initial explanation can usually be given on the first visit. Helpful descriptions (unfortunately without much objective pathophysiological evidence) include:

- Explaining that small volume, hard faeces cause the bowel muscle to contract harder
- Describing the pain as bowel spasm, similar to muscle cramp
- Suggesting that the bowel is more sensitive than normal, and that some foods may trigger spasm in many patients (Section 12.4, p. 389)
- Describing the typical features of an irritable bowel (often recognised by the patient, with relief) and relation to stress in some people (like pre-examination diarrhoea)
- A diagram illustrating colonic segmentation (haustra) may assist explanation
- Explaining that the results of any investigations that have been arranged are expected to be normal

Subsequent

On a subsequent visit, with the results of normal investigations, it is important to make a definitive diagnosis of IBS, to acknowledge the symptoms and explain the likely pattern of symptoms.

- Symptoms often continue for months or years, but ultimately usually resolve
- Symptoms can be relieved, but not always cured
- There is no increased risk of cancer or serious disease
- Explain that there is something wrong, but that it is not a disease and the bowel is 'out of tune' or 'more sensitive' than normal
- Emphasise that a combination strategy (dietary manipulation, fibre, antispasmodics, anticholinergic agents) is often needed, rather than to expect a single treatment to work. For intractable symptoms, aim to help the patient cope with the symptoms rather than expect a cure

Diet

Clinical evidence is limited due to the considerable difficulty in trial design of dietary intervention studies in IBS. Nevertheless, dietary modification should be considered first in all patients

- Modifying the *pattern of eating* (regular, balanced meals compared to hasty snacks) may be as important for symptom control as the content
- Excess coffee, tea, milk, or alcohol may exacerbate diarrhoea
- Sorbitol, mannitol, xylitol, or fructose (which occur both naturally and are used as artificial sweeteners in drink, jams or chewing gums) act as laxatives when consumed on a regular basis or in large quantities
- Digestion-*resistant starches* (often from modified wheat flour, contained in convenience foods, dried pasta, potato salads, toasted bread) promote colonic fermentation, gas, bloating and flatulence (p.389)
- Blanket recommendations for dairy-free, wheat-free, or gluten-free diets are rarely helpful as first-line treatment for IBS

• Exaggerated gastro-colic response may be reduced by eating smaller meals containing less fat

Identify specific food intolerances with the aid of a dietitian

Role of fibre

• *Increasing* dietary fibre is only indicated when constipation is a prominent feature. A *reduction* in fibre helps some (maybe half) patients with diarrhoea
• Fibre (properly known as *non-starch polysaccharide*) is broadly divided into soluble and insoluble forms:
  • *Soluble fibre*, contained in ripe fruits, increases stool weight and accelerates whole gut transit
  • *Insoluble fibre*, contained in dried bran, may increase pain, flatulence, diarrhoea, or bloating, because short-chain fatty acids and gas are produced by colonic fermentation. Recognise that some sources of fibre are initially insoluble and evolve to soluble forms (e.g. fruit ripening)
• Fibre intake should be increased gradually. Mixed sources of fibre (fruit, pulses, cereals and grains) are more palatable than adding bran to food (p. 388). Encourage an increase in fluid intake and activity simultaneously
• Polyethylene glycol 3350 (Movicol 1–2 sachets/day) cannot be metabolised by bacteria, produces less gas and therefore may be better tolerated, as well as having an osmotic effect to increase stool water

Food intolerance

• Some patients have a specific food intolerance (terminology explained on p. 229) that can be identified by trials of dietary exclusion and reintroduction (p. 392). Dietary manipulation may appreciably improve two-thirds of patients. Formal *exclusion diets* help a minority (10–15%) but are not easy to implement in practice, are time-intensive and need support from a motivated dietitian (p. 390)
• Once the food(s) has been identified (often wheat, milk, caffeine, onions, chocolate, or salad vegetables), avoidance brings relief. The food can often be reintroduced without relapse after 12 months, for unexplained reasons. Small quantities are best tried on a 3-monthly basis
• 'Food allergy' tests waste time and money

Drugs

• Drugs are only used to treat symptoms and none are universally successful
• Clinical evidence is hampered by poorly conducted trials, lack of definitive endpoints and adequately defined disease entities
• The placebo rate is high and about one-third to one half of patients will get better on any particular drug. Many patients prefer to manage without drugs. The efficacy of one drug in an individual often varies with time
• Drugs should be used sparingly, targeting the symptom of most concern

Pain

- Antispasmodics have an anticholinergic action and offer, at best, a modest benefit for predictable, post-prandial pain. They are less effective with chronic use or when constipation predominates
- Mebeverine 135–270 mg three times daily is dramatically effective in a few, gives some relief to many, but may have no effect. Other drugs (alverine citrate 60–120 mg, dicyclomine 10–20 mg hyoscine 10–20 mg three times daily) may help different patients
- Peppermint oil (1–2 capsules three times daily) may be useful for patients who have constipation and bloating, since it has no anticholinergic action, or for those patients who dislike 'drugs'
- It is worth trying different drugs, because benefit is often temporary, or unpredictable
- Amitriptyline 10–50 mg daily, or Motival 1–3 tablets daily are helpful for persistent pain, especially when associated with diarrhoea

Constipation

- An osmotic laxative (lactulose 30–100 mL/day or magnesium hydroxide, e.g. Phillips Milk of Magnesia 15–60 mL/day) can be added if increasing soluble fibre in the diet is ineffective, but often makes bloating worse. Movicol (above) is an alternative. Stimulant laxatives (p. 295) may make pain worse
- Serotonin reuptake inhibitors increase gut transit and are occasionally helpful
- Tegaserod, a novel partial *5-HT$_4$ agonist*, is currently only licensed in the USA and Canada for women with constipation-predominant IBS. It accelerates small bowel and colonic transit and may induce intestinal fluid secretion. Studies have demonstrated improved global symptom relief, increased stool frequency and consistency

Diarrhoea

- Loperamide (2–16 mg daily) is an opioid analogue that does not cross the blood–brain barrier. It improves diarrhoea and urgency by retarding intestinal transit, enhancing water absorption and increasing resting anal sphincter tone. It is useful for preventing predictable diarrhoea. Liquid loperamide contains a high concentration of sorbitol
- Codeine phosphate is best avoided, because long-term use may cause dependency
- Amitriptyline, imipramine, or nortriptyline 10–30 mg, or Motival 1–3 tablets daily, may help persistent diarrhoea, partly through their anticholinergic effect (NNT-3). It is important to explain their peripheral effect on enteric nerves despite being originally developed as 'antidepressants', to start with small, 'paediatric' doses and to increase the dose gradually. Side-effects still limit their use in practice
- Diarrhoea that is not readily controlled is an indication for investigation (Fig. 7.1, p. 211)
- Alosetron, a *5-HT$_3$ antagonist*, was approved for women with diarrhoea-predominant IBS until it was temporarily withdrawn in 2000, because of adverse associations (including colonic obstruction and ischaemic colitis) when inappropriately used in constipated patients. It delays colonic transit and reduces colonic sensation in IBS patients with diarrhoea

Probiotics
- Preliminary studies suggest that probiotics (*Lactobacillus* spp.) may be useful for improving flatulence associated with IBS
- Specific recommendation cannot be made, but live yoghurt, or commercial drinks containing probiotic mixtures (such as Actimel) may help

Complementary therapy
- There are some patients who remain symptomatic, or who cannot tolerate or will not take conventional medication
- It is often helpful to discuss the limits of conventional ('Western' medicine) in these poorly understood disorders and to acknowledge the possible role of complementary medicine
- Complementary treatments enjoy widespread acceptance and cannot be summarily dismissed, particularly as many of the more traditional drugs lack evidence; they also have the advantage in that they allow patients to feel that they are taking more control of their symptom management
- Some treatments (*hypnotherapy*, *acupuncture*) have been subjected to comparative trials and benefit some patients with intractable symptoms. It is unclear how reproducible the response is with different practitioners using different techniques, but the trials with medically qualified hypnotists indicate that prolonged remission can be induced. Not everyone can be hypnotised. Treatment is time-consuming and not widely available
- The website http://www.quackwatch.com provides up-to-date evaluation to help doctors (and patients) on latest 'treatments' touted in the press
- Aloe vera or slippery elm have their advocates, but care should be taken with herbal medicines that may contain senna or ephedra, which may worsen diarrhoea

Prognosis
- Long-term follow-up studies are few
- Symptoms disappear or improve in about half after 12 months. < 5% become worse and the remainder remain unchanged
- Intermittent symptoms are likely, but these are usually due to identifiable stress or a change in diet and can be controlled
- There is no increased mortality

10.5 Post-infective irritable bowel syndrome

- Up to 20% of IBS patients date the onset of their symptoms to a bout of enteric infection (Table 10.1)
- Typically IBS symptoms follow the initial diarrhoeal episode despite eradication of the causative organism
- At least two of the following are required for diagnosis: an acute episode of fever, vomiting, diarrhoea, or a positive stool culture immediately before the onset of symptoms of IBS

Table 10.1 Risks for development of post-infective IBS after gastroenteritis

Factor	Risk, or relative risk (RR), of IBS
Duration of diarrhoea	
1–2 weeks	RR = 2.9
2–3 weeks	RR = 6.5
> 3 weeks	RR = 11.4
Organism	
Camplylobacter sp. or *Shigella* sp.	Risk 10%
Samonella sp.	Risk 1%
History of hypochondriasis	RR = 2.0
Concomitant adverse life event	RR = 2.0
Female gender	RR = 3.4, but may not be independent of other factors

- In post-infective IBS, increases in small bowel permeability, mucosal T lymphocytes and enteroendocrine cells have been reported. An increase in serotonin-containing secretory granules in enteroendocrine cell may contribute to looser, more frequent stools
- Transient lactose intolerance, transient bile salt malabsorption and microscopic colitis may all complicate gastroenteritis. These may coexist with postinfective IBS, should be considered and treated independently
- Prognosis of post-infective IBS may be better than other types of IBS. About 40% have fully recovered within 6 years. Poor prognosis is associated with female gender or a psychiatric history

10.6 Clinical dilemmas

Persistent symptoms
- Usually due to a failure to treat constipation adequately, or to alter the diet
- Personality is important. Psychologically distressed patients select themselves by presenting for treatment. Explanations to provide insight and assistance in coping with symptoms are more likely to reduce visits than a dismissive approach. Clinical depression may be present and should be treated
- Further investigation is not justified unless the symptom pattern has changed or clinical signs (such as weight loss) have developed
- IBS should not be considered a psychological disorder, but some patients are particularly anxious, or have symptoms as a feature of bereavement, or stress-related illness
- A high prevalence of sexual abuse in childhood has been reported. Time to develop a rapport is essential before these issues are explored. It may be best done by the patient's general practitioner, although some patients who know their general practitioner particularly well may prefer to discuss such problems outside the primary care setting
- Referral to a clinical psychologist for relaxation, cognitive behavioural therapy or brief psychotherapy depends on individual interest, local availability and resources. Sensitive discussion about psychological factors that are exacerbating symptoms should identify most patients likely to be helped by referral

- Some general practice surgeries have a stress counsellor to help teach coping strategies

Symptoms with identifiable disease
- Features of IBS remain common in patients with identifiable gastrointestinal disorders, such as gallstones, gastro-oesophageal reflux, ulcerative colitis or Crohn's disease
- Whilst judgement is necessary to decide which symptoms are related to the known disease, continuous abdominal discomfort, bloating or symptoms that do not fit with the common pattern of the disease are more likely to be due to an irritable bowel and are best treated with sympathetic explanation, dietary modification and reassurance

10.7 Somatisation disorder

Somatisation disorder is a term used to denote a chronic condition characterised by a history of numerous, recurrent physical complaints that begin in early life (before age 30) and persist for many years. If no single person takes responsibility for overall management of the patient, then the complaints are likely to continue, with multiple unnecessary referrals, investigations and treatment.

Diagnosis
Establishing the diagnosis is time-consuming, requiring careful scrutiny of hospital and primary care notes. All four criteria (A, B, C and D) in Table 10.2 must be present for diagnosis.

An alert clinician will recognise the 'frequent attender' and a liaison psychiatrist, working alongside the clinical colleagues in the main hospital, is best placed to confirm

Table 10.2 Diagnostic criteria for somatisation disorder

Criterion	Explanation or examples
A A history of many physical complaints beginning before age 30 years	
B Four pain symptoms	Pain in four sites (e.g. head, abdomen, back, joints, chest, or rectum)
and two gastrointestinal symptoms	Symptoms other than abdominal pain (e.g. nausea, bloating, diarrhoea, food intolerance)
and one sexual symptom	Not dyspareunia (e.g. sexual indifference, impotence, irregular menses)
and one neurological symptom	(e.g. impaired coordination/balance, dysphonia, numbness without neuropathy)
C *Either* none of the symptoms can be explained by disease or drug misuse *Or* when disease exists, the symptoms or disability are greater than explicable by the organic findings	
D The symptoms are not intentionally produced or consciously feigned	

the diagnosis as well as helping with management. General psychiatrists frequently find no treatable psychiatric disorder, which then makes management more difficult, because the patient cites this as 'evidence' that symptoms are not psychological.

Management

After establishing the diagnosis, the general practitioner and psychiatrist should implement a care plan to reduce hospital and primary care visits.

- Proactive care, with arrangements to see the patient at fixed intervals
- The doctor and not the patient should determine the frequency of these visits
- Make the patient feel understood, with the help of supportive listening, acceptance and interest
- Broaden the agenda by discussing previously elicited psychological and social factors (e.g. 'I am reminded of the troubles at home that have been worrying you')
- Make a possible link between symptoms and psychological problems (e.g. 'over-breathing can cause chest pain', 'depression lowers the threshold for pain')
- Negotiate graded withdrawal of psychotropic and/or analgesic drugs
- Treat any coexisting psychiatric disorder in the normal way
- Interview nearest relative and try to involve him/her as a therapeutic ally
- Minimise contact with other specialists to avoid overinvestigation and iatrogenic harm
- Talk to the patient in terms of 'coping' and not 'curing'

11 Gastrointestinal Infections

11.1 Acute gastroenteritis

Gastroenteritis is caused by infection in the gastrointestinal tract, which usually results in diarrhoea and abdominal pain of acute onset and short duration, commonly with vomiting. It is often not possible or necessary to identify the organism, but it is important to recognise when investigation is indicated (p. 351).

Causes

In the UK and USA pathogens are isolated in less than half of gastroenteritis cases. The most frequently identified organisms (Table 11.1) are:
- Viruses, in particular Norwalk-like viruses—50% (norovirus, p. 355)
- *Campylobacter* spp.—20% (> 80% are estimated to be food-borne)
- *Salmonella* spp.—15% (zoonotic organisms, spread from infected animals to humans, not those causing enteric fever)
- *Shigella* spp.—5%
- *Cl. difficile*—5%
- Miscellaneous—5%

Clinical features

- History of travel, or eating unusual or suspect food (reheated chicken, seafood, take-away food, mass catering, conference dinners)
- The incubation period depends on the cause (Table 11.2)
- Other people are often affected
- Diarrhoea—may be bloody (*Shigella* spp., *Campylobacter* spp., enteroinvasive *E. coli*, Box 7.1, p. 214)
- Crampy abdominal pain—often severe in the young or elderly, especially with *Campylobacter* spp.

Table 11.1 Common causes of acute gastroenteritis

Bacterial	Viral	Toxins	Other
Salmonella spp.	Norovirus	*E. coli*	*G. lamblia*
Shigella spp.*	Rotavirus	*Staphylococcus aureus*	*Cryptosporidium* spp.
Campylobacter spp.	Echovirus	*Cl. difficile*	*Isospora belli*
Y. enterocolitica*		*Vibrio cholerae*	Alcohol[†]
Clostridium perfringens*		*B. cereus*	Heavy metals[†]
E. coli		*Vibrio parahaemolyticus*	
Aeromonas spp.		*Cl. botulinum*	
		G. breve	

*Action partly through toxin production.
[†]Symptoms may be similar to infective causes.

11 Gastrointestinal Infections
11.1 Acute gastroenteritis

Table 11.2 Bacteria involved in food poisoning

Organism	Incubation (h)*	Food at risk	Duration
B. cereus†	1–5	Fried or reheated rice	12–24 h
Staphylococcus aureus	2–6	Unrefridgerated meat, milk	6–24 h
Vibrio parahaemolyticus	12–18 (< 48)	Crabs, shellfish	2–5 days
Clostridium perfringens	8–22	Cooled stewed meat	12–48 h
Salmonella spp.	12–24 (< 48)	Undercooked poultry, eggs	1–7 days
Clostridium botulinum‡	18–36 (< 96)	Fermented canned food	Months

*All times are very approximate.

†A non-vomiting type, causing diarrhoea, has a longer (8–20 h) incubation and may be acquired from ice cream, meat or vegetables.

‡Paralysis progresses rapidly after initial gastrointestinal upset. Antitoxin 20 mL intramuscular injection and 20 mL intravenously, after an intradermal test dose of 0.1 mL, is given when the diagnosis is suspected, with intravenous penicillin 2 MU four times daily to kill remaining bacteria. Ventilation is indicated if vital capacity < 1000 mL.

- Vomiting—particularly with *Bacillus cereus*
- Systemic features (fever, headache, myalgia) are common in *Shigella* spp., *Campylobacter* spp., or *Y. enterocolitica* infections
- Resolution usually within 24–96 h

Susceptible patients
- Elderly or very young
- Hypogammaglobulinaemia
- Gastric hypoacidity—but does not appear to be a major problem with H_2-receptor antagonists, or PPIs
- Total gastrectomy
- Immunocompromised—chemotherapy, AIDS (p. 363)
- Hyposplenic—invasive salmonellosis is more common

Sequelae
Sequelae are uncommon.
- Persistent diarrhoea may be due to:
  - secondary hypolactasia (especially postviral, in children)
  - persistent infection (*Giardia lamblia*, immunocompromised)
  - unmasked latent disease (ulcerative colitis, coeliac disease)
  - post-infective irritable bowel syndrome (most often, p. 343)
- Asymptomatic carrier-following *Salmonella* spp. enteritis
- Reactive arthritis:
  - or a full Reiter's syndrome (asymmetrical polyarthritis, orogenital ulceration, conjunctivitis) can occur after *Y. enterocolitica* or *Campylobacter* spp. infection and may be confused with ulcerative colitis or Crohn's disease
  - may also occur after *Salmonella* spp. and rarely after *Shigella* spp. infection in the susceptible
  - *Salmonella* spp. osteomyelitis may occur in hyposplenic patients

- Erythema nodosum:
  - after *Y. enterocolitica*
  - after *Campylobacter* spp. infection
- Haemolytic uraemic syndrome—renal failure and haemolysis is caused by the Shiga toxins secreted by *E. coli* 0157:H7
- Septicaemia:
  - in the immunocompromised, elderly or functionally hyposplenic (sickle-cell disease, coeliac disease, splenectomy)
  - usually the cause of *Salmonella*-associated deaths
  - focal infections (cholecystitis, meningitis) are very rare
- Infective colitis:
  - diffuse mucosal changes may mimic ulcerative colitis, but glandular architecture is preserved
  - *Campylobacter* spp., *Y. enterocolitica*, *Shigella* spp. or *E. coli* 0157 are often the cause
- Toxic dilatation—more commonly due to undiagnosed ulcerative colitis than *Campylobacter* spp., *Y. enterocolitica* or *E. coli* 0157 enteritis
- Neuropathy—may complicate *Cl. botulinum* (12–72 h), tetrahydropurine toxin (*Gymnodinium breve*) from shellfish or heavy-metal poisoning. Guillain–Barré syndrome rarely complicates *Campylobacter* spp.

Investigations

Uncomplicated acute gastroenteritis does not need investigation, because it usually resolves rapidly and spontaneously. When investigation is indicated (see below), stool culture and microscopy for cysts and trophozoites of *G. lamblia* and *Entamoeba histolytica* must be performed, with subsequent tests depending on the circumstances. Formed stool is unlikely to harbour pathogens. Investigation may be necessary for public health reasons (such as contact with a *Salmonella* carrier in the food industry).

Indications for investigation

- The elderly
- More than one person affected
- Symptoms persisting for more than 4 days
- Associated bleeding or other sequelae (see above)
- Acute gastroenteritis in a residential establishment or institution

Subsequent investigation

- Stool culture should be performed on fresh stool. If stool cannot be plated within 2 h, it should be refrigerated or placed in a transport medium. If the first culture is negative and symptoms persist, the stool culture should be repeated
- Most laboratories now use rapid enzyme immunoassays for the detection of *Campylobacter* sp., *Cl. difficile* toxins, and shiga-like toxins produced by *Shigella* sp. and EHEC. PCR-based detection techniques are likely to appear in service laboratories in the new future
- Stool examination for virus by electron microscopy is not necessary, except in outbreaks of culture-negative diarrhoea in institutions, or in children

- Persistent diarrhoea (> 2 weeks) is an indication for sigmoidoscopy, biopsy and referral to a gastroenterologist (Fig. 7.1, p. 211)
- Arthritis is an indication for joint aspiration if there is a fever or leucocytosis; rheumatoid factor to confirm a seronegative arthropathy, antibodies to *Y. enterocolitica* and X-ray if a large joint is involved
- Severely ill patients need admission to hospital, full blood count, electrolytes to assess dehydration, blood cultures and plain abdominal X-ray to exclude colonic dilatation

General management
- Encourage fluid intake
- Oral rehydration solutions (Dioralyte/Gastrolyte/Pedialyte, 500–3000 mL/day) for the elderly, very young, or if diarrhoea and dehydration is severe
- Meticulous hand hygiene and a personal towel
- Personal eating and drinking utensils probably do little to prevent the spread of infection, except in *Shigella* spp. infections, but remains customary advice
- Antidiarrhoeal agents should be avoided if possible, although clearance of pathogens is probably not delayed. Loperamide 4 mg, then 2 mg after each loose motion, usually relieves diarrhoea if symptom control is needed, but should never be given to children because fatal paralytic ileus has been reported
- Metoclopramide 10 mg intramuscular injection up to three times a day controls vomiting. Dystonic reactions (more common in the elderly and adolescents) do not occur with rectal domperidone 30–60 mg three times daily where available
- Intravenous 0.9% saline, alternating with 5% dextrose, each with 20 mmol/L KCl, is indicated for rehydrating severely ill patients. Judge adequate hydration by good urine output, but watch for possible fluid overload in the elderly
- Empirical antibiotic therapy (Ciprofloxacin 500 mg twice daily for 5 days) may be considered for patients at risk of severe or disseminated infection (advanced age, immunocompromised, diabetes, cirrhosis, intestinal hypomotility, or hypochlorhydria). Alternatives to quinolones (e.g. co-trimoxazole) may be appropriate for children, patients with quinolone sensitivity or in quinolone-resistant areas
- Suspected food poisoning is a notifiable disease in most jurisdictions (p. 367)

Management of specific infections

Campylobacter spp.
- Antibiotics are usually reserved for patients with prolonged (> 1 week), or deteriorating symptoms, immunocompromised patients and pregnant women (because of the effects on the fetus). Ciprofloxacin (750 mg twice daily for 1 week) reduces the duration of clinical symptoms if started early in the infection but there is increasing resistance: currently 15% in the UK, but over 60% in parts of Europe and > 90% in parts of South-East Asia. Erythromycin (500 mg four times daily for 1 week) is an alternative
- Excretion often continues for weeks after recovery, but no treatment is needed

Salmonella spp.
- Standard advice is *not* to give antibiotics, unless there is extraintestinal infection, as antibiotic therapy may prolong enteric carriage. Ciprofloxacin is appropriate for

severe disease in patients at risk of extraintestinal disease (the elderly, immunocompromised or young)

- *Salmonella* spp. strains resistant to a number of antibiotics are now emerging. There is some evidence linking this resistance to the agricultural use of antibiotics
- Faecal excretion continues for 4–8 weeks and very rarely up to 6 months, usually from a gall bladder reservoir of infection. This is part of the natural history of infection and antibiotics for acute infection, including ciprofloxacin, may prolong excretion
- Repeat stool samples are no longer advised, even in jobs such as food handlers or nurses. The risk of cross-infection from a patient with formed stools is negligible. Good education in personal hygiene is equally important
- Septicaemia or invasive salmonellosis is treated with ciprofloxacin 750 mg twice daily for 1 week (or intravenous 200 mg twice daily over 30 min if too sick for oral medication). Trimethoprim 200 mg twice daily (orally, or by slow intravenous infusion) is the alternative drug of choice
- Treatment of asymptomatic carriers is unnecessary because such patients represent a very small risk to public health and no risk to themselves. Gallstones may be a nidus of infection in < 1% of patients and cholecystectomy is then advisable, with antibiotic cover (ciprofloxacin 500 mg twice daily, for 48 h)

Shigella spp.
- It is often possible to manage patients without antibiotics
- Ciprofloxacin (500 mg orally twice daily) is appropriate for adults infected with virulent species (*Sh. shigae* or *Sh. dysenteriae*)
- Repeat stool samples are needed for the same reasons as *Salmonella* spp. enteritis
- Bacteria can survive for several hours on hands or towels. Outbreaks in residential establishments are an indication for disposable towels, and disinfection of hands, lavatory seats and taps

Yersinia enterocolitica
- Stool culture is positive in the acute stage, but antibody titres are necessary to confirm the diagnosis if presentation is delayed for more than 2 weeks (titres > 1 : 128 in a previously healthy individual are suggestive). It may closely mimic Crohn's disease
- Tetracycline (250 mg four times daily for 2 weeks) is indicated (but not in pregnancy, lactation or childhood), but this does not affect established post-infective arthritis

Escherichia coli 0157 : H7
- Haemorrhagic colitis caused by this organism is treated with ciprofloxacin 750 mg twice daily (or 200–400 mg intravenously over 30 min twice daily in the severely ill)
- 8% of infected patients (predominately children) develop haemolytic–uraemic syndrome (HUS). Antibiotic therapy may increase the risk of HUS by stimulating toxin secretion. Alternative drugs that bind toxin are being developed

Clostridium difficile
- Gram-positive, spore-forming anaerobic bacillus that is widely distributed in the environment. Hospitals in particular are heavily contaminated by spores that are

relatively resistant to standard disinfectants. Transmission in hospital is primarily by contaminated hands and equipment

- Causes acute, persistent, or recurrent diarrhoea after antibiotic treatment, primarily in elderly hospitalised patients (when it leads to an additional average inpatient stay of 21 days). The spectrum of disease ranges from asymptomatic carriage (2% of healthy adults) to diarrhoea without systemic upset (*Cl. difficile*-associated diarrhoea, CDAD), to colitis (pseudomembranous colitis, PMC, p. 379) and death. Community-acquired infection is probably underdocumented
- Risk factors for *Cl. difficile* infection include: age (> 65 years), class of antibiotic (see Table 11.3), PPIs, chemotherapy and comorbidity
- Combinations of risk factors have an additive effect
- Mortality is high in hospital patients (up to 30%, due to comorbidity), but lower in community-acquired CDAD (10%)
- Diagnosis is based upon the detection of *Cl. difficile* toxins (A&B). Assays that target both toxins are preferable as 3–5% of strains are toxin A negative/toxin B positive, but some laboratories only test for toxin A; it is important to know the assay provided by the local laboratory
- Initial management involves stopping the precipitating antibiotic(s) where possible. Oral metronidazole (1.0–1.5 g in divided daily doses for 7–10 days) is required if there is evidence of colitis, PMC or persistent symptoms despite stopping the antibiotic
- Recurrent infection is common (30%), often with increasing severity. Controlled trials show that vancomycin (125 mg four times daily for 2–4 weeks) is more effective than metronidazole for clearing recurrent *Cl. difficile*
- Cholestyramine, probiotic therapy with *Saccharomyces boulardii*, or intravenous gammaglobulin to treat those who cannot mount an antitoxin response (common in recurrent CDAD) are indicated if CDAD persists in spite of vancomycin
- *Cl. perfringens* and *Staphylococcus aureus* are less frequent causes of antibiotic-associated diarrhoea

Listeria monocytogenes
- *L. monocytogenes* grows at a wide range of temperatures. Outbreaks have been linked to wide variety of foods including refrigerated dairy products, unpasteurised cheese and ready-made meals

Table 11.3 Antibiotic risk of *Cl. difficile* infection

High Risk	Medium Risk	Low risk
Cephalosporins	Ampicillin/Amoxycillin	Aminoglycosides
Clindamycin	Co-trimoxazole	Metronidazole
	Macrolides	Antipseudomonal penicillins +/− beta-lactamase inhibitor
	Tetracyclines	Fluoroquinolones
		Rifampicin
		Vancomycin

- Causes self-limiting gastroenteritis in otherwise healthy people, but generalised sepsis and meningitis in specific high-risk subgroups (elderly, immunocompromised, fetuses, pregnancy) in which the mortality rate is high (20%). Such individuals should avoid high-risk foods

Norovirus

- The commonest cause of non-bacterial gastroenteritis in industrialised countries is norovirus (previously termed small-round-structured viruses, Norwalk-like viruses or human caliciviruses)
- Norovirus causes outbreaks of acute-onset vomiting and diarrhoea lasting for a median of 5 days. It accounted 85% of all non-bacterial outbreaks reported from 10 European countries. Prevalence is increasing (2002/3), possibly due to new strains
- A periodic cause of large outbreaks of diarrhoea in institutions, including hospitals
- Norovirus is transmitted by contamination of uncooked foods by food handlers. Certain foods, notably oysters and raspberries may be contaminated at source
- Treatment is supportive (fluids, antidiarrhoeal agents or antiemetics if clinically necessary)
- Prevention depends upon the elimination of faecal contamination of fruits and vegetables and adequate enteric precautions (hand washing) in institutions such as hospitals, day care facilities, and nursing homes

Cryptosporidium spp.

- No treatment is needed, since infection is usually self-limiting except in the immunocompromised

Cyclospora spp.

- Increasingly recognised cause of persistent diarrhoea after foreign travel
- Sulfamethoxazole/Trimethoprim (Co-trimoxazole/Septra) 800 mg/160 mg twice daily for 1–2 weeks is usually effective

Giardia lamblia

Tinidazole 2 g (not available in North America) as a single dose (p. 364) or metronidazole 750–800 mg three times daily for 3 days.

11.2 Other gastrointestinal infections

Post-infective and tropical enteropathy

A variety of infections, including *G. lamblia*, *E. coli*, *Klebsiella pneumoniae* and some viruses, may be followed by enterocyte damage that can be asymptomatic. It may progress to partial villous atrophy and cause malabsorption (postinfective tropical malabsorption or tropical sprue), but this is not due to any specific organism (p. 225).

Tuberculosis

- 1–4% of patients infected with tuberculosis have intestinal involvement. The diagnosis is often delayed or overlooked. Disease is caused by *Mycobacterium tuberculosis* or

M. bovis after direct ingestion (swallowed sputum or infected milk), by haematogenous spread from another focus, or rarely by direct extension from adjacent organs. Atypical mycobacterium (such as *M. avium-intracellulare*) is an AIDS-defining infection
- Differentiation from Crohn's disease is extremely important, as treatment with prednisolone or monoclonal antibody to tumour necrosis factor (Infliximab) will dramatically worsen the course of tuberculosis

Clinical features
- Immigrants comprise the largest and fastest-growing group of patients. The diagnosis should always be considered in Indian, African, South-East Asian, Eastern European or South/Central American patients with chronic gastrointestinal symptoms, even in second-generation immigrants. Presentation several years after the patient arrives from abroad is common. Other populations at risk include the homeless, prisoners, intravenous drug users, residents of long-term care institutions and the immunosuppressed, particularly patients with HIV infection
- The peak incidence occurs at age 25–44 years
- Tuberculosis can occur at any location in the gastrointestinal tract, but the following are the most frequent locations:

Ileocaecal tuberculosis
- Clinically similar to Crohn's disease (p. 252), with recurrent abdominal pain, pyrexia, weight loss or diarrhoea
- A mass is palpable in 40% and lymphocytosis is common, but by no means always present
- 12–16% of patients with an acute abdomen due to tuberculous appendicitis, small bowel obstruction, and perforation
- Colonic tuberculosis is very rare

Tuberculous peritonitis
- Ascites, weight loss and ill health. A 'doughy' feeling on abdominal palpation is classically described but is not commonly detected
- Clinical suspicion and a diagnostic tap are essential, although laparotomy is often needed to establish the diagnosis (p. 252)

Tuberculous adenitis
Mesenteric adenitis may cause acute abdominal pain, similar to appendicitis.

Perianal tuberculosis
Similar to Crohn's disease but very rare.

Diagnosis
- About 30% have an abnormal chest X-ray; sputum samples may then be diagnostic. Most have no active pulmonary disease
- A positive Mantoux test simply indicates previous exposure or vaccination. A strongly positive test (> 10 mm induration following 0.1 mL 1 : 10 000 tuberculin) favours active infection, but is often negative in peritonitis

- Ascitic fluid when present is typically cloudy yellow. Analysis reveals an exudate and a high lymphocyte count. Sensitivity of ascitic fluid for acid-fast bacilli staining and culture is low but may be increased by analysis of a large volume. Adenosine deaminase levels (p. 148), or peritoneal biopsy with an Abrams' needle, may be diagnostic for tuberculous peritonitis, but laparotomy is often necessary to establish the diagnosis
- Small bowel radiology will demonstrate ileocaecal tuberculosis, but cannot distinguish this from Crohn's disease, lymphoma, or severe *Strongyloides stercoralis* infection
- CT may reveal free or loculated ascites (high attenuation fluid due to high protein content), lymphadenopathy (peripheral enhancing ring with central hypodensity corresponding to region of caseation necrosis), peritoneal enhancement, small bowel abnormalities (thickening, strictures and mass lesion)
- Colonoscopic features are non-specific. Multiple biopsies should be taken for histology, culture and PCR. PCR offers a sensitivity of 64–75% and specificity of 100% with results obtained within 24 h
- Laparoscopy or laparotomy is indicated to establish the diagnosis when doubt exists. In an African or Indian patient with radiological ileocaecal distortion, tuberculosis can be assumed to be the cause unless there is no response to treatment after 2 months

Management
- The same regimen as for pulmonary tuberculosis is used, although evidence for efficacy is not as certain. Culture of biopsy specimens and ascites is necessary to determine drug sensitivities
- Triple therapy for 2 months (isoniazid 300 mg/day, rifampicin 600 mg/day, pyrazinamide 2 g/day, for an average patient), followed by isoniazid and rifampicin alone for 4 months
- If resistance is suspected based on local statistics, origin from a country with high resistance rates, or exposure to a drug-resistant case, ethambutol should be added, and continued until sensitivities are available
- *M. bovis* is insensitive to pyrazinamide and should be treated with rifampicin and isoniazid for 9 months, and ethambutol for the initial 2 months
- Pyridoxine 10 mg/day is unnecessary, unless higher doses of isoniazid are used or paraesthesia occurs
- Response is judged by clinical improvement, weight gain, reversal of anaemia and fall in ESR. Intestinal parasites often coexist and may contribute to anaemia
- Routine liver function tests are unnecessary during antituberculous chemotherapy, unless there is pre-existing liver disease, or results are borderline at the start of treatment
- Abnormal liver function tests may be due to drugs (isoniazid, rifampicin), tuberculosis or other disease (cirrhosis). Drugs should be continued unless deterioration occurs (threefold elevation in AST). Biopsy is then indicated to establish the cause
- Surgery is recommended for complications such as obstruction, perforation, massive bleeding, and in patients with large necrotic lesions into which the penetration of antibiotics may be poor
- Follow-up for 2 years after recovery and stopping treatment is recommended, in case of relapse
- Notification of public health authorities and contact tracing are essential (p. 367)

Typhoid and paratyphoid (enteric fever)

The disease occurs predominately in the developing world where sanitary conditions remain poor. It is a sporadic disease in developed countries that occurs mainly in returned travellers. In the UK there are about 200 cases a year of *Salmonella typhi*, *S. paratyphi A* or *S. paratyphi B* infection. Paratyphoid produces similar but less severe features than typhoid.

Clinical features

- Most people presenting to hospital are aged 5–25
- Patients typically present after 7–14 days with influenza-like symptoms, including fever (stepwise progression is characteristic, but rare), headache, malaise, anorexia, myalgia and cough
- Constipation—initially, but diarrhoea develops later
- Relative bradycardia—rarely in brucellosis too
- Rash ('rose-spots')—usually on the abdomen and chest appear after a few days. They are easily missed in dark-skinned patients
- A tender abdomen and hepatosplenomegaly are common
- Complications occur in 10–15% of patients typically in the third week. The most important are intestinal haemorrhage (due to erosion of a necrotic Peyer's patch through an enteric vessel wall), perforation, encephalopathy and death (< 1%)

Diagnosis

- Leucopenia is common, but may also occur with dengue fever and rarely in brucellosis
- Blood cultures in the first week, but bone marrow culture is the most reliable test and may be positive even after prior antibiotic treatment
- Urine or faecal culture in the second week
- Serology (Widal test) is of no value in acute illness

Management

- Ciprofloxacin 750 mg twice daily (or 400 mg by slow intravenous injection twice daily)
- Chloramphenicol 1 g (oral or intravenous) four times daily for 2 weeks. Multiple antibiotic resistance is increasing, especially from the Indian subcontinent. Care is necessary in children, for whom alternatives are trimethoprim or amoxicillin
- Dexamethasone reduces the mortality associated with encephalopathy
- Isolation of excreta (urine, faeces), to prevent cross-infection
- Notification of public health authorities is necessary (Table 11.7, p. 368) and contacts must be traced
- Three negative stool cultures are necessary before the patient returns to work. The district consultant for communicable diseases or public health authorities will advise (p. 367)
- Relapse occurs in 5–10% of patients, usually after 2–3 weeks
- 10% of patients continue to excrete the organism for up to 3 months
- 1–4% become long-term asymptomatic carriers (risk factors include the elderly, women, and patients with gallstones). Such patients should be offered

ciprofloxacin 750 mg twice daily for 28 days and a cholecystectomy if gallstones are present
- The Ty21a and Vi vaccines are recommended for travellers to endemic areas, household contacts or laboratory workers likely to handle the organism

Amoebiasis (Entamoeba histolytica *infection*)

In Europe and the USA amoebiasis is most commonly seen in immigrants from, and travellers to, developing countries. The disease is more severe at extremes of age and in patients receiving corticosteroids. Disease follows ingestion of faecally contaminated food or water. Asymptomatic cyst excretion is common (> 10% worldwide, 1% in Europe)

Clinical features
- > 90% of infections are asymptomatic
- Amoebic dysentery—clinically similar to ulcerative colitis (p. 266), with proctocolitis. In 0.5% of cases a fulminant, necrotising course with toxic megacolon is observed; this form of the disease carries a mortality of > 40%
- Non-dysenteric colonic disease is less common and may mimic Crohn's disease or carcinoma. Features include strictures, an inflammatory mass (amoeboma), appendicitis, abscesses, perianal, fistulating disease, and skip lesions
- Amoebic liver abscess—10 times more common in men and rare in children. A short history (2–4 weeks) of constant dull right upper quadrant pain, fever and cough associated with focally tender hepatomegaly is typical. Associated gastrointestinal symptoms are present in 10–35% of patients. Complications of hepatic abscesses include rupture into the pleural, peritoneal or pericardial cavities. Extrahepatic amoebic abscesses in the lung, brain and skin are rare

Diagnosis
- Diagnosis is based upon the detection in stool of *E. histolytica*-specific antigen or DNA, and by the detection of antiamoebic antibodies in serum. The addition of serology helps exclude patients with asymptomatic carriage (antibodies are present in 70–90% of patients with active disease but absent in asymptomatic carriage), but remains positive for years after infection
- Microscopy of fresh, warm stools to identify red cell–consuming (haematophagous) amoebae is diagnostic and is still used. Cyst excretion alone may be incidental. The drawbacks of this method include its low sensitivity and false-positive rate due to the presence of *E. dispar* or *E. moshkovskii* infection
- Biopsies or mucosal scrapings should also be examined for trophozoites (amoebae with pseudopodia adjacent to the mucosa), and classic flask-shaped focal ulcerations extending into the submucosa
- Diagnosis of amoebic liver abscess depends on the presence of appropriate epidemiologic risk factors, imaging by ultrasound, CT or MR (usually single lesions in the right lobe) and elevated antibodies to *E. histolytica*. Patients characteristically have focal tenderness over one area of the liver. Hiccups indicate diaphragmatic irritation and impending rupture. Percutaneous aspiration is occasionally required to rule out a pyogenic abscess. Viscous, reddish ('anchovy sauce') fluid is characteristic of an

amoebic liver abscess. Amoebae are visualised in the abscess fluid in only a minority of patients

Management
- Metronidazole (750–800 mg three times daily for 5 days) is effective for all types of amoebiasis, but should always be followed by paromyocin (25–35 mg/kg/day in three divided doses for 7 days) or diloxanide furoate (500 mg three times daily for 10 days) to eradicate luminal parasites that remain in 40–60% of patients
- Three repeat stool specimens, to confirm clearance, are advisable
- Asymptomatic cyst excretors should receive treatment with paromyocin or diloxanide furoate
- Ultrasound-guided drainage of a hepatic abscess should be considered in patients who have no response to drug therapy within 7 days or those with a high risk of rupture (diameter > 5 cm, left lobe lesions, hiccups)

Schistosomiasis
Schistosomiasis is endemic in Asia, much of the Middle East, Africa, the Caribbean and South America. Chronic schistosomiasis usually affects the indigenous population, who may then travel and present to doctors in non-endemic areas.

Visitors to endemic areas do not develop severe chronic schistosomiasis as a heavy worm burden takes many years to accumulate, but may suffer schistosome dermatitis, or rarely acute schistosomiasis (Katayama fever). Swimming in sea water or chlorinated swimming pools is safe, even in endemic areas, because the parasite needs the freshwater snail to develop. It is not infectious, for the same reason.

Diagnosis is made by detecting excretion of ova in faeces. As a rule schistosomiasis does not cause symptoms unless there is heavy excretion of ova, even if serological tests are positive, which only indicates previous exposure.

Schistosome dermatitis
An itchy papular rash affects exposed skin (swimmers' itch) within 24 h and resolves within 72 h, but is most unusual after primary exposure.

Acute schistosomiasis (Katayama fever)
- Fever, rigors, anorexia, myalgia, bloody diarrhoea, tender hepatosplenomegaly and cough develop 20–60 days after heavy initial exposure
- Diagnosis is suspected because of eosinophilia and confirmed by finding schistosome ova in faeces. Three stool specimens may be required as shedding may be intermittent. Formalin-based sedimentation and concentration techniques may increase the yield. Serology is both less sensitive and specific, remaining positive after successful treatment. Chest X-ray may show interstitial pneumonitis

Chronic schistosomiasis
- Disease results from the granulomatous immune reaction evoked by antigens secreted by the schistosome eggs
- *Schistosoma japonicum* in Asia, and *S. mansoni* in other areas, may cause bloody diarrhoea and in < 10% of patients hepatosplenomegaly and portal hypertension

- *S. haematobium* in the Middle East predominantly affects the urinary tract manifesting as haematuria 10–12 weeks after infection. Late manifestations include proteinuria, calcifications in the bladder, ureteric obstruction and renal failure. Vulval and perineal disease is seen in approximately one-third of women
- *Schistosoma* colitis causes bloody diarrhoea. Granulomatous inflammatory nodules may be visible on sigmoidoscopy and confirmed by rectal biopsy, which also shows ova. Chronic inflammation may lead to stenoses and inflammatory masses that may mimic carcinoma
- Portal hypertension may cause recurrent haematemesis, but not encephalopathy, except in the terminal stages, because hepatic fibrosis is presinusoidal and hepatocellular function is preserved until very late in the disease (p. 151)
- Co-infection of *S. mansoni* with HBV or HCV is not uncommon. Chronic liver disease in an Asian patient with light excretion of ova may still be due to hepatitis B, but granulomas on liver biopsy suggest schistosomiasis. Co-infection is associated with an accelerated deterioration of hepatic function and a higher risk of hepatocellular carcinoma

Management
- Treatment is indicated for schistosomiasis with praziquantel, but is best undertaken by specialists, preferably following quantitative egg counts. Praziquantel 40 mg/kg as a single dose is effective in *S. mansoni*, and 25 mg/kg for 3 days in *S. japonicum*. Re-examination of faeces or urine, 1 month after treatment is recommended in order to assess efficacy
- Portal hypertension is likely to improve and surgical portosystemic shunting should be a last resort, although surgery gives a better prognosis than in patients with cirrhosis

11.3 Other parasitic infections

Infection by parasites, often several, is the norm in many parts of the world. Classification can be confusing (Table 11.4).

Table 11.4 Classification of common gastrointestinal parasites

Protozoa	Nematodes	Cestodes	Trematodes
G. lamblia	Roundworm	Tapeworm	Liver flukes
Cryptosporidium spp.	*A. lumbricoides*	*T. solium*	*Clonorchis sinensis*
	Hookworm	(*cysticercosis*)	*Opisthorchis viverrinis*
E. histolytica	*Necator americanus*	*T. saginata*	*Fasciola hepatica*
Leishmania spp.	*A. duodenale*	*Hymenolopsis nana*	*Schistosoma* spp.
	Threadworm		*S. mansoni*
	E. vermicularis	*D. latum*	*S. japonicum*
	Whipworm	Hydatid	
	T. trichiura	*E. granulosus*	
	S. stercoralis		
	Trichinella spiralis		

Clinical features

General
- Infections are usually asymptomatic, but can cause low-grade debility or specific features (see below)
- Gastrointestinal upset—nausea, bloating or diarrhoea are common but non-specific when symptoms occur; this affects a minority only
- Weight loss—indicates heavy infection or a complication, but this is unusual

Specific
- Anaemia: iron deficiency (*Necator americanus, Ancylostoma duodenale, Trichuris trichuria*), B_{12} deficiency (*Diphyllobothrium latum*, from raw fish)
- Asthma—during larval migration (*Ascaris lumbricoides, Str. stercoralis*)
- Colitis—often with granulomas (*E. histolytica, T. trichiura, S. mansoni* or *S. japonicum*)
- Cutaneous: urticaria (*Str. stercoralis* 'cutaneous larva migrans'), dermatitis (*Schistosoma* spp. 'swimmer's itch')
- Encystment—muscle, brain (*Taenia solium, Trichinella spiralis*)
- Fever: transient (*T. spiralis, Schistosoma* spp.) fulminant septicaemia (*Str. stercoralis* hyperinfection in immunocompromised patients)
- Obstruction: intestinal, biliary (*A. lumbricoides*, hydatid)
- Portal hypertension: *Schistosoma* spp., *Clonorchis sinensis*
- Pruritus ani: *Enterobius vermicularis*
- Steatorrhoea: *Str. stercoralis*

Visible faecal worms
This may be the only manifestation of infection and usually prompts a rapid visit to the doctor in the UK. The worm may have been retained for inspection.
- 0.5 cm long and 0.1 cm diameter, thicker at one end than the other: *T. trichuria* (whipworm) or *Ent. vermicularis* (threadworm)
- 10–30 cm long, like a white earthworm: *A. lumbricoides*
- From 2 to over 20 cm long, segmented: *Taenia saginata* or *T. solium. D. latum* is a single, long (up to 25 m) worm that is very rare in Britain
- All other worms excreted in faeces are microscopic

Diagnosis

Eosinophilia
- $> 0.44 \times 10^9$/L. The number of eosinophils should be expressed in absolute terms, not as a percentage
- Common marker of infection, usually $> 0.8 \times 10^9$/L in active infection
- Other causes include:
  - drug hypersensitivity
  - atopy
  - bronchopulmonary aspergillosis
  - pulmonary infiltrates and eosinophilia

- vasculitis (polyarteritis)
- lymphoma (rarely)
- chronic active hepatitis (rarely)
- Crohn's disease (rarely)
- ulcerative colitis (very rarely)
- eosinophilic gastroenteritis
- eosinophilic leukaemia (exceptional)

Examination of faecal sample

- Faecal examination of ova or cysts is the only way of differentiating infections, but ova or cyst excretion may be difficult to detect. Repeated stool samples and concentration techniques should be discussed with the laboratory
- Perianal skin is heavily infected during *Ent. vermicularis* infection, which can be detected by a Sellotape slide (Sellotape applied to the anal margin and examined under a microscope for 0.5–1 cm long worms)

Serological tests

- Not available for most parasitic infections
- ELISA tests for *E. histolytica*, *Schistosoma* spp., *Echinococcus granulosus* (hydatid disease), *Leishmania* spp, and *T. spiralis* virtually exclude the disease if negative, except in the early stages
- Serological tests are not a reliable index of active infection. Treatment is, however, indicated in the UK and North America for patients with positive serology and a compatible clinical picture

Management of specific parasites

- The recommendations in Table 11.5 are for sporadic infection in non-endemic areas. General measures, including hand hygiene for nematode infections (especially *Ent. vermicularis*), or treatment of anaemia, are also important. Other members of the patient's family should have stools examined for parasites
- Treatment of complications (such as *Str. stercoralis* hyperinfection) should be in consultation with specialists

11.4 Immunocompromised patients

HIV-1 and -2 are now the predominant cause of acquired immune deficiency in all parts of the world, but other immunocompromised patients (following chemotherapy) are also susceptible to opportunistic gastrointestinal infections.

Detailed consideration of the gastrointestinal and hepatobiliary manifestations of HIV infection are beyond the scope of this text. Readers are referred to further reading (Appendix 2, p. 442).

AIDS

Acute HIV infection has unusual, specific gastrointestinal features, but most opportunistic infections that become pathogenic (*Cryptosporidium* spp., CMV, Tables 11.6 and 11.7) suggest AIDS.

Table 11.5 Drugs for gastrointestinal parasites

Parasite	First choice	Second choice
Protozoa		
G. lamblia	Tinidazole 2 g stat. or Metronidazole 750 mg t.d.s. 3 days	Mepacrine 100 mg t.d.s. 7 days
E. histolytica	Metronidazole 750–800 mg t.d.s. 5 days	Diloxanide furoate 500 mg t.d.s. 10 days
Cryptosporidium spp.	None	
I. belli	Co-trimoxazole (trimethoprim/ sulfamethoxazol(e) 960 mg b.d. 21 days	Metronidazole
Cyclospora spp.	Co-trimoxazole 960 mg b.d. 7 days	
Leishmania spp.	Sodium stibogluconate 20 mg/kg 20 days	Pentamidine[†]
Nematodes		
A. lumbricoides	Mebendazole 100 mg b.d. 3 days	Levamisole[†]
Necator americanus	Mebendazole 100 mg b.d. 2 days	[†]
A. duodenale	Same	[†]
E. vermicularis	Mebendazole 100 mg stat. (repeated after 2 weeks)	[†]
T. trichuria	Mebendazole 100 mg b.d. 3 days	Albendazole 4 mg/kg stat.*
S. stercoralis	Thiabendazole 1.5 g b.d. 3 days	[†]
Trichinella spiralis	Thiabendazole 25 mg/kg for 3 days	
Cestodes		
Taenia spp.	Niclosamide 2 g stat.	Praziquantel 10–20 mg/kg stat.*
D. latum	Same	[†]
Hymenolepsis nana	Same	[†]
Echinococcus spp.	Albendazole 800 mg Daily for 28 days[†]	Praziquantel[†]
Trematodes		
Clonorchis sinensis	Praziquantel 25 mg/kg t.d.s. 2 days*	
Opisthorchis viverrani	Same	
Fasciola hepatica	Same	
S. japonicum	Same	
S. mansoni	Praziquantel 40 mg/kg*[†]	

*Named patients only, from SmithKline Beecham (albendazole), or Bayer (praziquantel).
[†]Specialist advice required; general measures (hygiene) are as important.
Stat., immediately; b.d., twice daily; t.d.s., three times daily.

The term 'gay bowel syndrome', although no longer used, referred to infections causing proctocolitis or diarrhoea in homosexual men who were not necessarily immunocompromised. Any infection with an organism in Tables 11.6 or 11.7 is an indication for measuring immunoglobulins and HIV status, *after* counselling.

Specialist combination treatment for HIV infection with antiretroviral agents and protease inhibitors is appropriate.

HIV enteropathy

Diarrhoea for which no causative organism can be found is common in AIDS and AIDS-related complex (ARC). This is attributed to HIV enteropathy causing partial

Table 11.6 Differential diagnosis of diarrhoea in AIDS

Moderate	Severe/malabsorption	Bloody
G. lamblia	*Cryptosporidium* spp.	Herpes simplex virus
Salmonella spp.	*I. belli*	*Chlamydia trachomatis*
Campylobacter spp.	Cytomegalovirus	Cytomegalovirus
Mycobacterium spp.	*Enterocytozoon bieneusi*	*Campylobacter* spp.
Gonorrhoea	*Cyclospora* spp.	*E. histolytica*
HIV enteropathy		*Shigella* spp.

villous atrophy, with histological crypt malabsorption, weight loss or susceptibility to infection.

A lactose-free diet may diminish symptoms associated with hypolactasia, but general avoidance of dairy products is not usually required. There is no other specific treatment apart from antidiarrhoeal agents. Severe diarrhoea is usually caused by a superimposed infection.

Candida spp.

- Oropharyngeal candidiasis causes a sore mouth or painful dysphagia if there is oesophageal involvement (p. 73). It is the most common oesophageal infection in

Table 11.7 Gastrointestinal complications of AIDS

Clinical problem	Site	Cause
Sore mouth	Oropharyngeal	*Candida* spp.
		Gonorrhoea
		Herpes simplex
Mouth ulcer(s)	Oropharyngeal	*Herpes simplex*
		Syphilis
		Kaposi's sarcoma*
		Acute HIV infection
Painful dysphagia	Oesophageal	*Candida* spp.
		Cytomegalovirus*
Diarrhoea (Table 11.5)		Acute HIV infection
Constipation	Rectal stricture	*Chlamydia* spp.
		Lymphogranuloma venereum
Abdominal pain	Subacute obstruction	*Mycobacterium* spp.*
		Intestinal lymphoma*
		Kaposi's sarcoma*
	Gall bladder	Cytomegalovirus*
Rectal bleeding	Ulcer/tumour	Syphilis
		Lymphogranuloma venereum
		Kaposi's sarcoma*
		Anorectal carcinoma
	Other	Thrombocytopenia (drug-induced)
Jaundice	Liver	Hepatitis B, B + D or C Sclerosing cholangitis (microsporidia)
		Drugs

*Diagnostic of AIDS in the presence of immunodeficiency for which no other cause can be found.
†Systemic infection is common in immunodeficiency.

AIDS patients. It is associated with a low CD4 count, high HIV RNA level, prior zidovudine use and recent antibiotic use

- Diagnosis is by sight (white oral plaques, not to be confused with oral hairy leucoplakia) and confirmed by swab (hyphae, demonstrated by Gram stain)
- Oral candidiasis is treated with nystatin suspension 1 mL four times daily, or oral fluconazole 50–100 mg daily for 14 days, which should be given prophylactically in AIDS after an episode of oral candidiasis
- Oesophageal or systemic candidiasis is treated with oral fluconazole 50–100 mg daily for 14 days, ketoconazole 200 mg daily for 14 days, or voriconazole 200 mg twice daily for 2–6 weeks. Specialist advice is recommended

Cryptosporidium spp.
- *C. parvum* is the species most commonly associated with disease in humans. In immunocompetent humans parasites locate primarily to the distal ileum and cause self-limiting abdominal pain, diarrhoea and occasionally vomiting. There is some evidence that *C. parvum* may exacerbate irritable bowel disease. In immunocompromised patients the whole gastrointestinal tract may be involved producing intractable watery diarrhoea malabsorption, weight loss and dehydration
- Diagnosis is traditionally based upon detection of oocysts in stool. Both ELISA and PCR-based methods to detect *C. parvum* antigen are now available
- There is no consistently effective therapy for cryptosporidiosis, but spiramycin 1 g three times daily for 3 weeks (not available on UK market) is sometimes effective. Trimethoprim/sulfamethoxazole (co-trimoxazole/Septra 800/160 mg twice daily for 2–3 weeks is indicated for *Isospora belli*

Cyclospora cayetanensis
- Symptoms are similar to those of cryptosporidiosis and is an increasingly common cause of diarrhoea from abroad that does not respond to ciprofloxacin or metronidazole
- Complications include infection of the biliary tree, Guillain–Barré syndrome and Reiter's syndrome
- Detection of organisms in stool samples is difficult but may be facilitated by concentration methods and by the use of ultraviolet microscopy as *Cyclospora* sp. oocysts autofluoresce
- The drug of choice for all patients is trimethoprim/sulfamethoxazole (co-trimoxazole 960 mg twice daily for 2–3 weeks)

Isospora belli
- Causes chronic high-volume diarrhoea in immunocompromised patients and mild self-limiting watery diarrhoea lasting < 2 weeks in immunocompetent individuals
- Detection of organisms in stool samples may require concentration methods. Villous atrophy and eosinophil infiltrates on duodenal biopsy may provide helpful clues
- Treatment is as for *Cyclospora cayetanensis*

Microsporidia
- Causes chronic diarrhoea in immunocompromised patients. Parasite dissemination may occur including spread to the bile ducts, which causes a progressive cholangitis

- Electron microscopy is the gold standard for diagnosis
- Albendazole is effective in treating *Encephalitozoon intestinalis*, but does not reliably eradicate *E. bieneusi*, which should be treated with fumagillin. Specialist advice is appropriate

Herpes simplex virus type 1

- Proctitis occasionally occurs. Extensive oropharyngeal ulceration or disseminated herpetic infection is more common in the immunocompromised. There is often a past history of genital herpes (herpes simplex virus type 2)
- Nuclear inclusion bodies in a rectal biopsy specimen distinguish herpetic proctitis from Crohn's disease
- Antibodies to *Herpes simplex* virus (and other viruses, including hepatitis B) may be absent in immunodeficiency. This is a poor prognostic sign
- Oral acyclovir (200–400 mg five times daily for 5 days) is effective, but intravenous treatment (5–10 mg/kg over 1 h, three times daily) is needed for sick patients. Maintenance therapy (same oral dose, long term) is indicated for frequent relapse

Cytomegalovirus (CMV)

- Proctocolitis is recognised by bloody, watery diarrhoea and superficial mucosal ulceration at sigmoidoscopy, in association with choroidoretinitis or pneumonitis. Oesophagitis causes odynophagia and may be complicated by strictures following treatment (p. 73)
- Diagnosis is confirmed by multiple intranuclear eosinophilic inclusion bodies in a rectal biopsy specimen. An occasional inclusion body in a patient with colitis does not make the diagnosis
- CMV colitis should be considered a cause of deterioration in a patient with ulcerative colitis who is on azathioprine or other immunomodulators
- Intravenous ganciclovir (5 mg/kg every 12 h for 14 days) is potentially toxic and only indicated in immunocompromised patients with severe colitis, or sight-threatening infection. Specialist advice should be sought, including alternatives (valganciclovir, foscarnet or cidofovir). Disseminated infection is usually fatal

Chlamydia *spp*.

- Chlamydial proctitis closely resembles Crohn's disease
- Biopsy occasionally demonstrates chlamydial inclusion bodies, which can be distinguished from CMV or herpes simplex virus inclusion bodies by electron microscopy. Microimmunofluorescent antibody tests establish the diagnosis
- Tetracycline 500 mg four times daily is effective, but may have to be continued for several weeks

11.5 Notification

Diseases affecting the gastrointestinal tract that are notifiable by law are shown in Table 11.8. The Director of Public Health (telephone number and address on the notification form, or from the area health authority offices) should first be tele-

Table 11.8 Notifiable and prescribed gastrointestinal disorders in the UK

Common	Rare
Hepatitis—any type*	Tuberculosis*
Food poisoning—any type or suspected	Leptospirosis*
Dysentery—bacillary (*Shigella* spp.)	Amoebiasis
	Typhoid
	Paratyphoid
	Cholera
	Lead poisoning*
	Toxic jaundice (hydrocarbons)*
	Ancylostomiasis[†]
	Brucellosis[†]
	Vinyl chloride portal fibrosis[†]
	Hepatic angiosarcoma[†]
	Beryllium (hepatic granuloma)[†]
	Arsenic and other heavy metals[†]

*Statutorily notifiable, but a prescribed disease in certain occupations. Notifiable diseases vary between jurisdictions, especially in the USA and Canada: seek advice from the Public Health Authority.
[†]Prescribed disease in certain occupations.

phoned and then sent the notification form, for which a small fee is payable. Some districts in Britain now have a consultant in communicable diseases, about which the local microbiology department will know. The environmental health department of local councils in Britain deal with commercial establishments, rather than patients.

Reporting requirements vary between jurisdictions within the USA and Canada. Contact with the local Public Health authorities should be made if there is any possibility that a disease is reportable.

Prescribed diseases have an industrial origin for which compensation may be payable, if the claimant has worked in a specified occupation. The Employment Medical Adviser at the Health and Safety Executive (Appendix 1, p. 438) will advise.

12 Nutrition

12.1 Nutritional assessment

Nutritional assessment of any patient, particularly one with gastrointestinal disease, is essential. Inadequate dietary intake, disordered appetite and general or specific malabsorption all contribute to nutritional deficiency. Neglecting the nutritional status of ill patients compromises survival (increases hospital length of stay and increases complications). Starvation in hospital may follow surgery, prolonged investigation or gastrointestinal symptoms, combined with apprehension and unappetising food (see below).

The aim of assessment is to recognise general (protein–calorie) malnutrition (Table 12.1), as well as specific nutritional deficiencies (Tables 12.2–12.4).

General malnutrition
• No single measurement is sufficient

Table 12.1 Assessment of protein–calorie malnutrition

Readily assessed	Objective measurements
History	Weight loss > 10% in < 3 months
• anorexia	Blood tests
• dietary history (dietitian)	• albumin < 35 g/L
• calorie intake (dietitian)	• lymphocytes < 1.5 × 10⁹/L
• food and fluid chart (inpatient)	• transferrin < 2 g/L
Examination	Skin fold tests
• muscle wasting	• mid-triceps skin fold
• oedema	• < 8 mm (M)
• angular stomatitis	• < 17 mm (F)
Weight and height (Appendix 3, p. 450)	• mid-arm muscle circumference
• below minimum weight for height	• < 30 cm (M)
• BMI < 19 kg/m²	• < 26 cm (F)
	• negative tuberculin test (anergy)

F, female; M, male.

Table 12.2 Recognition of fat-soluble vitamin deficiencies in adults

Substance	Clinical	Diagnostic tests
Vitamin A	Night blindness Xerophthalmia, keratomalaci	Dark adaptation time
Vitamin D	Bone pain, proximal myopathy	Alkaline phosphatase Low calcium, low phosphate Pelvic X-ray (Looser's zones), bone biopsy
Vitamin K	Bruising	Prothrombin time, or INR > 1.3
Vitamin E	Spinocerebellar degeneration	White cell vitamin E

Table 12.3 Recognition of water-soluble vitamin deficiencies in adults

Substance	Clinical	Diagnostic tests
Thiamine (B_1)	Neuropathy, ophthalmoplegia, psychosis, cardiac failure All alcoholics admitted to hospital	Red cell transketolase
Riboflavin (B_2)	Angular stomatitis, mucosal fissures (lips, genitalia) Normochromic anaemia, apathy, ataxia	Red cell glutathione reductase activity
Pyridoxine (B_6)	Sideroblastic anaemia, neuropathy, hyperoxaluria	Aminotransferase activity
Nicotinamide (Niacin)	Dermatitis, diarrhoea, dementia, weight loss	Urinary metabolites
Folate	Macrocytic anaemia Alcoholic patients	Red cell folate < 120 ng/L
B_{12}	Macrocytic anaemia, painful neuropathy, ataxia, poor proprioception, paresis	Serum B_{12} < 150 ng/L
Vitamin C	Poor wound healing, gum hyperplasia, bleeding, perifollicular or subperiosteal haemorrhages	White cell ascorbic acid, or urinary excretion < 10% after 1 g ascorbate

Table 12.4 Recognition of mineral deficiencies in adults

Substance	Clinical	Diagnostic tests
Iron	Microcytic anaemia, glossitis, cheilosis, koilonychia	Serum iron < 11 µmol/L (F) < 14 µmol/L (M), iron binding capacity >75 µmol/L, serum ferritin <15 µg/L
Calcium	Weakness, proximal myopathy, perioral paraesthesiae, tetany, Chvostek (jaw), Trousseau (arm) signs	Serum calcium <2.20 mmol/L add 0.02 × (40-serum albumin) to correct for albumin level)
Phosphate	Proximal myopathy	Serum phosphate < 0.80 mmol/L
Magnesium	Myopathy not responding to calcium replacement	Serum magnesium < 0.70 mmol/L
Zinc	Anorexia, crusting red rash, diarrhoea, depression, anaemia, candidiasis	Serum zinc < 6 µmol/L(may be low in any acute illness)
Copper	Hypochromic anaemia not responsive to iron, low white cell count, osteoporosis	Red cell superoxide dismutase activity
Selenium	Cardiac failure	Glutathione peroxidase activity, serum Se

F, female; M, male.

- The % change in body weight correlates most closely with malnutrition. An unintended weight loss > 10% within 1 month is an indication for nutritional support
- Height, weight and serum albumin (or total protein) may be the simplest measures available, but do not accurately reflect nutritional status. Infection, hepatic, renal or intestinal

disease may contribute to a low albumin or total serum protein independent of poor nutrition

- Malabsorption, which may occur in the absence of diarrhoea, must not be overlooked (p. 217)
- The BMI, or Quetelet index, is a crude but simple measure of overall nutritional status. It is calculated according to the formula: BMI = weight (kg)/height^2 (m)
- In general, a healthy BMI is defined as 20–25 kg/m^2, malnutrition is manifest at BMI 14–17 and a BMI < 14 is potentially life-threatening. A BMI > 30 kg/m^2 defines obesity and > 40 kg/m^2 morbid obesity (see Appx 3, p. 450)
- The relation to mortality for high BMI (obesity) is shown in Fig. 12.1
- It is important to recognise that overweight/obese patients can be (and frequently are) malnourished in hospitals, during periods of no oral intake, surgery and sepsis, and should be treated accordingly

Malnutrition in hospital patients

- Frequently not recognised, although treatment of malnutrition has a major effect on length of hospital stay, postoperative complications and survival. Malnutrition demonstrably affects the immune response wound healing, respiratory function and comorbidity in surgical patients
- Six studies on hospital admissions have shown a 20–53% prevalence of malnutrition
- In one study of 112 patients (Appendix 2, p. 448) assessed on discharge from hospital, 78% had lost weight by discharge and those undernourished on admission had lost a greater proportion of weight whilst in hospital
- In another study of 501 patients with a fractured neck of femur, those receiving oral nutritional supplements stayed in hospital 24 days, compared to 40 days in a control group receiving no supplements. Mortality was also reduced by 19% in those receiving supplements

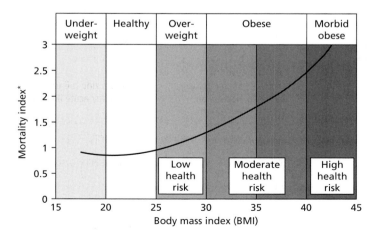

Fig. 12.1 Relationship between obesity and mortality. BMI is explained in the text. Adapted from Bray GA. *International Journal of Obesity* 1978; 2: 99–114, with permission. *Excess mortality from life insurance statistics.

- A nutritional support team is a cost-effective way of reducing complications related to total parenteral and enteral nutrition in hospital, ensuring appropriate referral and resource utilisation and educating hospital staff

Specific deficiencies
- Deficiencies of vitamins and minerals are usually mixed, so clinical presentation is rarely classic (Tables 12.2–12.4, pp. 371-372)
- Diagnosis depends on the clinical context. Clues to the type of nutritional deficiency may be provided by chronic hepatic disease, malabsorption or malnutrition due to inadequate diet in housebound elderly, alcoholics, vegans (B_{12}) or poor milk intake and/or sun exposure (vitamin D)
- Normal values of many of the less common tests vary between laboratories and the technique used. It is often unnecessary to do specific vitamin or trace element tests, but simply to treat suspected deficiency generously (Tables 12.5 and 12.6)
- Requirements increase during periods of prolonged stress (such as catabolic states due to infection, or intestinal failure). Measurement of trace elements and vitamin concentrations at 2–3-month intervals to monitor replacement is then appropriate

Indications for nutritional support
The decision to provide nutritional support depends on the nutritional status (Table 12.1, p. 371) and nature of the illness (Table 12.5). Consideration of nutritional support is mandatory if eating has not been possible for 3–5 days or dietary intake has been inadequate for 5–7 days. A dietitian should be involved in this decision-making process.

Nutritional requirements
- Five factors must be considered:
  - fluid balance
  - energy (from fat and carbohydrate)
  - nitrogen

Table 12.5 Indications for nutritional support

General	Specific
Weight loss > 10%	Multiple injuries/critical care
Albumin < 35 g/L	Burns
No food intake > 3 days	Inadequate dietary intake > 5 days
	Chronic sepsis (abscess)
	Acute pancreatitis
	Intestinal fistulae
	Short bowel syndrome
	Crohn's disease
	Complications of major surgery
	Dysphagia
	Persistent vomiting
	Malignancy
	Children or adolescents with chronic disease

Table 12.6 Daily nutritional requirements

Catabolic states	Low	Intermediate	High
Energy			
• kJ/kg/24 h*	125	125–150	150–250
• kcal/kg/24 h	30	30–35	35–60
Nitrogen			
• g/kg/24 h	0.16	0.2–0.3	0.25–0.35
Potassium (mmol/L/g N)	5	5	7
Phosphate (mmol/24 h)	20	20–30	30–50
Requirements for all catabolic states		Enteral	Parenteral
Electrolytes			
Sodium	1 mmol/kg/24 h	1 mmol/kg/24 h	
Potassium	5 mmol/kg/24 h	5 mmol/kg/24 h	
Calcium	20 mmol/24 h	7–14 mmol/24 h	
Magnesium	14 mmol/24 h	3–28 mmol/24 h	
Trace elements (μmol/24 h)			
Iron	180–320	20–70	
Zinc	230	100	
Manganese	45–90	5–10	
Copper	30–45	20	
Chromium	1–4	0.2–0.4	
Fluorine	80–200	50	
Iodine	1–2	1	
Selenium	0.6–2.6	0.4	
Molybdenum	0.2	0.2	

*Energy is also measured in kilocalories (1 cal = 4.2 J), but kcal is frequently shortened to cal, which is confusing.
†The non-protein energy: nitrogen ratio is not widely used any more, but is approximately 1000 kJ/g N (250 kcal/g N) in low catabolic and 550 kJ/g N (135 kcal/g N) in high catabolic states.

- electrolytes
- trace elements/vitamins
- The nutritional status of the patient, severity of disease and catabolic rate determine the energy/nitrogen balance required (Table 12.6). High energy and nitrogen intakes are not needed in most situations, unless the patient is profoundly catabolic or has major nutrient losses, as in burns
- In low catabolic states such as starvation, paralysis or disease preventing an adequate oral intake, replacement with a normal energy/nitrogen balance is needed, with electrolyte, trace element or vitamin supplements if specific deficiencies are present
- In high catabolic states, including fever, sepsis, major surgery, trauma and burns, energy expenditure and hence requirements are increased by 10–100%
- Protein is 16% nitrogen, so 1 g N = 6.25 g protein. Nitrogen requirements increase in catabolic states

Feeding route

Artificial nutrition support is indicated when the nutritional intake via the oral route remains suboptimal after 5–7 days and is likely to remain so for a prolonged period. The dietitian and the patient and their family need to be involved with medical and nursing staff in this decision process to ensure optimum care/appropriate nutrition support.

- Enteral feeding is the preferred method and should always be used if the gut is functioning, by whatever access is possible (sip feed supplements, fine-bore nasogastric tube, percutaneous endoscopic gastrostomy or surgical jejunostomy)
- Parenteral feeding should only be used when enteral feeding is impossible due to gut failure (Table 12.8, p. 380)

12.2 Enteral feeding

Enteral feeding includes feeding with specially formulated sip feeds, fine-bore nasogastric tube or by enterostomy (gastro- or jejunostomy).

Indications (See Box 12.1)

Choice of feed

- There are either polymeric (the nitrogen source is whole protein), semi-elemental/peptide or elemental (pure amino acids) monomeric feeds, with many proprietary preparations. Elemental feeds are indicated for severe malabsorption (short bowel, pancreatic insufficiency)
- Energy and nitrogen balance (Table 12.6, p. 375), volume, osmolality, palatability and cost must be considered
- Most preparations contain appropriate amounts of vitamins (except folate) and trace elements, when given in quantities to meet macronutrient (energy, protein) requirements of the patient, unless there are specific deficiencies, when supplements will be needed. Most are also gluten- and lactose-free. Check with the dietitian
- Other modifications include variations in fat content (for steatorrhoea), fibre (purported to reduce the incidence of feed-associated diarrhoea) and glutamine content (ostensibly to enhance small intestinal integrity) and other immune nutrients

---

Box 12.1 Indications for enteral nutrition

Gastrointestinal disease
   malabsorption
     liver disease
   short bowel
     inflammatory bowel disease
Catabolic states
   burns
     critical care
   sepsis
     trauma
Anorexia
   any prolonged (> 5 days) illness
   especially after a stroke (dysphagia)
   other neurological illness (bulbar palsy, motor neurone disease)
   before/after surgery
   cancer and its therapy

- Disease-specific formulas have been marketed for patients with hepatic, renal or pulmonary disease for various theoretical reasons, but are expensive and are currently of little demonstrable benefit above standard feeds
- Careful studies have not shown any difference in nutrient absorption or clinical benefit between polymeric, oligomeric or monomeric feeds and it is difficult to show any consistent benefit from the various modifications
- The choice of feed can be limited to a polymeric feed for the majority of patients and is reasonably guided by a local prescribing policy taking cost into account

General purpose (polymeric) feeds
- Hospitals will usually have a local prescribing policy that defines the choice of enteral feeds and other preparations because of contractual agreements. The dietitians will advise
- Feeds usually come as different flavoured cartons of 250 mL (such as Ensure, Resource, Enlive, Fortisip) or as 500–1000 mL bottles for infusion (such as Osmolite, Clinifeed Favour). There is little to choose between the feeds on nutritional grounds and dietetic advice should be taken
- 1500–3000 mL/day is needed for fluid requirements; the dietitian modifies the type of feed, according to energy requirements (1.0, 1.2 or 1.5 kcal/mL)

Elemental feeds
- Elemental feeds are pre-digested, containing nutrients in a directly absorbable form
- Elemental feeds (such as Elemental 028) are often considered unpalatable, but some find them acceptable and take them as sole source of nutrition. They are all hyperosmolar and considerable advances have been made in palatability with Elemental 028 cartons and flavouring packets. They are expensive and the indications for their use are extremely limited (such as active Crohn's disease refractory to steroids, p. 254). However, active Crohn's disease has been shown to respond as well to polymeric feeds
- Oligomeric feeds (such as Peptisorb, Perative, Peptamen, Peptanex) may be better tolerated by those with persistent diarrhoea
- A fine-bore tube is usually needed and the feed must be introduced slowly to avoid side-effects (diarrhoea, abdominal cramps, nausea)

Method of delivery

Oral supplements, in addition to meals
- Suitable for most patients needing nutritional supplements. Proprietary preparations (such as Ensure, EnsurePlus, Resource, Boost, Enlive, Fortisip, Fortijuice, Fortimel, Clinutren, Build Up) have a wide variety of flavours. It is worth experimenting to find the most palatable preparation because poor compliance is likely to lead to higher costs. Dietitians, nursing staff and nutrition assistants all play a vital role in encouraging and supporting nutritional supplementation, with encouragement from the medical team
- Patients who cannot eat may not be able to drink sufficient liquid supplements (1500–3000 mL/day) for all their nutritional requirements. Encouragement and

counselling from a dietitian can improve compliance. Fine-bore nasogastric feeding or other forms of artificial nutritional support may be needed

Nasogastric and nasojejunal tube feeding
- Polyurethane tubes with a stylet are easily inserted (p. 413) and neither impair the swallowing reflex in patients with a stroke nor cause oesophagitis
- Nasogastric feeding can be used for up to 6 weeks, but if feeding is needed for longer than 4–6 weeks, then a percutaneous gastrostomy is usually appropriate
- Nasojejunal feeding should be considered for patients with gastroparesis or pancreatitis, but does not necessarily reduce the risk of aspiration or tube displacement. Tube placement can be difficult and may require endoscopic or fluoroscopic assistance. 'Self-propelling' tubes (such as the Bengmark) have yet to show that they reliably reach the jejunum
- Combined nasojejunal feeding tubes with a gastric aspiration channel are available and useful in an intensive care setting
- Tubes should be flushed before and after use to prevent blockage, which may occur due to protein precipitation from the feed, or from crushed medication. This is best prevented by flushing with water before and after feeding and between each bottle change. Proprietary preparations for unblocking tubes are available, although soda water, 5% sodium bicarbonate solution, or pancreatic enzymes mixed with sodium bicarbonate also work

Regimen
- Continuous drip feeding enhances absorption and reduces complications. A pump should be used to regulate the feed
- The starting rate is variable and should be advised by a dietitian. If advice is not available, starting at 30 mL/h is reasonable, but particular care should be taken over those at risk of refeeding syndrome (p. 383). Additional water to maintain fluid balance is better than diluting the feed
- Bolus feeding is generally avoided, because it promotes gastro-oesophageal reflux, risking aspiration, or diarrhoea. It is, however, sometimes appropriate in some home-fed patients
- Feed containers and giving sets should be changed every 24 h to prevent bacterial contamination

Gastrostomy and jejunostomy feeding

Percutaneous endoscopic gastrostomy
- PEG is the technique of choice for longer-term (> 4–6 weeks) feeding of patients. Common indications include neurological dysphagia (e.g. after a stroke), neoplastic diseases of the oropharynx, larynx or oesophagus and patients with head or facial injuries
- PEG-J is occasionally indicated for patients with gastroparesis, or in patients with repeated tube feeding–related aspiration. Their use is limited by the high incidence of retrograde migration, kinking and obstruction

- Major complications are reported in 0.5–8% of procedures, including wound infections, aspiration, bleeding, perforation, ileus and death (2%). Pneumoperitoneum is of no consequence unless accompanied by signs and symptoms of peritonitis
- If a PEG is inadvertently removed, a small Foley catheter can often be inserted through the track within the first few hours and feeding restarted until the PEG is replaced

Home enteral feeding
- Increasing exponentially, but needs careful liaison between hospital and community nurses, dietitians, doctors and the feed companies
- PEG feeding should be well established before discharge, unless there is specialist dietetic support in the community
- The dietitian will generally arrange for supplies of feed, plastic connectors and a feeding pump. A contact number for the carer to call if there are problems with the pump is essential, as well as agreement about who is to pay. Plastics and feed can usually be supplied by the local chemist or feed company after the dietitian has arranged the prescription with the general practitioner (GP). Dietitians usually provide the link between hospital and home for most patients

Complications (See Table 12.7)
It is important to check for other causes of diarrhoea before altering the feed rate. Diarrhoea with enteral feeding is often due to antibiotics, or other pathology (e.g. pseudomembranous colitis). It can be alleviated by treating the infection, checking medications (e.g. Sando K can cause diarrhoea), continuous feeding (if necessary at a slow rate to start with) and loperamide 8–16 mg/day, or codeine phosphate 60–180 mg/day.

Immunonutrition
- Enteral formulations enriched with arginine, omega-3 fatty acids and glutamine nucleotides are considered to enhance the immune response. They remain controversial and cannot currently be recommended

Table 12.7 Potential complications of enteral nutrition

Problem	Prevention
Aspiration	Feed in semi-recumbent position
Diarrhoea	Do not give feed directly from the refrigerator
	Introduce feed slowly (increase rate over 3 days)
	Stop antibiotics if possible
Abdominal distension	Reduce rate of infusion
Tube obstruction	Inject water (1 mL syringe), or replace tube
Tube misplacement	X-ray position in unconscious patients
Oesophagitis	Use a soft, fine-bore, polyurethane tube
Hyperglycaemia	Insulin s.c. (common in septicaemia)
Electrolyte imbalance	Check serum potassium weekly, phosphate and zinc after 3 weeks
Low folate	Folate supplements after 3 weeks

s.c., subcutaneous.

- A recent systematic review concluded that immunonutrition may reduce infectious complications and the length of stay in patients undergoing elective surgery, but in critical illness may be associated with increased mortality, possibly by excessive production of nitric oxide

12.3 Parenteral feeding

Parenteral feeding is much more demanding and hazardous than enteral feeding, unless it is done well. Meticulous asepsis and care of the catheter are essential, if life-threatening complications are to be avoided.

Indications
The gastrointestinal tract is inaccessible in unusual circumstances (Table 12.8). The indications for nutritional support are the same as for enteral feeding (Table 12.5, p. 374; Box 12.1, p. 376), when associated with gut failure.

Choice of feed

All-in-one (total nutrient admixture) bags
- All-in-one (total nutrient admixture) bags should be standard (volume varies depending on the company or pharmacy supplying the feed), since they are much safer and easier to use than separate bottles or bags of lipid emulsion and glucose/amino acid solutions. This is especially true for occasional users
- Many hospitals have a commercial supplier able to modify the constituents according to daily electrolytes

Individual constituents
Nitrogen is provided by an amino acid solution, and energy from glucose and a fat emulsion. There are four steps in calculating the constituents for an individual patient:

Table 12.8 Circumstances requiring parenteral nutrition

Problem	Comment
Complete dysphagia	Fine-bore tubes pass most strictures
	Tube placement with a paediatric endoscope is sometimes necessary, pending definitive treatment
Intestinal obstruction	
mechanical	Perioperative
ileus	Postoperative
short bowel	When enteral feeding is insufficient
Intestinal fistulae	
extensive disease resection	Elemental feeds may be an alternative for Crohn's disease (p. 254)
	Home parenteral feeding is for specialist centres
Acute pancreatitis	Fig. 1.4 (p. 31)

- Daily nitrogen requirements must be decided first (Table 12.6, p. 375). In broad terms, 11–14 g nitrogen/day is sufficient for most, but individual calculations by the dietitian are appropriate. Hypercatabolic patients or patients with excessive nitrogen losses may need 16 g nitrogen/day, but greater amounts of nitrogen are rarely utilised. Patients with renal failure may need less or more nitrogen per day depending on the type of renal support, so check with the renal dietitian
- The amount of energy required must then be calculated, depending on the weight of the patient, activity level and underlying disease (p. 376, and Table 12.6, p. 375). 20–30% of calories should be infused as fat at a rate that does not exceed 1.0 kcal/kg/h. Lipid emulsions should be used with caution in patients with hypertriglyceridemia or obese patients
- Additional electrolytes are added according to the daily results of electrolyte monitoring (Table 12.9). In unstable patients it is easier to use a separate intravenous line to infuse additional fluids and electrolytes
- Soluble insulin (1–2 U/h by separate subcutaneous infusion) may be needed if hyperglycaemic. Adding insulin to the bag is inappropriate in the acute care setting, since it prevents adjustment of the rate. As a general rule, *no* drugs should be added to the total parenteral nutrition (TPN) bag
- Vitamins and trace elements are added (e.g. Decan, Cerevit, Solvito N, 1 vial daily for water-soluble vitamins, Vitlipid N 10 mL/24 h for fat-soluble vitamins and Addamel or other trace element mix 10 mL/24 h for trace elements such as chromium, copper, zinc, selenium, manganese, iodine). Multi-12 contains water- and fat-soluble vitamins with the exception of vitamin K. Many amino acid solutions are low in phosphate and this needs to be corrected (Addiphos contains 40 mmol phosphate, but also contains 30 mmol K and 30 mmol Na/20 mL). The vitamin and mineral status should be checked and corrected as appropriate (increasing the vitamin and trace element additions to the TPN bag under the guidance of the pharmacist)

Table 12.9 Monitoring during parenteral nutrition

Measurement	Daily	Twice weekly	Weekly	Three-monthly
Sodium, potassium, phosphate, magnesium and calcium	+			
Creatinine	+			
Full blood count	+			
Glucose	+			
Check entry site	+			
Fluid balance	+			
Weight		+		
Albumin		+		
Liver function tests		+		
Zinc			+	
Iron				+
Folate				+
Trace elements				+

Techniques

Tunnelled central venous lines

- The cannula is inserted under local anaesthetic, in the operating theatre, anaesthetic room or side room. The catheter runs subcutaneously for about 5 cm before entering the subclavian or internal jugular vein
- The cannula is connected to a 10 cm extension tube, which is both sutured and taped onto the skin, to avoid tugging directly on the cannula
- The position is checked by X-ray (catheters are faintly radio-opaque). The tip should lie about 1 cm proximal to the right atrium
- Peripherally inserted central venous catheters (PICC lines) are appropriate when technically possible, since this avoids the risks of pneumothorax. The catheter is inserted into the basilic vein in the antecubital fossa or any other sufficiently large vein above the elbow and measured round to a location proximal to the atrium. A chest X-ray should be taken to confirm location in a major vein (superior vena cava or innominate vein) before use

Catheter care

- The skin entry site and any connections must be checked and cleaned aseptically daily
- 1 cm wide Elastoplast strips should be used to secure the extension tube, but should not cover the connections or entry site
- A dressing is unnecessary. Dressings hide the entry site, create a warm, moist environment for bacterial growth and, when changed, increase the risk of infection. Some transparent dressings (such as Opsite) adhere tenaciously to plastic tubing. No dressing at all is preferable if the site is checked and cleaned daily
- The catheter must only be used for parenteral feeding and *not* for giving drugs or taking blood. A triple-lumen catheter is advisable for sick patients, with one labelled, designated port for TPN. The giving set must be changed daily. A three-way tap should *not* be inserted between the extension tube and giving set to lock off the catheter, since this increases the temptation to inject drugs through this route. An in-line filter (1.2 μm) should be used to prevent particulate contamination
- Meticulous catheter care following defined protocols is the key to success. Doctors and other health care workers should be told to keep their hands off the TPN line unless a member of the nutrition or line-insertion team provides instruction or guidance
- Should fever develop, peripheral and retrograde line cultures should be sent. Only when other causes have been excluded should the catheter be removed and the tip sent for culture

Peripheral parenteral nutrition

- Peripheral intravenous nutrition is useful when it is desirable to maintain nutrition, but when enteral feeding is temporarily inappropriate and can be expected to start within the next 7–10 days. 75% of patients receive parenteral nutrition for < 14 days
- Lower osmolality and nitrogen in peripheral parenteral nutrition reduces thrombophlebitis, which is the main problem. Complications associated with central venous cannulation are avoided but the number of calories that can be provided is limited by the lower osmolality

- Special long, soft catheters (such as Hydrocath) inserted into the basilic vein have a good patency rate. A nitrate patch applied over the vein distal to the cannula may also decrease thrombophlebitis
- Additives cannot currently be given, although peripheral parenteral nutrition is much better than no nutrition at all

Monitoring

- Guidelines are shown in Table 12.9 (p. 381). Daily estimations of electrolytes, phosphate, magnesium and calcium are often necessary in the first week but for a minimum of the first 3 days. When feeding is stable, the frequency can be reduced to twice, then once weekly depending on the clinical situation
- Baseline measurements must be taken before treatment. Measurement of phosphate, magnesium, folate and zinc are often forgotten
- Microbiology specimens (sputum, urine, drains, blood, faeces, catheter tips) are prepared as clinically indicated
- Accurate fluid balance is vital
- Routine 24 h urine collection for nitrogen balance is no longer considered necessary. Nitrogen loss calculated from 24 h urinary urea (1 mol urea contains 28 g nitrogen) is inaccurate. Calculated balance has an error of up to 5 g/day. Nitrogen balance is, however, still useful in complex patients with sepsis, especially if stoma or laparostomy wound output is large. It helps confirm that nitrogen intake is adequate.

Complications

The complication rate depends on the experience of the person inserting the line, and especially on subsequent catheter care (Box 12.2). Designated people, as part of the nutrition support team, should be responsible for inserting feeding lines and checking catheter care.

Line sepsis

In the presence of suspected catheter sepsis the site should be inspected and swabbed for culture, blood cultures should be taken from the line and a peripheral vein, and empiric antibiotics started. Indications for catheter removal are given in Box 12.3.

Refeeding syndrome

- Refeeding syndrome is a complication induced by too rapid reintroduction of feed after a prolonged period of starvation. It is commonly overlooked
- Signs include fluid overload, congestive cardiac failure, electrolyte abnormalities (hypophosphataemia, hypokalaemia and hypomagnesaemia), cardiac arrhythmias and sudden death
- At-risk patients include those who have starved for > 7 days, or lost more than 20% of body weight in < 3 months and chronic alcoholics and patients with anorexia nervosa
- Dietitians should assess the risk

Management of refeeding syndrome

- Check biochemistry—phosphate, magnesium, potassium, calcium:

Box 12.2 Complications of parenteral nutrition

Mechanical
  pneumothorax
  air embolus
  catheter displacement
  major venous thrombosis
  pulmonary embolus
Septic
  septicaemia
  endocarditis
Metabolic
  refeeding syndrome
  fluid overload
  hyperglycaemia
  electrolyte imbalance
Hepatic
  abnormal liver function tests[*]
  steatosis
    steatohepatitis
    lipidosis
    cholestasis
    cirrhosis
Biliary
    acalculous cholecystitis
    cholecystitis
Deficiencies
    phosphate
    trace elements
    essential fatty acids (linoleic, arachidonic)
    vitamins, especially folate
Metabolic bone disease
    osteomalacia
    osteopenia

[*]Usually cholestatic.

Box 12.3 Infectious indications for catheter removal

Indications for immediate removal
• Purulent discharge or abscess at the site of insertion ('exit site' infection)
• Septic shock with no other focus of infection
Consider removal if
• Persistent fever for 72–96 h after initiating appropriate antibiotics, in the absence of any
  other focus of infection
• Persistent or recurrent bacteraemia
• Infection with *Candida* sp., *Staphylococcus aureus* or *Pseudomonas* sp.
• Polymicrobial infection

If phosphate < 0.3 mmol/L
If Mg < 0.5 mmol/L ⎫ correct levels before feeding starts (Table 12.12)
If K < 2.5 mmol/L ⎭
- Recheck biochemistry
- Start feeding 20 kcals/kg
  - highest risk should be started at no more than 10–15 kcal/kg/day
  - low to moderate risk should be started at 15–20 kcal/kg/day for 2–3 days, then increased gradually over the first week to full feeding
- Monitor phosphate, magnesium, potassium and calcium daily for first 2 weeks
  - a fall in electrolyte (particularly phosphate) concentration is a feature of refeeding syndrome. Electrolytes should be replenished as required
- Many hospitals now have a nutritional support team consisting of a doctor, nurse, dietitian and pharmacist (Appendix 2, p. 485). The advantages are that a nutritional team can agree on standard procedures and policy, as well as offering expertise, advice and training throughout the hospital

Cholestasis
- Cholestasis is common during TPN and the risk of gallstones is increased
- The cause may be excessive lipid, but other causes should not be overlooked
- If liver function tests become cholestatic, the drug chart should be checked for any culprit drugs and an abdominal ultrasound performed; sepsis can also produce significant cholestasis. If no other cause can be found, TPN is implicated and the lipid content of feeding bags can be reduced. This can be achieved by reducing the amount of lipid provided each day or by reducing lipid administration to 2–3 days/week after discussion of nutritional requirements with the dietitian
- If cholestasis continues, consider whether TPN is essential (enteral feeding or anastomotic surgery may be possible) and switch to a medium–chain triglyceride (MCT) mixture. Occasionally complete removal of lipid is necessary, but this causes fat-soluble vitamin and essential–fatty acid deficiency
  - Deficiency of a number of nutrients or metabolic cofactors have been suggested as contributing to TPN-associated liver disease. These include taurine, carnitine and choline. To date there have been no controlled trial data to support the use of supplements in patients with cholestasis or abnormal liver enzymes although a trial of choline is ongoing

Table 12.10 Refeeding syndrome: replacement of electrolytes before feeding

Electrolyte	Replacement
Low phosphate (serum < 0.3 mmol/L)	*Addiphos:* 40 mmol (20 mL vial) in 500 mL 5% dextrose over 6 h. Shake bag well. Oral phosphate causes diarrhoea. One vial of addiphos contains: Phosphate 40 mmol, potassium 30 mmol, sodium 30 mmol
Low magnesium (< 0.5 mmol/L)	*Magnesium sulphate 50%:* 6 g (24 mmol = 12 mL) in 500 mL 5% dextrose over 6–12 h. Oral magnesium is poorly tolerated due to gut side-effects at large doses
Low potassium (< 2.5 mmol/L)	*Sando K* (12 mmol/tablet): 2 tabs three times daily, or IV fluids containing potassium

Home parenteral nutrition
- The prevalence of home parenteral nutrition is increasing. In Europe the rate is 1–2/million residents, but is up to tenfold higher in the USA (predominately reflecting use in patients with cancer, for which evidence is lacking)
- The quality of life benefit varies according to the indication for home parenteral nutrition, but is comparable to that of haemodialysis patients. Cost utility analyses suggest that 1 quality-adjusted year of life costs £69 000 ($100 000)
- The incidence of complications per catheter year depend on the measure of support by an expert team. Figures from the USA are sepsis (34%), occlusion (7%) and central vein occlusion (3%). Sepsis rates for patients managed at specialist centres should be < 10%. The incidence of other problems including liver and bone disease and depression are unknown
- Trace elements (selenium, manganese, copper, vitamin concentrations) should be monitored every 3 months and adjustments made to the feed accordingly. Each individual patient needs to be assessed on a regular basis for the risk of developing nutrient deficiencies

12.4 Therapeutic diets

Badly planned and/or poorly understood diets result in poor compliance and are not worth prescribing. An imaginative and supportive dietitian is invaluable for helping patients maintain special diets.

Weight-reducing diet
In the USA > 50% of adults are obese or overweight and > 5% are severely obese (BMI ≥ 35). A similar trend is now emerging in the UK and Europe. Obesity contributes to osteoarthritis, diabetes, cardiovascular disease and many other diseases, directly increasing the risk of death (Fig. 12.1, p. 373). Mortality in patients > 25% overweight is increased by 500% in diabetics, and 160% in patients with ischaemic heart disease.

Principles
- Indicated for overweight (> 110% recommended weight for height; Appendix 3, p. 451) patients (BMI usually 25–30) and obese (> 120%) patients (BMI > 30 kg/m²)
- A realistic target weight should be set (Appendix 3, p. 451) and steady, moderate weight loss planned (about 0.5 kg/week) using a combined strategy of diet, exercise (3–7 sessions per week lasting 30–60 min) and behaviour therapy. Energy expenditure must exceed intake until the target weight is reached. Targeting advice for individuals is appropriate
- Low-calorie diets (LCDs; 800–1500 kcal/day) are recommended over very low-calorie diets (VLCDs; < 800 kcal/day), because LCDs are as effective as VLCDs at 1 year, with less risk of nutritional deficiency. Low fat and sugar, but high complex carbohydrate (fibre) intake is recommended. Fat has more than twice the energy density of protein or carbohydrate
- Sustained, steady dieting is necessary for any substantial loss of body fat. Early weight loss is largely due to loss of body water resulting from breakdown of glycogen.

Inappropriately low carbohydrate intake can lead to a breakdown of lean body mass (protein)
- Regular supervision, a weight chart posted in a prominent place, support from a skilled dietitian or slimming organisations (especially those that charge) improve success
- Patients > 120 kg usually have a *high* metabolic rate (> 8000 kJ) and even higher food intake, despite frequent denials about excessive eating

Constituents of 5040 kJ (1200 kcal) diet
- Daily allowance:
  - skimmed milk 11/2 pints (or equivalent in low-fat dairy products—yoghurt, cheese, custard)
  - butter or margarine 15 g, or low-fat butter substitute 25 g
  - as much vegetables/salad as wanted
  - unlimited water, tea, coffee, low-calorie fizzy drinks/squashes or sodas
- Protein—any two of the following, each day:
  - lean meat or poultry 100 g (liver, pork, veal, steak, beef, lamb, chicken, turkey—no fat)
  - fish or shellfish 100 g (not in batter)
  - beans or pulses 175 g
  - cottage cheese 100 g
  - hard cheese 50 g
  - two eggs (no more than six eggs/week)
- Carbohydrate (unrefined, high fibre—a total of 6–10 portions of any of the following:
  - one slice wholemeal bread
  - one medium-sized potato
  - 25 g breakfast cereal (not sugar-coated)
  - one Weetabix or Shredded Wheat
  - 1/2 cup cooked pasta or rice

Pharmacotherapy for obesity
- Dietary compliance is invariably required with any antiobesity drug treatment
- Sibutramine, a β-phenethylamine, acts as an appetite suppressant (through inhibition of serotonin and noradrenaline reuptake) and may also increase thermogenesis. The principal concern is a dose-related increase in heart rate and blood pressure. The most commonly reported adverse effects are headache, dry mouth, insomnia and constipation.
- Orlistat is an inhibitor of pancreatic, gastric and carboxylester lipases, which are required for the hydrolysis of dietary fat in the gastrointestinal tract. A therapeutic dose of 120 mg three times daily blocks the absorption and digestion of 30% of dietary fat. Weight loss is associated with improved glucose tolerance and reduces rate of progression of type II diabetes. Orlistat has additional independent beneficial effects on cholesterol and low-density lipoprotein concentrations. Side-effects relate to fat malabsorption (oily stool, increased evacuation) but improve as patients diminish their dietary fat intake

Surgical approaches to obesity
- Strategies aim to induce weight loss either by gastric restriction or intestinal malabsorption. Patients should be considered for surgery if they have failed attempts

at nonsurgical weight loss and have a BMI ≥ 35 with comorbidity, or a BMI ≥ 40 with or without comorbidity

- Restrictive procedures cause early satiety by the creation of a small gastric pouch and prolong satiety by the creation of a small pouch outlet. Dietary compliance is still required, as restrictive procedures do not prevent the intake of high-calorie drinks or soft foods. In Europe use of laparoscopic adjustable gastric bands is the preferred approach achieving a 40–60% excess weight loss at 3–5 years. Mean hospital stay is < 2 days and mortality is low. Major complications include band slippage (2–10%), port complications (1–11%) and band erosion (0.5–2%)
- Malabsorptive procedures (biliopancreatic bypass, distal gastric bypass) involve some degree of gastric volume reduction but primarily act by bypassing a length of small intestine. Benefits include greater sustained weight loss, which is not dependant on dietary compliance. Disadvantages include increased risk of malnutrition and vitamin deficiencies
- In the USA the preferred surgical procedure is the Roux-en-Y gastric bypass that combines both restrictive and malabsorptive actions to achieve long-term excess weight loss of 50–65%. Complications include pulmonary embolus (3%), anastomotic leak (5%) or stricture (10%), hernia (24%), and marginal ulcers (10%). A laparoscopic approach is increasingly being adopted but few follow-up data are available

High-fibre diet

Indicated for diverticulosis, most patients with constipation and some with IBS. The potential for reducing the risk of colorectal cancer, cardiovascular disease or gallstones has yet to be confirmed. A higher-fibre intake (aiming for 30 g/day) is suitable for most Western people as a pattern of healthy eating. See also p. 341.

Principles

- Fibre provides bulk, absorbs water and satisfies hunger. Intake should be increased gradually to minimise adverse symptoms, e.g. flatulence or bloating
- Insoluble fibre is characteristically particulate and is found in cereal husks, bran, etc. It is particularly effective in regulating colonic function by increasing stool bulk
- Soluble fibre is viscous in the form of gums and mucilages, derived mainly from legumes and oats and some fruits and vegetables. It modifies digestion and absorption, thus helping lower cholesterol and assisting glycaemic control
- Excessive flatulence from bacterial fermentation is the main disadvantage from some fibrous foods, but only intestinal strictures or neurogenic constipation (p. 292) are contraindications
- Additional bran is rarely needed if fibre-rich foods are eaten regularly and in sufficient quantity
- Fluid intake must be increased (to 1500 mL/day or more) to compensate for water retained by increased fibre

Guidelines

- Good sources of fibre are:
  - wholemeal/wholegrain (not ordinary brown) bread

- wholegrain cereals (muesli, All Bran, Bran Flakes, Weetabix, Shredded Wheat)
- porridge oats
- wholemeal flour
- wholemeal pasta
- fresh vegetables (beans, peas, green leafy vegetables)
- pulses (dried beans, lentils)
- fresh/tinned/dried fruit
- Vegetables should be lightly cooked
- Unprocessed coarse bran can be added if dietary changes are insufficient: 1 tbsp/day, added to soups, cereals, stewed fruit, home baking
- Bran tablets are available, but not prescribed. Isphagula husk granules (Regulan, Fybogel) are more convenient and expensive than dietary changes or unprocessed bran, but much less preferable and may interact with iron absorption with long-term use

Modified resistant-starch diet
Indicated for IBS where bloating and wind predominate.

Principles
- Digestibility of starch, especially wheat starch, varies according to the source and preparation. Toasted bread, dried pasta, or precooked meals have a higher content of resistant starches than white bread or fresh pasta
- The undigested carbohydrate component is fermented in the colon to produce short-chain fatty acids (that influence colonic motility) and gas (associated with bloating)

Guidelines
- Reduce intake of bread, pasta, cakes and other wheat-based products
- Avoid sorbitol (effervescent drinks, gum, low-calorie sweeteners or drinks)
- Avoid toasting, or reheated food (including precooked meals)
- Use white bread or fresh pasta in preference to brown or granary bread and dried pasta

Gluten-free diet
Indicated for coeliac disease (p. 219).

Principles
- An *absolute* gluten-free diet is the only way to treat coeliacs. Non-compliance is the commonest cause of persistent symptoms (p. 221). Support and regular dietetic input aids compliance
- Gluten ingestion increases the risk of lymphoma and ulcerative jejunitis in coeliac disease, so the diet must be continued for life
- The Coeliac Society (Appendix 1, p. 437) provides an excellent Food and Drink directory, which greatly enables patients in their food selection

Guidelines
- Avoid:
  - wheat, barley, rye
  - any products of these cereals (bread, cakes, biscuits, pastry, crisp bread)

- wheat cereals (Weetabix, Puffed Wheat)
- pasta
- packet soups
- beer
- gravy, Oxo cubes, curry powder, mustard, sauces
- some chocolate, ice cream, sweets, crisps
- Allowed:
  - oats
  - any fish, meat, poultry, game (no breadcrumbs/batter)
  - any cheese, eggs, milk, dairy products
  - potatoes, rice, corn
  - any fruit and vegetables
  - cornflakes, rice Krispies
  - bread, cakes or biscuits made from gluten-free flour
- Essential gluten-free products may be prescribed in some jurisdictions. These foods include bread (Juvela, Rite Diet), pasta (Aglutella, Aproten), biscuits (Nutricia) and flour (see British National Formulary or equivalent for a comprehensive list)

Lactose-free diet

Rarely indicated and often overprescribed for hypolactasia after acute gastroenteritis (p. 349), Crohn's disease (p. 245), ulcerative colitis (p. 266) or coeliac disease (p. 219). Inappropriate lactose restriction severely limits calcium intake. Most people with hypolactasia can tolerate up to 10 g lactose daily. This is often only a temporary restriction.

Principles
- Milk and liquid milk products are the only appreciable source of lactose. Many dairy products contain insufficient lactose to cause symptoms
- Hypolactasia may be temporary, so milk can be reintroduced later
- Variable tolerance to milk is often due to changes in colonic absorptive capacity (p. 207)
- Supplemental calcium is necessary (e.g. calcium and vitamin D forte, Caltrate with vitamin D, Os-Cal or Calcichew 2 tabs daily) when adhering to a lactose-free diet

Guidelines
- Avoid:
  - milk of any sort (cows, goats, sheep, cream), except soya milk
  - yoghurt
  - cottage cheese
  - ice cream
- Allowed:
  - anything else, including butter and cheese

Elemental diet (See pp. 257 and 377)

Low-fibre diet

Indicated when intestinal strictures cause symptoms, or in preparation for investigations (colonoscopy, barium enema, small bowel radiology), or colorectal surgery. Occasionally beneficial in patients with poor anal sphincter control.

Principles
- Indigestible fibrous foods are kept to a minimum
- Nutritional supplements (p. 377) are often necessary for strictures in association with Crohn's disease

Guidelines
- Avoid high-fibre foods (p. 388)
- Allowed any meat, fish, poultry or game (no stuffing), dairy products

Low-fat diet

Indicated for steatorrhoea due to chronic pancreatitis, cholestasis or severe malabsorption, as well as hyperlipidaemia. No benefit has been shown for other types of hepatobiliary disease, although avoiding fatty foods (rather than a specific low-fat diet) decreases postprandial discomfort in some patients with gallstones or hepatitis. Needs to be commenced on appropriate patients only—it is not the standard of care for all patients with cholestasis/cholelithiasis.

Principles
- Reduce total fat intake to 30–50 g/day, or until steatorrhoea is controlled
- Substitute unsaturated for saturated fats in hyperlipidaemia
- Fat is important for palatability and the diet must be prescribed carefully. Medium-chain triglyceride supplements are indicated if calorie intake is insufficient following fat restriction (shown by continued weight loss)

Guidelines
- Avoid:
  - all fried food
  - butter, margarine (in moderation)
  - cheese in large amounts (> 30–40 g/day), except cottage cheese
  - whole, evaporated or condensed milk, cream
  - fatty meat (goose, duck, sausages, pâté)
  - salad cream, mayonnaise, salad dressing
  - any pastry or cakes
  - chocolate, marzipan, Ovaltine, nuts, olives
- Allowed:
  - skimmed milk and low-fat dairy products
  - low-fat spreads
  - cottage cheese
  - lean meat and poultry (beef, lamb, pork, chicken, turkey, not roasted)
  - fish

- any vegetables or fruit
- any bread or pasta and most cereals
- Marmite, Oxo, herbs, spices

Low-protein diet

Indicated for incipient or established chronic renal failure, but no longer indicated for acute hepatic encephalopathy (p. 145).

Principles

- The aim is an intake that maintains adequate nutrition, but avoids accelerating renal impairment (usually 40–50 g/day). This needs to be guided and converted into practical terms for the patient by a specialist renal dietitian.

Exclusion diet (See Table 12.11)

Exclusion diets are used to identify food intolerance and they require the guidance and support of a skilled and interested dietitian (p. 341). An experienced dietitian is needed to motivate the patient and to provide a systematic approach. They may be used in IBS to confirm/refute the role of food intolerance in their symptoms.

Table 12.11 Constituents of an exclusion diet

	Exclude	Allowed
Meat	Beef, processed/preserved tinned meats Corned beef, pâté, salami Bacon, sausages	All other meats/poultry Chicken, lamb, pulses
Fish	Battered fish Shellfish (mussels, prawns)	All other fish
Vegetables	Potatoes (any kind) Onions (fresh or dried) Sweetcorn	All other vegetables Cabbage, sprouts, beans, carrots, peas
Fruit	Citrus (lemons, grapefruit, oranges, limes), including citrus fruit juice	All other fruits
Cereals	Wheat (bread, cakes, biscuits) Rye (crispbreads) Oats (porridge) Corn (cornflakes, cornflour)	Rice Tapioca Millet, buckwheat
Oils	Corn, vegetable	Sunflower, olive, soya
Dairy	Cows' milk Butter Cheese Eggs Yoghurt	Goat's milk, soya milk and yoghurts Goat's and sheep's milk cheese
Drinks	Tea Coffee (fresh, decaffeinated) Alcohol Squashes	Apple, pineapple, grape, tomato, cranberry juices Rooibos (redbush) tea Herbal teas
Others	Chocolate Yeast Marmite Nuts Preservatives	Spices Herbs Sea salt

Principles
- The diet is followed for 2 weeks, with a diary recording food eaten and symptoms experienced
- Foods are reintroduced one at a time after 2 weeks, if improvement has occurred. Further items are introduced at intervals of 2 days
- Foods should be fresh or frozen, since many tinned or packet foods contain preservatives
- Intelligent cooperation by the patient is clearly essential
- If no effect is observed by dietary exclusion, the patients normal diet is resumed

12.5 Mineral and vitamin supplements

Indicated when there are specific deficiencies (Table 12.4, p. 372) or unexplained symptoms in association with severe malabsorption. Prophylaxis is indicated in profound cholestasis (primary biliary cirrhosis), short bowel syndrome or parenteral nutrition. Optimum amounts are often uncertain, but Recommended Nutrient Intake Guidelines (Tables 12.12–12.14) provide guidance.

Table 12.12 Treatment of fat-soluble vitamin deficiencies in gastrointestinal disorders

Substance	Acute deficiency	Prophylaxis
Vitamin A	Retinol 100 000 U i.m. weekly	100 000 U i.m. monthly
Vitamin D	Calciferol 100 000 U i.m. weekly	Calciferol 100 000 U i.m. monthly
	Oral alfacalcidol 1 µg daily is indicated in severe primary biliary cholangitis	
Vitamin K	Phytomenadione 10 mg i.v. for 3 days	10 mg i.m. monthly
Vitamin E	Vitamin E suspension 5 mg daily	No parenteral preparation

i.m., intramuscular; i.v., intravenous; o.d., once daily; b.d., twice daily; t.d.s., three times daily

Table 12.13 Treatment of water-soluble vitamin deficiencies in gastrointestinal disorders

Substance	Acute deficiency	Prophylaxis
Thiamine (B$_1$)	Pabrinex 1+2 vials i.v. for 3 days (see also p. 178)	Parentrovite weak 4 mL i.m. monthly
Riboflavin (B$_2$)	Same	Same (although deficiency still possible despite Parentrovite)
Pyridoxine (B$_6$)	Same	Parentrovite weak 4 mL i.m. monthly, or oral pyridoxine 10 mg
Nicotinamide (niacin)	Same	Parentrovite weak 4 mL i.m. monthly
Folate	Folic acid 15 mg daily for 1 month, then 5 mg for 3 months to replenish stores	5 mg daily; 15 mg daily in malabsorption; no parenteral preparation
B$_{12}$	Hydroxycobalamin 1000 pg i.m daily for 5 days	1000 µg i.m. every 3 months
Vitamin C	Ascorbic acid 300 mg i.m. daily	Parentrovite weak 4 mL i.m. monthly

Table 12.14 Treatment of mineral deficiencies in gastrointestinal disorders

Substance	Acute deficiency	Prophylaxis
Iron	Ferrous sulphate 200 mg t.d.s. for 3 months Total dose iron infusion if oral iron not absorbed or tolerated	200 mg daily
Calcium	Calcium gluconate 10 mL i.v. (tetany) then 40 mL i.v./day	Calcium gluconate 2 tabs* t.d.s.
Phosphate	50 mmol/L i.v. over 12 h	Phosphate-Sandoz 2 tabs o.d.†
Magnesium	50 mmol $MgCl_2$ i.v. over 12 h	Magnesium glycerophosphate 1 g twice daily
Zinc	125 mg zinc sulphate effervescent tab t.d.s. for 2 weeks	125 mg daily
Trace elements (see above)		

*Effervescent calcium tablets contain 4.5 mmol Na. Calcium should be monitored every 2 weeks, especially if vitamin D is given as well.
†Rarely required.

Parenteral administration may be necessary, since deficiencies in gastrointestinal disease are due to failure of absorption (p. 248).

Principles
- Diagnostic tests are complicated or unreliable for many substances (Table 12.3, p. 372). Iron, B_{12} and folate are exceptions
- Mixed deficiencies are common
- Fat-soluble vitamins are deficient in cholestasis, but all vitamins and some trace elements become deficient in severe malabsorption
- Vitamin A or D, iron, calcium, zinc and copper are toxic in overdose, so response should be checked every 1–2 weeks

Guidelines for trace elements
- Copper, manganese, iodine, fluoride, chromium, selenium, molybdenum, nickel, cobalt, vanadium are ubiquitous
- Additrace 10 mL contains the daily requirements (including calcium, magnesium but not phosphate, and relatively deficient in iron) for parenteral nutrition; Multi-12 is an alternative source of trace elements
- Supplementation is rarely necessary even in severe chronic malabsorption, but copper, iodine or selenium deficiency may occur
- If zinc or magnesium supplements are required, monthly infusions (40 mL Addamel/L over 12 h) are justifiable
- 500 mL Intralipid 20% should then also be given to provide essential fatty acids

13 The Gut in Systemic Disorders

The Gut in Systemic Disorders

Most systemic disorders have gastrointestinal manifestations, which may sometimes be the presenting feature of the condition. More commonly, gastrointestinal symptoms present in a patient with a known condition, which, in turn, influences the investigation or management of the gastrointestinal symptoms. This chapter draws attention to problems that are often a cause for referral to gastroenterologists from other specialists.

13.1 Pregnancy

The most serious gastroenterological diseases in pregnancy are hepatic (HELLP syndrome and acute fatty liver, p. 142), but luminal disorders are far more common. Pregnancy alters visceral anatomy, oesophagogastric and intestinal motility, and impairs the omental response to peritoneal inflammation. Pregnancy also influences the choice of investigations or treatments because of potential effects on the embryo or fetus. Breastfeeding influences choice of treatments in the postpartum period.

Nausea and vomiting
- Nausea and vomiting affect up to 50% of pregnant women between 5 and occasionally up to 20 weeks
- Hyperemesis gravidarum is defined as persistent severe nausea and vomiting in the first trimester, leading to 5% loss of body weight; it can rarely persist throughout pregnancy
- Consider other provoking factors, including urinary infection, gastroenteritis, gastro-oesophageal reflux, prodromal phase of hepatitis and biliary disease. Peptic ulcers are rare
- Conservative treatment is initially advisable, with reassurance, fluids and frequent small meals. Metoclopramide (10 mg three times daily) or prochlorperazine (25 mg three times daily) have been widely used and appear to be safe; Diclectin has also been widely used and appears to be safe
- Endoscopy and treatment of reflux is appropriate for refractory cases, because a cycle of vomiting, reflux, oesophagitis and further vomiting becomes established

Gastro-oesophageal reflux
- A majority experience heartburn during pregnancy, often deteriorating in the third trimester
- General measures include elevating the head of the bed, frequent small meals, avoiding lying down after eating and symptom relief with alginates (Gastrocote or Gaviscon)
- Although not absolutely known to be safe in pregnancy, both H_2-receptor antagonists and PPIs have been widely used and appear to be safe and effective for refractory symptoms

Acute abdominal pain (See p. 21)

- In the absence of labour, biliary or renal colic, appendicitis and pancreatitis should be considered
- Amylase, full blood count and liver function tests should be checked and ultrasound arranged. If ultrasound is inadequate and cross-sectional imaging is needed to look for an abscess, then MR scanning is appropriate
- Management depends on the stage of pregnancy and severity of illness. The most experienced advice should be sought. Early surgery is appropriate if appendicitis is suspected
- ERCP and sphincterotomy have been performed successfully during pregnancy for gallstone-related pancreatitis or obstructive jaundice, but definitive management of gallstones in uncomplicated biliary colic is best delayed until after delivery if possible
- If pancreatitis occurs for the first time in pregnancy and if there are no gallstones, then it is likely to recur in subsequent pregnancies

Jaundice and abnormal liver function tests (See p. 156)

- Consider coincidental illness (incubating hepatitis before pregnancy or gallstones), drugs (including recreational), pre-existing disease, cholestasis of pregnancy, HELLP syndrome and acute fatty liver of pregnancy. Liver function tests, viral serology, autoantibodies and abdominal ultrasound should be arranged. Specialist advice should be sought
- *Cholestasis of pregnancy* occurs in the third trimester, with itching, cholestatic liver function tests and resolution after delivery (p. 193 and p. 142). It commonly recurs with subsequent pregnancy and is associated with increased fetal mortality/morbidity. Ursodeoxycholic acid appears to improve fetal outcome but has not been tested in a randomised controlled trial
- *HELLP syndrome* has a spectrum of severity up to acute liver failure (p. 142). It occurs in the third trimester often associated with pre-eclampsia and early delivery is essential
- *Acute fatty liver of pregnancy* is potentially fatal, presents with vomiting and abdominal pain in the third trimester, with elevated AST, bilirubin and INR, but no haemolysis. Early delivery is essential
- *Pre-existing liver disease* usually reduces fertility. Primary biliary cirrhosis may present in pregnancy. Bleeding from varices is a real risk, especially when varices have previously bled. Liver biopsy is appropriate when abnormal liver function tests persist for 3–6 months after delivery

Inflammatory bowel disease (See pp. 265 and 279)

- *Fertility* is usually normal except in women with active disease, or severe Crohn's disease, who may have tubal obstruction or menstrual irregularities and anovulatory cycles. Sulphasalazine causes reversible oligospermia in men
- *Pregnancy* is best planned during a period of sustained remission (> 6 months). Folate supplements are appropriate as for all planned pregnancies, to reduce the risk of neural tube defects
- *Maintenance therapy* should be continued, to reduce the risk of relapse. The risks from active disease are higher than any side-effects of medication. Azathioprine is a

special case: wide experience now suggests that it is safe, and it is often inappropriate to stop the drug in patients with previously refractory disease. The advantages (maintaining remission) and disadvantages (theoretical concerns of immunosuppression on the fetus) should be carefully discussed with the patient and a joint decision (usually in favour of continuing treatment) made

- *Active disease* should be promptly treated with corticosteroids as for other patients. Severe or refractory disease increases fetal mortality. Cyclosporin is probably best avoided in favour of colectomy for refractory severe colitis but its use has been reported in pregnancy. Decision-making is difficult, but should not be delayed and specialist advice should be sought

13.2 The elderly

About 15% of the population of the UK and USA are aged over 65 years, compared to 5% in the Far East. Demographic predictions indicate that in the UK, the proportion is not going to change appreciably, although a greater percentage will be aged > 85 years (currently 2%). At age 65 life expectancy is 12 years, with an even chance of living another year at age 85.

Investigations

Classical symptom patterns rarely occur in the elderly. Cholangitis (p. 200), for example, may present as confusion and abnormal liver function tests, without pain or fever. Prompt investigation by an alert clinician allows definitive treatment such as endoscopic sphincterotomy with good results. Delay in diagnosis and treatment in the elderly compromises already diminished nutritional and functional reserves.

Technological advances in less invasive imaging techniques particularly benefit the elderly. Abdominal CT scanning (especially with spiral CT) has a diagnostic accuracy for colonic neoplasms of about 85–90%. Whilst this is less than contrast radiology (95%), or colonoscopy (98%), the minimal preparation and non-invasive nature of CT scans make it the best technique for frail, elderly patients. In contrast, colonoscopy may offer a therapeutic as well as diagnostic opportunity (such as polypectomy or stenting, obstructing colorectal tumours). Clinical judgement is needed, guided by the need to make a diagnosis and achieve symptom relief with minimum distress to the patient.

Dysphagia

- Peptic oesophageal strictures and oesophageal cancer (p. 62) are common, but so are age-related pharyngeal and neuromuscular disorders (pharyngeal pouch, xerostomia, stroke or Parkinson's disease, Table 2.1, p. 51). Motility disorders are common, but the ageing oesophagus ('presbyoesophagus') is no longer considered a distinct entity
- A barium swallow is the initial investigation of choice, before endoscopy, to exclude a high stricture or pharyngeal pouch
- Treatment of motility disorders is difficult. Small, solid meals, avoiding drinking and eating at the same time, or prokinetic agents (domperidone 10–20 mg before meals) may help

Constipation (See p. 287)

- Inadequate fibre and poor mobility are common causes
- Exclude drugs (analgesics, tricyclics, calcium antagonists), hypothyroidism, hypercalcaemia and local disease (fissure, prolapse)

Diarrhoea

- Gastroenteritis (including *Cl. difficile*) and faecal impaction with overflow should not be overlooked. Send stool culture, request *Cl. difficile* toxin assay and do a rectal examination
- Apart from malignancy, ulcerative or ischaemic colitis may cause bloody diarrhoea
- Flexible sigmoidoscopy after phosphate enema preparation takes a few minutes, is well tolerated and rapidly provides a definitive diagnosis in many instances
- Barium enema is often worse than useless: preparation may be detrimental, inadequate pictures are common due to poor mobility or faecal residue, and significant mucosal disease can be overlooked
- Jejunal diverticulosis, bacterial overgrowth, thyrotoxicosis or microscopic colitis may cause watery or malodorous diarrhoea. An empirical course of metronidazole 400 mg three times daily for 1 week may give rapid symptomatic relief from bacterial overgrowth

Abdominal pain (See p. 27)

- Serum amylase, abdominal ultrasound, then CT scan are the most useful diagnostic tests
- Appendicitis or perforation (diverticulum or duodenal ulcer) have a high mortality, because signs of peritonitis can be minimal
- Mesenteric ischaemia should always be considered when pain is severe and signs are few
- Early laparotomy is advisable if there is doubt. Delay increases mortality when there is serious pathology and if there is not, laparotomy is usually well tolerated

Inflammatory bowel disease

- Malnutrition, especially in elderly patients with colonic Crohn's disease, is common
- Early diagnosis by flexible sigmoidoscopy and adequate treatment with corticosteroids are fundamental (p. 273)
- Joint care with a gastroenterologist is advisable, especially when patients are ill enough to be admitted. The severity of ulcerative colitis is readily underestimated (p. 273) and if colectomy is inappropriately delayed, mortality is high

13.3 Endocrine disease

Diabetes

Gastroparesis, autonomic neuropathy and concomitant disease need to be considered.

Gastroparesis
- Causes fullness, postprandial vomiting and a succussion splash
- Endoscopy or barium meal identifies food residue in the stomach and also excludes pyloric stenosis. The diagnosis may be obvious in these circumstances, but lesser degrees of delayed gastric emptying can be detected by isotope studies
- Prokinetic agents (metoclopramide or domperidone up to 60 mg daily, or erythromycin 500 mg before meals) occasionally help. In the most severe cases, percutaneous endoscopic gastrostomy with a jejunal extension (PEG-J) helps maintain nutrition, reduces massive swings in glycaemic control and may improve gastric emptying. Surgical Roux-en-Y anastomosis has been advocated, but specialist advice should be sought

Autonomic neuropathy
- Can present with watery diarrhoea, but often causes constipation or even pseudo-obstruction
- Concomitant disease (villous atrophy, thyrotoxicosis, hypolactasia, microscopic colitis) should be excluded
- Postural hypotension and peripheral neuropathy are clues to autonomic dysfunction
- Bacterial overgrowth or decreased adrenergic tone may cause the diarrhoea
- Meticulous diabetic control is crucial to delay progression and may improve autonomic dysfunction
- Metronidazole 400–500 mg three times daily (repeated if necessary for explosive, malodorous diarrhoea) or clonidine 500 μg three times daily (for diarrhoea, but rarely tolerated) can be tried
- Pseudo-obstruction with constipation and severe abdominal pain can be intractable. Prokinetic agents, stool softening laxatives and meticulous diabetic control may help

Concomitant disease
Diseases associated with diabetes include coeliac disease (iron deficiency is a clue), acute pancreatitis (may present with ketoacidosis), chronic pancreatitis (consider alcohol or haemochromatosis), fatty liver (10% of diabetics have abnormal liver enzymes) and mesenteric ischaemia.

Thyrotoxicosis
- Diarrhoea is a well-recognised feature and can be the presenting feature
- Mildly abnormal liver function tests are also common and return to normal when euthyroid
- Occasionally frank malabsorption, abdominal pain or jaundice can occur
- Ulcerative colitis is said to be associated

Hypothyroidism
- Constipation of recent onset should always raise the possibility of myxoedema. Pseudo-obstruction or spurious diarrhoea due to faecal impaction may occur in hypothyroidism

- Ascites occurs in extreme cases, but hypothyroidism is also associated with primary biliary cirrhosis

Acromegaly

- The risk of colorectal polyps is increased, but debate remains whether deaths from colorectal cancer are also increased. A plausible mechanism is an increased secretion of trophoblastic hormones (growth hormone and insulin-like growth factor)
- Colonoscopic screening has been advised (Table 9.5, p. 310), but procedures are often challenging owing to organomegaly affecting the colon. Survival benefit has yet to be demonstrated

Addison's disease

Anorexia, weight loss and diarrhoea or abdominal pain are common non-specific symptoms in gastroenterology outpatients. If common causes are excluded, Addison's should be considered before symptoms are attributed to a functional disorder. Symptoms are often long-standing, so pigmentation (watch out for a surprising 'suntan') may be present

Multiple endocrine neoplasia (See p. 105)

13.4 Neoplastic and paraneoplastic disorders

- Intestinal metastases occur in up to 20% of all non-gut cancers. Breast, lung, ovarian cancer and melanoma are the commonest source. Serosal metastases may cause pain, ascites, obstruction or recurrent gastrointestinal bleeding
- Paraneoplastic pseudo-obstruction is a rare feature of small cell lung cancer
- Chemotherapy can cause diarrhoea due to *Cl. difficile* (especially with neutropenia, also termed 'typhlitis'), mucositis (malnutrition may be critical and require parenteral nutrition) or autonomic neuropathy

13.5 Connective tissue disease

- Abnormal liver function tests, particularly a raised ALP, are commonly elevated in patients with connective tissue disease including elderly patients with polymyalgia/temporal arteritis and respond to treatment of the underlying condition.

Rheumatoid arthritis

- Dysphagia may be due to impaired mastication (temporomandibular arthritis) or oesophageal dysmotility
- Anaemia is common. Consider NSAID-induced peptic ulceration (p. 110), enteropathy or colitis, coincidental colonic pathology (such as caecal carcinoma) or small intestinal villous atrophy (very rarely due to NSAIDs), anaemia of chronic disease, and drug-induced haemolysis or marrow suppression (sulphasalazine, penicillamine, gold). Essential investigations include iron studies, serum and RBC folate, serum

B12, reticulocyte count and Coombs' test, endoscopy with distal duodenal biopsy, and colonoscopy. CT colonography (p. 304) may be more appropriate than colonoscopy in patients with limited mobility

- Abdominal pain may be due to a peptic ulcer, but acalculous cholecystitis, appendicitis and mesenteric vasculitis must be considered. Small intestinal obstruction can very rarely be caused by NSAID-induced strictures, which are best detected by small bowel enema
- Abnormal liver function tests, usually ALP and GGT, are commonly elevated in active rheumatoid arthritis and normalise with treatment of the underlying arthritis. It is important to exclude coexistent primary biliary cirrhosis. Rarely a raised ALP may be due to regenerative nodular hyperplasia, which can also cause presinusoidal portal hypertension
- Malabsorption may rarely be caused by amyloidosis, or drugs (NSAIDs, gold)
- Bloody diarrhoea may be due to ischaemic colitis, gold or NSAID-induced colitis, or infection (*Cl. difficile*). Stool culture, toxin assay, plain abdominal X-ray, colonoscopy and serial biopsies should identify the cause

Systemic sclerosis

- Dysphagia is characteristic, often with severe oesophagitis, a peptic stricture and aperistalsis on oesophageal manometry. High-dose omeprazole (40–80 mg daily) usually helps. Specialist advice should be sought. Surgery (Roux-en-Y anastomosis) is a last resort
- Diarrhoea may be due to bacterial overgrowth and often responds to antibiotics on an intermittent or cyclical basis (p. 227). Small bowel radiology shows characteristic pseudosacculation
- Constipation is also due to intestinal dysmotility and is often progressive, ultimately causing pseudo-obstruction. Treatment is difficult. Stool softening and stimulant laxatives are often needed in combination
- Malnutrition is common, often due to dysphagia and intestinal dysmotility. Nutrition supplements are appropriate at an early stage. A smaller mouth may need a smaller spoon. Any decision to start parenteral nutrition should be carefully considered, since by this stage the patient usually has poor manual dexterity and is entering the terminal phase of a progressive disease

Systemic lupus erythematosus

- Dysphagia, abdominal pain and bloating are common, due to oesophageal and intestinal dysmotility. Active disease should be controlled and prokinetics, antispasmodics or tricyclic agents may help
- Mesenteric vasculitis affects about 2%. Severe pain (exclude pancreatitis), intestinal haemorrhage or peritonitis suggests the diagnosis. Mortality is high. Cyclophosphamide may be more effective than steroids as an adjunct to surgery for perforation or ischaemic bowel

Polymyositis

- Dysphagia is common and may be the presenting feature. The association of dysphagia with a systemic illness suggests the diagnosis, confirmed by elevated muscle enzymes (creatine kinase, aldolase)

- Up to 10% of patients with polymyositis–dermatomyositis have an underlying malignancy, which may be gastric or colonic

Vasculitis

- Behçet's syndrome is a rare cause of ileocolic disease. An abdominal bruit suggests a vasculitis rather than Crohn's disease, but the two conditions can be similar and occasionally overlap. Infliximab appears to be highly effective treatment, but specialist advice should be sought
- Henoch–Schönlein purpura is characterised by abdominal pain, purpuric rash on the extensor surfaces and renal impairment. Melaena or rectal bleeding may occur; adults of any age, as well as children, may be affected

NSAIDs and dyspepsia (See p. 109)

13.6 Renal disease

Chronic renal failure

- Anorexia, dyspepsia and reflux are common, often with a normal endoscopy, although peptic ulcers are more common in patients on haemodialysis. Acid suppression or domperidone can be tried for symptomatic relief if a peptic ulcer is excluded
- Gastrointestinal bleeding is common. Once a peptic ulcer has been excluded, angiodysplasia and uraemic platelet dysfunction are common causes. Anecdotal reports suggest that oestrogen therapy (p. 14) may help. Colonic haemorrhage may be due to isolated caecal or rectal ulcers, diverticula or stercoral ulcers and may be life-threatening. Active resuscitation, diagnosis and definitive treatment should be the approach. The temptation to delay colonoscopy or surgery (because the patient is 'too ill') should usually be resisted, because delay increases mortality
- Diarrhoea is commonly due to *Cl. difficile* ('uraemic colitis' is an obsolete term, before the prevalence of pseudomembranous colitis was recognised). Occasionally, chronic diarrhoea can be due to bile salt malabsorption. Cholestyramine is worth trying, but consider other systemic causes of renal failure that may affect the gut (vasculitis, amyloid)
- Beware COX-2 inhibitors (prescribed instead of standard NSAIDs for 'gastroduodenal protection') as a cause of renal failure

Transplantation

- Up to half of early post-transplant deaths are gastrointestinal-related. Haemorrhage from peptic ulcer is frequent, but perforation and enteritis occur
- CMV oesophagitis, enteritis or colitis should be considered. Diagnosis is by endoscopy (aphthoid or diffuse ulceration), biopsy (inclusion bodies) and serology
- Colonic or small bowel perforation is common, possibly due to ischaemia, immunosuppression or faecal impaction

Anaemia
Anaemia should not be attributed to renal failure without considering gastrointestinal blood loss. Active investigation (endoscopy, distal duodenal biopsy, barium enema or colonoscopy) is cost-effective, since treatment of blood loss reduces the dose of expensive erythropoietin.

13.7 Cardiorespiratory disease

Myocardial infarction and acute gastrointestinal bleeding
- Haematemesis or melaena in the immediate postinfarct period is not that uncommon (between five and ten cases per year in a hospital serving 500 000). Active resuscitation is essential, but endoscopy is potentially dangerous, since it may provoke dysrrhythmias. If the bleeding is minor and self-limiting, endoscopy is best delayed for 6 weeks after infarction and empirical acid suppression (PPI) given meanwhile
- If bleeding continues, endoscopy should be performed by an experienced endoscopist on the coronary care unit, with supplemental oxygen, adequate sedation, ECG, blood pressure and oximetry monitoring. The cardiology registrar should be present to monitor the ECG during the procedure. The aim is to find and inject a bleeding point. A combination of 1 : 10 000 adrenaline and thrombin appears to be most successful. Surgery is avoided if possible, because mortality in the postinfarct period is very high

Chronic gastrointestinal bleeding
- An association between aortic stenosis and intestinal angiodysplasia has long been speculated. Portal hypertension in tricuspid regurgitation is another unusual cause
- Gastroduodenal and colonic lesions must be excluded by endoscopy and colonoscopy, in the first instance, followed by a small bowel enema (Fig. 9.8, p. 326)
- Valve replacement with a xenograft that will not require anticoagulation is usually advisable, but has an unpredictable effect on blood loss. If regular iron does not maintain the haemoglobin, oestrogens can be tried (p. 14)

Thrombolysis or anticoagulation in dyspeptic patients
- Dyspepsia or a history of peptic ulceration is *not* a contraindication to thrombolysis or starting heparin, *unless* there has been a documented ulcer within the past month
- Endoscopy is sensible prior to starting warfarin if there is a history of dyspepsia

Reflux and asthma
Nocturnal asthma may be a symptom of reflux (p. 54), but the association is often difficult to define. An empirical trial of a PPI for 4 weeks with monitoring of peak flow rates is appropriate when treating nocturnal symptoms.

13.8 Miscellaneous disorders

Osteoporosis
- Coeliac disease, ulcerative colitis, Crohn's disease and cirrhosis all increase the risk of osteoporosis independently of corticosteroids, although steroids hasten bone loss within 3–6 months of use
- Exercise and a good calcium intake (often inappropriately restricted) are sound advice for everyone
- HRT delays or abolishes bone loss in controlled trials of women with inflammatory bowel disease or malabsorption. This is sufficient indication for advising HRT in postmenopausal women with these conditions
- Calcium supplements have a debatable role in preventing osteoporosis. Premenopausal women should be encouraged to maintain an 'adequate' calcium intake, but recommended daily allowances are confusing. 50–100 mmol calcium/day (1–2 g calcium) is often advised when there is intestinal disease. Milk is the only appreciable source of calcium and contains 1.02 g/L, or 0.58 g/pint. Very few patients will drink or tolerate 1–2 L of milk/day. A sensible balance is to supplement clearly inadequate intake (< 15 mmol/day, or < 250 mL milk/day)
- Bone densitometry (dual emission X-ray absorptiometry, DEXA) is the best way of evaluating osteoporosis and is indicated in men or premenopausal women who have taken or are likely to take steroids for long periods (6 months or more). If bone density is more than 2.5 standard deviations below the mean for a young adult (i.e. osteoporotic), bisphosphonates should be considered. There are no adequate controlled trials of bisphosphonates in intestinal disease, because the pharmaceutical companies are wary about side-effects (nausea, diarrhoea and ulceration). However, bisphosphonates are often well tolerated
- Guidelines on investigation and treatment of osteoporosis for luminal and hepatic disease have been published (Appendix 2), but the area remains controversial. Population-based studies in patients with inflammatory bowel disease or coeliac disease in both Europe and the USA have shown that the actual fracture rate is only minimally increased, despite the prevalence of osteoporosis

Bone marrow transplantation
- Three principal causes of intestinal and hepatic disease after transplantation are chemotherapy, infections and graft-versus-host disease
- *Pretransplant chemo/radiotherapy* causes symptoms (diarrhoea, abdominal pain) by day 10 due to 'mucositis' damaging crypt-cell proliferation, but resolves by day 30. It may also cause veno-occlusive disease, with painful hepatomegaly and jaundice, especially in patients with pre-existing hepatitis B or C. Post-transplant chemotherapy (cyclosporin, methotrexate) may promote intestinal lymphoma
- *Infections* occur during the recovery phase from transplant—bacterial or fungal before day 30, viral thereafter. Diarrhoea due to *Cl. difficile*, *Candida* sp. oesophagitis, CMV, colitis or hepatitis are among the common infections
- *Graft-versus-host disease* is an immunological phenomenon causing rashes, diarrhoea with sloughing of the intestinal mucosa, protein-losing enteropathy, or cholestasis in

the acute phase (1–3 months). Chronic graft-versus-host disease at 3–15 months causes cholestasis with bile duct obliteration and malabsorption due to submucosal fibrosis and a scleroderma-like syndrome. Diagnosis is made by hepatic or endoscopic intestinal biopsy. Treatment with nutritional support and immunosuppression is difficult

Blood coagulation disorders

- Haemophiliacs may bleed from a peptic ulcer or develop acute abdominal pain from intramural haemorrhage, but HIV infection (p. 363) and chronic liver disease due to hepatitis C (p. 166), are more serious problems
- von Willebrand's disease quite frequently causes chronic iron deficiency without an identifiable source of blood loss. Iron supplements are appropriate, with oestrogen therapy for women, or tranexamic acid for men if anaemia persists. Desamino-D-arginine vasopressin (dDAVP) is rarely effective for chronic loss
- Thrombotic thrombocytopenic purpura causes thrombocytopenia, microangiopathic haemolytic anaemia, fever, renal insufficiency and confusion, often with abdominal pain. Pancreatitis, mesenteric infarction and acalculous cholecystitis are complications. Plasmapheresis and FFP or cryosupernatant (with high molecular weight von Willebrand factor removed) infusion are appropriate

Neuromuscular disease

- Dysphagia commonly complicates cerebrovascular or progressive neurological disease. Endoscopy is often normal, but necessary to exclude other pathology. Prokinetic agents rarely help. When nutrition is compromised, percutaneous gastrostomy is appropriate (p. 378)
- Constipation is a major problem after spinal injury, or progressive neuromuscular disease such as motor neurone disease, Parkinson's disease, mitochondrial myopathy, other myopathies or multiple sclerosis. Fibre often makes symptoms worse. Early use of stool-softening agents and occasional stimulant laxatives should be given. When constipation is intractable, vigorous bowel clear-out with Picolax (or bisacodyl 5–10 mg) and high doses of polyethylene glycol (Movicol 2–4 sachets daily) to prevent silting up again may help. Spurious diarrhoea from constipation is best treated by keeping the rectum empty with a Micralax or glycerine suppository on alternate days.
- Faecal impaction can be a cause of confusion or apparent neurological deterioration. Faecal impaction can also be treated with polyethylene glycol (Movicol 8 sachets in 6 h) (p. 295)
- Chronic abdominal pain and pseudo-obstruction can become intractable. Treatment is unsatisfactory. Analgesics, laxatives, tricyclic agents or serotonin reuptake inhibitors can be tried, often without success.

Autonomic dysreflexia

Severe hypertension and tachycardia with subsequent subarachnoid haemorrhage or seizures in tetraplegic patients can be provoked by faecal impaction or urinary retention. Prevention by avoiding constipation and routine catheterisation is the key.

14 Procedures and Investigations

14.1 Practical techniques

Rectal examination

Rectal examination is an essential part of every complete physical examination and fundamental when there is a history of rectal bleeding, melaena, abdominal pain, altered bowel habit, anaemia or symptoms of anorectal disease. It is all too often cursorily performed.

- Explain the procedure. It often helps to sympathise with the embarrassment and discomfort
- Position the patient in the left lateral position
- Part the buttocks to inspect the perineum for skin tags (violaceous and oedematous in Crohn's) or excoriation. Look for fistulous openings. If there is a history of incontinence or neurological disorder, test perineal sensation for light touch and discrimination between sharp and dull
- Gently insert the lubricated, gloved right index finger and assess anal sphincter tone, then introduce it to its fullest extent
- Sweep the finger round in a full circle, consciously feeling anterior, lateral and posterior walls of the rectum. Cancer of the rectum (15% of all colorectal cancers can be felt on digital examination) is felt as an indurated ulcerating lesion, a stenosis or proliferating tumour. Faecal residue may sometimes be confused with polyps. A villous tumour has a characteristic feel, somewhat like plastic bubble packing
- Clean the anus after examination. Inspect the material on the glove, which can also be used for microscopy or testing for occult blood

Rigid sigmoidoscopy

Proctosigmoidoscopy should always be performed before referring a patient for barium enema. Rigid sigmoidoscopy is still widely performed because it is simple, rapid and convenient, but flexible sigmoidoscopy (p. 417) after phosphate enema preparation is preferable if readily available.

- Before starting, check that the light source fits the instrument and works, that the air insufflator is connected, that the obturator fits, that there are biopsy forceps, formalin, gloves, tissues and lubricant jelly
- Explain sympathetically to the patient that the procedure may cause some discomfort and a desire to defecate, but should not be painful. Deep breathing often relieves the discomfort. No bowel preparation is necessary
- Position the patient in the left lateral position, lying almost transversely across the bed or couch. Unsuccessful examination is often the consequence of faulty positioning
- Perform a careful rectal examination before introducing 5 cm of the lubricated sigmoidoscope through the anal sphincter in the direction of the umbilicus

- Remove the obturator and close the eyepiece. Gently insufflate air and introduce the sigmoidoscope under direct vision. The tip has to point posteriorly along the sacral curve, so the examiner's head must move forward
- If mucosa occludes the lumen, withdraw the sigmoidoscope 1 cm, insufflate a little more air (too much is uncomfortable and can be dangerous), then move the tip further posteriorly, or laterally. Faecal residue can be moved out of the way with the tip of the sigmoidoscope, but if stool occludes the lumen, it can usually be displaced by swab-holding forceps or a swab on a stick inserted through the sigmoidoscope. Remember to close the eyepiece after removing the swab
- Examine the mucosa up to the rectosigmoid junction (15 cm) and beyond if not too uncomfortable for the patient
- Biopsies should routinely be taken if the patient has had diarrhoea, because they may detect unexpected pathology and also provide an objective record of the procedure. The St Mark's pinch biopsy forceps with 2 mm cups are safest and easiest to use. Most other biopsy forceps with larger cups (e.g. alligator forceps) were originally designed to remove rectal polyps or tumour tissue and take too deep a biopsy from flat mucosa. Following a biopsy with these larger forceps, a barium enema should be delayed for 3 days to reduce the risk of perforation
- Continue to inspect the mucosa when withdrawing the instrument. Clean the anus and document in the notes the distance examined, appearance of the mucosa and stool, and whether a biopsy was taken

Abdominal paracentesis

Diagnostic paracentesis ('ascitic tap') is essential in any patient with ascites (p. 146). Therapeutic paracentesis is increasingly used in the management of tense ascites (p. 150).

Diagnostic paracentesis

- An aseptic technique performed at the bedside
- Clean the right flank around the site midway between the umbilicus and the anterior superior iliac spine. Cover the area with a dressing towel with a hole cut out in the middle, over the paracentesis site. The left lower quadrant can also be used for diagnostic or therapeutic paracentesis. Guidance from ultrasonography is indicated if the initial tap is 'dry'
- Infiltrate 2 mL 2% lignocaine through a 21-gauge needle intradermally and more deeply to anaesthetise the peritoneum. Some consider anaesthetic unnecessary, but reflect on how you would like the procedure performed on yourself
- Aspirate ascites through a 19-gauge needle attached to a 20 mL syringe. If unsuccessful, ask the patient to lie a little further on the right side, or use a longer needle (lumbar puncture needle). Inspect the fluid (Table 5.8, p. 148) send it for protein estimation, culture and cytology (p. 149)

Therapeutic paracentesis

- Performed in the same site as diagnostic paracentesis
- The simplest technique is to use the soft (Bonanno) catheter designed for suprapubic bladder aspiration. A wide-bore intravenous cannula (minimum 16 French diameter)

can also be used but this may block unless cautiously held in position. A peritoneal dialysis catheter is another option but this has the disadvantages of being large and rigid with connections designed not to fit catheter bags or ordinary intravenous giving sets
- After cleaning and anaesthetising the skin, insert the catheter into the right or left flank midway between the umbilicus and anterior superior iliac spine, remove the trocar, connect the catheter bag or vacuum bottle and secure the catheter with tape
- Give 100 mL 20% salt-poor albumin (or 500 mL 4.5% albumin) for every 5 L of ascites drained, to avoid intravascular volume depletion
- Remove the catheter as soon as the ascites has drained, or within 2 h. Longer dwell times increase the risk of infection

Nasogastric tube insertion
Fine-bore (8 French gauge) nasogastric feeding has transformed enteral nutritional support (p. 374) and does not interfere with the swallowing reflex in stroke patients. Fine-bore tubes have a wire stylet to help introduction and the procedure is explained below; ordinary nasogastric tubes (12 or 14 French gauge) do not have a stylet, but are otherwise inserted in a similar way.
- Explain the procedure to the patient
- Sit the patient up, with neck slightly flexed
- Ensure the stylet can be inserted and removed easily from the tube (lubricate with water)
- Lubricate the end of the tube with gel and gently insert through the nose into the back of the throat (nasopharynx)
- Allow the patient to rest and give a sip of water to hold in the mouth
- Ask the patient to swallow and gently advance the tube
- If coughing occurs, stop and withdraw the tube into the nasopharynx before starting again
- Once the tube is half-way down, withdraw the stylet a few centimetres to make sure it runs freely
- Continue insertion until about 10 cm remains. Withdraw the stylet. If it sticks, carefully pull the tube back until the stylet can be withdrawn before reintroducing the tube
- Confirm the tube is in the stomach by aspirating gastric contents or the bubble test (sharply inject 20 mL air whilst listening for bubbling over the epigastrium with a stethoscope)
- Obtain an X-ray to check position if the consciousness level is impaired or if there is any doubt about position after aspirating or using the bubble test
- Tape the tube securely to the nose and along the skin under the cheek bone

14.2 House Officer's checklist

The explanation given in each section is designed to help those unfamiliar with the procedures to describe them to patients. The history and examination must be documented in the notes before any invasive procedure. Resuscitation equipment must be immediately available for any procedure that involves sedation.

Upper gastrointestinal endoscopy

Indications

Diagnostic
- Dyspepsia or abdominal pain with alarm symptoms (p. 78)
- Haematemesis or melaena (p. 9)
- Weight loss
- Iron-deficiency anaemia (always take distal duodenal biopsies to look for villous atrophy, p. 327)
- Persistent vomiting (p. 84)
- Biopsy of gastric lesions detected by barium meal
- Biopsy of distal duodenal mucosa for coeliac disease (p. 220)
- Follow-up of gastric ulcer (p. 94)

Therapeutic
- Sclerotherapy of bleeding oesophageal varices (p. 15)
- Injection, thermocoagulation or laser photocoagulation of other bleeding lesions (p. 14)
- Dilatation of oesophageal or pyloric strictures
- Palliation of oesophageal cancer with plastic or self-expanding metal stents, alcohol injection or laser therapy (p. 65)
- Positioning of percutaneous gastrostomy or nasojejunal feeding tubes

Preparation
- Nil by mouth for at least 4 h (longer after a large meal)
- Water only for 12 h and nil by mouth for 8 h, if pyloric obstruction is suspected
- Delay for 24 h after any upper gastrointestinal barium study (such as a barium swallow for dysphagia): barium can block the suction channel of the endoscope
- Written consent, after explanation

Explanation
- Intravenous sedation (often midazolam 2.5–10 mg) is usually given. The procedure can readily be performed without sedation, only using local anaesthetic spray to the pharynx, but requires good cooperation between endoscopist and patient. Many patients prefer light sedation; some choose heavier sedation so that they have no recall
- The pharynx is usually sprayed with lignocaine (lidocaine) 1% to reduce the gag reflex
- The flexible endoscope, the diameter of a small finger, is gently passed into the oesophagus and steered through the stomach into the duodenum (a diagram helps patients to understand)
- Breathing is not impaired, but a probe (from a pulse oximeter) is strapped to a finger to measure blood oxygen saturation. Supplemental oxygen is provided through a nasal cannula
- The procedure takes 5–10 min

- Eating or drinking is allowed 60 min after the procedure if local anaesthetic spray has been used, when pharyngeal sensation has recovered
- Findings and instructions should be given after the procedure in the presence of a friend or family member, or written down, because amnesia often follows sedation

Complications
- Sore throat may occur, but is transient. Occasionally nasal oxygen dries out the nasal mucosa, resulting in a runny nose from hypersecretion for 24 h
- Amnesia following sedation sometimes persists for hours, even though the patient appears to have recovered. Patients must not be allowed to drive or perform a responsible job without assistance for 24 h (looking after children, driving, operating machinery, signing legal documents)
- Perforation or bleeding (< 0.1%)
- Cardiorespiratory arrest or death (< 0.01%) are very rare and mainly affect the very sick or elderly, but remain a risk that must be considered when requesting the procedure

Antibiotic prophylaxis for endoscopy, sigmoidoscopy, colonoscopy and barium enema

Indications
- Prosthetic heart valves
- Previous endocarditis
- Synthetic vascular graft < 1 year old
- Severe neutropenia (< 100×10^9/L)
- Surgically constructed systemic–pulmonary shunt

Recommendations

Patients not allergic to penicillin
Patients not allergic to penicillin, and who have not had penicillin more than once in the previous month:
- Adults: 1 g amoxycillin and 120 mg gentamicin intravenously over 3–4 min before the procedure
- Children under 10 years: 500 mg amoxycillin and gentamicin 2 mg/kg body weight intravenously as above

Patients allergic to penicillin
Patients allergic to penicillin, or who have had penicillin more than once in the previous month:
- Adults: vancomycin 1 g infusion over 2 h followed by gentamicin 120 mg intravenously before the start of the procedure; or teicoplanin 400 mg and gentamicin 120 mg before the start of the procedure
- Children under 10 years: vancomycin 20 mg/kg infusion and gentamicin 2 mg/kg as above; or teicoplanin 6 mg/kg and gentamicin 2 mg/kg as above

Patients with severe neutropenia

Add metronidazole 7.5 mg/kg intravenously to any of the above regimes.

Jejunal biopsy

- Four distal duodenal biopsies (from the third part of the duodenum) at upper gastrointestinal endoscopy are satisfactory for most purposes (p. 218). Whilst a normal biopsy excludes coeliac disease, duodenal villi can appear stunted when overlying Brunner's glands: repeat biopsy is then indicated if there is any doubt about the diagnosis, sometimes using a paediatric colonoscope instead of a gastroscope to reach the jejunum
- Unusual causes of malabsorption, including giardiasis, lymphoma, Whipple's disease or amyloidosis can also be diagnosed by jejunal biopsy (p. 235)
- The Crosby/Watson biopsy capsule must now be considered obsolete. The Quinton hydraulic instrument that allows multiple biopsies remains a research tool

Indications

- Diagnosis of coeliac disease and repeated, after 3–6 months on a gluten-free diet, to confirm response (p. 222)
- Iron-deficiency anaemia, or folate deficiency, at the time of the first upper gastrointestinal endoscopy
- Persistent diarrhoea (Fig. 7.1, p. 211)
- Weight loss
- Diagnosis of *G. lamblia* infection, if stool examination is normal (p. 226)
- Preparation, explanation and procedure are as for upper gastrointestinal endoscopy

Colonoscopy

Indications

Diagnostic

- Investigation of bloody diarrhoea, always in preference to a barium enema
- Rectal bleeding, especially when recurrent, or after a normal or inadequate barium enema
- Persistent diarrhoea (Fig. 7.1, p. 211), to obtain serial mucosal biopsies
- Assessing the distribution of disease in patients with Crohn's disease (p. 248) or ulcerative colitis (p. 268). Colonoscopy is generally *not* required in severe colitis and risks perforation. *Flexible sigmoidoscopy* (p. 417) is almost always sufficient for management decisions
- Biopsy of a lesion detected by barium enema
- Iron-deficiency anaemia (p. 327)
- Surveillance for colorectal cancer in selected patients (p. 308)

Therapeutic

- Polypectomy
- Diathermy or laser photocoagulation of angiodysplasia or rectal tumours
- Dilatation of colonic strictures in selected patients (p. 306)

Preparation

Regimens vary enormously between endoscopy units. The following is a simple and widely available approach:

- Low-residue diet (no fruit, vegetables or bread) for 48 h and liquids only for 24 h before the procedure. Stop iron supplements
- Sodium picosulphate and magnesium citrate (Picolax), 1 sachet at 8 AM and another at 4 PM on the day before the procedure, with a cup of water every hour to ensure a good fluid intake (inadequate fluid is usually the cause of poor preparation) *or* polyethylene glycol (PEG) solution (GoLytely, Colyte, KleenPrep, LytePrep) 4 L taken over a 3–4 h period on the afternoon or evening prior to the procedure
- Consent, after explanation

Explanation

- Sedation is given (such as intravenous midazolam 2.5–5 mg with intravenous fentanyl 50–100 µg); an antispasmodic (intravenous hyoscine 20 mg) may be given to reduce colonic spasm
- The flexible colonoscope (diameter of an index finger) is passed per rectum, around the colon. Fluoroscopy is sometimes helpful
- The procedure takes 10–20 min
- The patient goes home accompanied, 1 or 2 h after the procedure

Complications

Complications are best *avoided* by ensuring that *inappropriate* procedures are not performed. Examples include colonoscopy for isolated abdominal pain, repeat procedures for metaplastic polyps, or surveillance on elderly patients with comorbidity. Each unit should, ideally, have its own patient information leaflet giving local information, including procedures performed and complication rates.

- Electrolye imbalance (hyponatraemia) from bowel preparation in elderly patients (age > 80). Other imaging, such as CT colonography (p. 304) is preferable
- Abdominal discomfort after the procedure is common, but rarely persists for more than a few hours. It can be reduced if air, which is insufflated during the procedure, is aspirated during withdrawal of the colonoscope, or if carbon dioxide is used instead of air for insufflation
- Incomplete examination occurs in 5–20%, depending on operator experience. A barium enema, CT colonography or repeat examination is then indicated
- Perforation is rare (0.1%), but more common after hot biopsy, snare polypectomy (0.5%), severe diverticulosis, acute colitis, or ischaemic colitis. The latter are relative contraindications to colonoscopy. Haemorrhage after biopsy or polypectomy is less common

Flexible sigmoidoscopy

Indications

- Investigation of bright red rectal bleeding, especially in young patients (< 40 years), when a distal source of bleeding is suspected and full examination of the colon is unnecessary

- Investigation of choice in acute colitis in hospitalised patients, when full colonoscopy is unsafe
- An alternative to rigid sigmoidoscopy for initial examination of the distal colon in outpatients, if the equipment and facilities for preparation are available. Up to 75% of colorectal tumours are accessible at flexible sigmoidoscopy

Preparation
- Phosphate enema 30–60 min before the procedure
- Can be performed without any preparation at all, but views are usually suboptimal and a phosphate enema is safe and reasonably well tolerated even in acute colitis

Explanation
- Usually performed without sedation, although sedation can be given if necessary as long as appropriate facilities are available
- An ordinary colonoscope (see above) is usually used to examine the rectum and sigmoid colon. Short (60 cm) flexible sigmoidoscopes are available, but are less versatile than a colonoscope and cost only slightly less
- The procedure takes 5 min

ERCP

Indications
(See p. 196; Fig. 4.2, p. 118; Fig. 6.5, p. 197)

Preparation
- Platelet count $> 100 \times 10^9/L$
- Coagulation studies (INR < 1.3, prothrombin time < 22 s)
- Nil by mouth for 4 h
- Premedication policy differs between units. Some always use parenteral sedative and antibiotic premedication; others only use oral antibiotics and perform diagnostic ERCP as an outpatient
- Oral ciprofloxacin 750 mg 60–90 min before the procedure is as effective as intravenous antibiotic prophylaxis
- Consent, after explanation

Explanation
- The procedure is performed in the X-ray department
- Effective sedation (intravenous midazolam 5–10 mg with pethidine/meperidine 50–100 mg or fentanyl 50–100 μg) is given, depending on premedication and individual needs of the patient
- A side-viewing endoscope is passed into the duodenum. A fine catheter is inserted through the ampulla, into the pancreatic duct and then into the bile duct. Contrast is injected and X-rays taken
- Therapeutic procedures include sphincterotomy (5–10 mm incision through the ampulla), precut sphincterotomy (when the bile duct cannot be cannulated), stent

insertion (through a stricture) or stone retrieval (by basket, balloon, lithotripsy or occasionally dissolution)
• The procedure takes 20–60 min
• The patient can go home the same day, unless a therapeutic procedure has been performed

Complications
The overall complication rate of ERCP is 5% and mortality 0.4% (Table 1.6, p. 32). Endoscopic sphincterotomy has 10–40% complications, similar to coronary artery bypass surgery. Complications are best *avoided* by not performing *inappropriate* procedures. With the advent of MR cholangiography and contrast-enhanced spiral CT scanning, there is little role for diagnostic ERCP.
• Complete examination is possible in > 90%, but more than one attempt may be needed, especially for therapeutic procedures
• Acute pancreatitis (2%; the serum amylase always rises after ERCP, but in the absence of abdominal pain and vomiting can be ignored). The risk is increased three-fold in young females, if the bilirubin is normal, or if a precut sphincterotomy is necessary to gain access to the bile duct (Table 1.6, p. 32)
• Haemorrhage after sphincterotomy (1%), requiring prompt surgery since it rarely stops spontaneously. If haemorrhage is haemodynamically significant, it is rarely possible to obtain adequate views to perform effective endoscopic haemostasis
• Cholangitis (2%)
• Death (0.5%)

Video capsule enteroscopy

Indications
• A novel technique, not yet widely available, involves swallowing a disposable video capsule (2 cm × 1 cm) that images the small intestine. It has captured the imagination of patients and doctors
• Principal indication is occult gastrointestinal bleeding or recurrent anaemia when the source cannot be defined by other techniques. Other indications (almost any reason for small bowel imaging) are evolving
• Contraindicated in the presence of partial intestinal obstruction and best used with caution in Crohn's disease, because laparotomy is necessary to retrieve the capsule if it impacts on a stricture

Explanation
• The procedure takes 4–8 h and interpretation of the images by a skilled endoscopist takes a couple of hours, even with computer-assisted analysis. The capsule is evacuated with stool and flushed away
• If the cause of bleeding is identified, definitive treatment will often mean surgical resection of the lesion
• Coincidental lesions (small ulcers, red spots) may be identified, of unknown or irrelevant significance

Liver biopsy

Indications

Diagnostic

- Persistently elevated (> twofold) liver enzymes 6 months after viral hepatitis (p. 140)
- Asymptomatic elevation of liver enzymes (Fig. 5.9, p. 183), especially in alcohol abuse (p. 183)
- Clinical suspicion of cirrhosis (p. 152), chronic active hepatitis (p. 167) or carcinoma (p. 178)
- Biopsy of hepatic lesions detected by ultrasound or CT scan
- Abnormal liver function in relatives of patients with familial hepatic disease (haemochromatosis, Wilson's disease)
- Contraindications include a bleeding diathesis, ascites, extrahepatic biliary obstruction, suspected hydatid disease, hepatic peliosis or haemangioma, or emphysema

Preparation

- Platelet count $> 100 \times 10^9/L$
- Coagulation studies (INR < 1.3, prothrombin time < 22 s). Give a single dose of vitamin K 10 mg and recheck clotting 48 h later if coagulation is disordered; otherwise infuse 2–4 units of FFP immediately prior to biopsy
- Consent, after explanation
- Liver biopsy is best performed before 2 PM, so that observations can be made when staff are readily available and complications recognised
- Ultrasound or CT scan guided liver biopsy is helpful for focal lesions, but need to be discussed and coordinated with a radiologist. Needle biopsy is best avoided if hepatocellular carcinoma is suspected, since tracking of the tumour can occur. Surgical biopsy is preferable
- Biopsy can safely be performed on an outpatient before 12 AM (to allow 6 h observation), in patients who have normal coagulation and platelet count, and who live within 10 miles of the hospital, as long as the biopsy is successful in a single pass

Explanation

- The procedure may be performed on the ward, but in some hospitals is always performed by a radiologist under ultrasound control. Sedation is not usually necessary
- Lignocaine/lidocaine 2% is carefully infiltrated down to the capsule between the eighth and tenth ribs, where there is dullness to percussion in the mid-axillary line. Effective local anaesthesia is essential. Always use at least 10 mL 2% lignocaine/lidocaine and use a long needle (sometimes a spinal needle) in obese patients. The patient should not experience pain and this dose of lignocaine will not cause cardiac depression
- A 2 mm nick in the skin is made with a scalpel
- Breathing is rehearsed (breath must be held in full expiration during biopsy)
- Biopsy with a fine needle (Trucut or Menghini) takes a few seconds
- After the biopsy the patient lies on the right side for 2 h and then stays in bed for 6 h. Pulse and blood pressure are measured every 15 min for 1 h, every 30 min for 2 h and then hourly up to 8 h

- If being performed on an outpatient, the patient must be seen by a doctor before discharge and given the ward telephone number to call if there are problems overnight
- Transjugular biopsy is a specialist technique performed by interventional radiologists when percutaneous biopsy is contraindicated due to disordered coagulation or ascites

Complications
- Local pain (often pleuritic or in the shoulder) is common, but usually relieved by oral paracetamol/acetaminophen 2 tablets every 4 h. Severe pain may indicate a subcapsular haematoma: ultrasound will detect a significant haematoma, but resolution of pain with analgesics within 24–48 h is usual
- Pneumothorax is rarely clinically apparent and does not need drainage unless breathing is compromised
- Bleeding, requiring transfusion (< 0.5%) or operation (very rarely)
- Death (< 0.1%) may follow inappropriate biopsy (colon, pancreas, gall bladder, inferior vena cava), or a tear in the liver capsule

Percutaneous biliary procedures
Percutaneous transhepatic cholangiograms are rarely performed now that ERCP is the procedure of first choice. The technique is, however, occasionally useful.

Indications

Diagnostic
Cholestatic jaundice with a dilated biliary tree (Fig. 6.4, p. 191) when ERCP is unavailable or impossible (p. 196)

Therapeutic
- Insertion of a percutaneous self-expanding metal stent across biliary strictures (especially at the bifurcation), which cannot be cannulated at ERCP
- When ERCP is initially unsuccessful in cannulating an obstructed biliary tree: performed in conjunction with ERCP by insertion of a wire, which is then retrieved endoscopically, so that a stent can be inserted (p. 196)

Preparation
As for ERCP.

Explanation
- The procedure is performed by a radiologist under local anaesthetic. Sedation is often helpful
- A fine needle is inserted into the liver, in the eighth or ninth intercostal space. Contrast is gently injected as the needle is withdrawn under fluoroscopy, until an intrahepatic duct is delineated. Contrast is then injected to outline the biliary tree and X-rays taken
- The procedure takes 15–30 min
- Observation after the procedure is the same as for liver biopsy

Complications
- Local pain is relieved by paracetamol
- Biliary leak is rare, even in obstructive jaundice, and usually resolves spontaneously. Analgesia (intramuscular pethidine/meperidine 50–100 mg) may be necessary
- Cholangitis is very rare, except when an external drainage catheter is left *in situ*

14.3 Radiology

Requests
Salient clinical features, rather than a statement of the suspected diagnosis, help the radiologist interpret X-rays. Stating the specific question to be answered by the radiological investigation is also helpful. Potential complicating factors (diabetes, epilepsy, allergies, pacemakers) should be mentioned, especially for contrast or invasive procedures.

Discussion with the radiologist about the most appropriate imaging technique saves the patient unnecessary investigation and allows the radiologist to proceed at his or her discretion, depending on the findings (e.g. from ultrasound to CT scan). A visit to the X-ray department and 'please' or 'thank you' on the request form are simple courtesies that pay dividends!

Plain film checklist
Plain, supine abdominal and erect chest X-rays are indicated for any patient with acute abdominal pain (p. 28). Erect abdominal X-ray rarely adds diagnostic information to a supine film and should not be requested.

On a plain abdominal X-ray
Look for:
- Subdiaphragmatic gas, or clear delineation of liver, kidneys or spleen (perforated viscus, p. 31)
- Faecal distribution:
  - throughout the colon (constipation)
  - distal extent (identifies the proximal distribution of active ulcerative colitis, or stricture)
- Intestinal diameter:
  - small intestine > 2.5 cm (obstruction)
  - colon > 5.5 cm (obstruction, toxic dilatation, Fig. 1.6, p. 41)
- Mucosal pattern:
  - thickened wall (acute ulcerative colitis or Crohn's disease)
  - mucosal islands (small radio-opaque projections into the lumen in acute colitis, p. 41)
  - thumbprinting (large radio-opaque projections, ischaemic colitis, Fig. 9.7, p. 322)
  - gas in the wall (impending perforation, pneumatosis coli)
- Gas pattern:
  - displaced or separated loops of small bowel (mass effect, inflammation)
  - segment of jejunum ('sentinel loop' in acute pancreatitis)
  - fluid levels (obstruction, on an erect abdominal film)

- central distribution of normal small bowel (ascites)
- gas in the biliary tree (cholangitis, recent passage of stone)
- Calculi:
  - along the line of the transverse processes (renal/ureteric)
  - right upper quadrant (gallstones)
  - phleboliths, calcified lymph nodes, foreign bodies or artefacts may be included in the differential diagnosis

Contrast studies

In a double contrast study, barium coats the mucosa and gas provides the contrast. Effervescent tablets are swallowed, or air is insufflated, to put the mucosa under slight tension. Barium is used unless perforation is suspected, when Gastrografin or non-ionic agents are indicated. Single contrast studies have few indications (p. 423).

Endoscopy (p. 79) is usually preferable to a barium meal except when pyloric stenosis is suspected, and colonoscopy is the procedure of choice instead of a barium enema for investigating bloody diarrhoea or visible rectal bleeding (p. 210). In elderly patients, abdominal CT scan is usually more appropriate than a barium enema (p. 399). For small bowel imaging, MR enteroclysis or capsule enteroscopy (p. 419) are likely to replace some contrast studies, but techniques are evolving and not yet widely available

Oesophagus
(See Figures 1.1 (p. 6), 2.3 (p. 60), 2.4 (p. 63), 2.5 (p. 66))

Small bowel (see also p. 426)
- Barium follow-through is better tolerated and more widely used than small bowel enema, but gives inferior mucosal definition
- Films of the abdomen are taken at intervals until barium reaches the caecum (2–4 h). Enhanced films of areas of interest (terminal ileum) are then taken (Fig. 7.3, p. 215; Fig. 8.1, p. 249). Much depends on how closely the procedure is supervised by a radiologist if lesions are not to be missed
- Small bowel enema is more troublesome and needs bowel preparation and duodenal intubation, but produces better mucosal definition. It is indicated when mucosal changes may be subtle (Crohn's disease, polyps), or if a follow-through examination is unsatisfactory

Large bowel
- Barium enema should only be done after digital rectal examination, sigmoidoscopy and biopsy. It is sensible to wait for 72 h after rectal biopsy before a barium enema, but the risk of perforation with modern biopsy forceps is minimal
- Preparation is the same as for colonoscopy. Elderly (> 80 years) or frail patients should be considered for CT colonography (p. 304) in the first instance
- A smooth muscle relaxant (intravenous hyoscine butylbromide 20 mg or glucagon 1 mg) are sometimes administered to decrease colonic spasm
- Large films are taken every 10–15 min until the barium reaches the caecum, followed by films of areas of interest (lateral views to show the rectum and posterior rectal space, enhanced views of the flexures or caecum). The procedure takes 20–30 min

- A single contrast enema, without preparation ('instant enema'), is only indicated when mechanical large bowel obstruction needs to be distinguished from pseudo-obstruction. Flexible sigmoidoscopy is more appropriate to define the type of colitis

Abdominal and endoscopic ultrasound

Abdominal ultrasound
- Indicated for the investigation of abdominal pain (gallstones, pancreatitis), jaundice, abnormal liver function tests (Fig. 5.9, p. 183), hepatomegaly, ascites or abdominal masses. Doppler examination of blood flow in portal or hepatic veins is appropriate in portal hypertension (p. 152) and of mesenteric blood flow when intestinal ischaemia is suspected (p. 320). These are specialist techniques. Diagnostic biopsy or therapeutic aspiration can be performed under ultrasound control
- An ideal, non-invasive investigation for thin patients
- Whilst reliable in experienced hands, the interpretation is subjective and intestinal gas can prevent adequate views, especially of retroperitoneal structures including the pancreas
- Preparation involves nothing to eat for 4 h if the gall bladder is to be imaged. Failure of the gall bladder to contract after a fatty meal suggests chronic cholecystitis (p. 190) and influences non-surgical management of gallstones (p. 193)
- Ultrasound of other areas of the abdomen needs no preparation, apart from the pelvis, when the bladder should be full

Endoscopic ultrasound
- Endosonography of the rectum and oesophagus have become standard techniques for the evaluation of malignancy before surgery
- EUS gives accurate and complementary information about the margins of tumour infiltration or nodal involvement compared with CT scanning, but in the UK is still confined to specialist centres
- Biopsy of lymph nodes is possible, depending on the type of instrument
- EUS is also useful for preoperative staging of small pancreatic carcinomas, detection of common bile duct calculi (to avoid unnecessary sphincterotomy), percutaneous drainage of pancreatic pseudocysts and guiding endoscopic biopsy of submucosal lesions
- Rectal ultrasound is more widely available and is part of the standard evaluation of anal sphincter integrity for patients with faecal incontinence
- Intraoperative ultrasound is particularly useful in hepatic resection of tumours or in identifying pancreatic lesions (such as endocrine tumours)

CT scan

Standard CT scanning
- Indicated when ultrasound is not technically possible (fat patients, excessive bowel gas), when doubt about the diagnosis persists (Fig. 4.1, p. 114), for percutaneous biopsy or drainage of intra-abdominal lesions and abscesses, and as alternative to contrast radiology for frail patients (p. 399)
- CT scan is better than ultrasound for demonstrating retroperitoneal structures, common bile duct stones or for fat patients, but needs skilled interpretation

- Contrast (5 mL oral Gastrografin on the evening before the procedure) is given to facilitate definition. Intravenous contrast to define vascular structures is given at the discretion of the radiologist
- Preparation is otherwise the same as for ultrasound
- Spiral (helical) CT scanning has become standard in many centres. The table moves continuously through a rotating image field, so images may be viewed from different angles and at different intervals, instead of being confined to 1 mm or 5 mm axial 'cuts'. This improves resolution, allows better spatial orientation (including three-dimensional reconstruction of lesions)
- Other advantages include rapid scanning (complete abdominal or thoracic imaging in a single breath-hold of 15–18 s), which makes it more suitable for sick patients, and ability to image luminal structures ('virtual colonoscopy')

CT colonography

- CT is potentially a non-invasive way of colonic imaging. Terminology is confusing and evolving
- *CT colonography* is suitable for excluding colorectal carcinoma in elderly or frail patients. It avoids the need for purgative bowel preparation. A small dose of oral contrast is given 24 h before the procedure and a helical (spiral) scanner is needed. It detects around 85% of colorectal carcinomas, compared to 95% by barium enema
- *CT colonoscopy* involves full bowel preparation and oral contrast. Using the helical scanner it is possible to reconstruct three-dimensional images and detect 75–90% of polyps > 1 cm compared to colonoscopy. It is non-invasive, but the radiation dose is appreciable and if polyps are detected, colonoscopy is still necessary

MRI

Implants of magnetic materials (clips, prosthetic valves, pacemakers) are contraindications, depending on the type of implant. Unlike CT scanning it can be performed immediately after contrast radiology. Claustrophobic patients may find the procedure unacceptable, because they are enclosed in the scanner. Most scans take 15–30 min.

Pelvis

- MR is the procedure of choice for pelvic imaging to evaluate recurrent perianal fistulae, perianal Crohn's disease or for staging rectal carcinoma. Patients being investigated for pelvic pain should have a pelvic ultrasound first
- The high signal in perianal fistulae or abscesses allows good definition of complex fistulae (Fig. 8.2, p. 262), potentially avoiding the need for examination under anaesthetic
- In rectal carcinoma, it is complementary to CT scanning for staging prior to surgery. It accurately defines tumour margin in relation to the mesorectal plane

Abdomen

- Depending on available software and enhancing agents (gadolinium), MR is normally indicated for the evaluation of isolated hepatic lesions to distinguish adenomas from focal nodular hyperplasia, or tumour (Fig 5.2, p. 139). It is helpful when investigating

suspected pancreatic lesions not identified by CT scanning (particularly neuroendocrine tumours)
- Secretin-stimulated MR is an evolving technique that may become the procedure of choice for evaluating chronic pancreatitis. Injection of secretin stimulates pancreatic flow to provide high resolution contrast in the pancreatic ducts (Fig 4.3, p. 118)

Magnetic resonance cholangiography
- Indicated before diagnostic ERCP for suspected common bile duct stones or investigation of biliary pathology (p. 191). A normal scan may avoid the need for (and risks of) an ERCP. Modern scanners need only a single breath-hold to acquire images and avoid movement artefact (Fig. 6.5, p. 197)

Magnetic resonance enteroclysis
- An evolving technique that may replace some small bowel contrast radiology (Fig 7.4, p. 220 and Fig. 8.1, p. 250). Nasojejunal intubation is still needed for optimal images

Other imaging techniques

Mesenteric angiography
(See Fig. 1.3, p. 20)
- Intra-arterial digital subtraction angiography needs less contrast than conventional techniques, for equivalent definition. Low ionic contrast media (such as Omnipaque) cause fewer side-effects and do not contain iodine
- Indicated for profuse gastrointestinal bleeding when the source cannot be identified by endoscopy or colonoscopy (p. 19), investigation of recurrent iron-deficiency anaemia when an intestinal arteriovenous malformation is suspected (although may be replaced by capsule enteroscopy), and investigation of chronic mesenteric ischaemia after Doppler ultrasound studies (p. 321)
- Mesenteric anatomy is shown in Fig. 9.5 (p. 314)

Isotope studies
- The ^{13}C- or ^{14}C-urea breath test are one of the most useful tests for confirming effective eradication of *Helicobacter pylori* (p. 86)
- Potentially useful minimally invasive techniques for identifying intestinal inflammation (white cell scan), blood loss (red cell scan), or Meckel's diverticulum and some other conditions (Table 14.1). Unfortunately, results are open to interpretation and all too frequently fail to achieve the diagnostic sensitivity and specificity of published series
- Discussion with the nuclear medicine department is advised, because not all tests may be locally available
- No preparation is necessary, but isotope studies should be avoided in children, or women of childbearing age, especially if they may be pregnant

14.4 Function tests

The reliability of results depends on familiarity with the procedure and if such tests are thought necessary, the patient is best referred to a centre where they are regularly

Table 14.1 Indications for gastrointestinal isotope studies

Condition	Scan	Page
Acute cholecystitis	^{99}Tc HIDA	24
Active bleeding	^{99}Tc sulphur colloid	18
Obscure bleeding	^{99}Tc red cell	
	^{51}Cr red cell	329
Meckel's diverticulum	^{99}Tc pertechnate	263
Protein-losing enteropathy	^{125}I-albumin	218
Steatorrhoea	^{14}C triolein	429
Crohn's disease activity	^{111}In white cell	251
	^{99}Tc-HMPAO	251
Terminal ileal absorption	^{75}SeHCAT	429
	$^{57/58}$Co B$_{12}$	
Budd–Chiari syndrome	^{99}Tc pertechnate	155
Gastric emptying	^{99}Tc scrambled egg	431

performed. Details of the tests are available in larger textbooks (Appendix 2, p. 442) and only an outline is given here.

Breath tests

Lactose hydrogen breath test
- *Indication*: diagnosis of hypolactasia
- *Principle*: lactose is normally digested (into glucose and galactose), then absorbed. In hypolactasia, lactose is incompletely digested and undigested lactose is fermented when it reaches the colon. Hydrogen is then released, absorbed and exhaled in breath
- *Method*: 50 g lactose is ingested after an overnight fast. Exhaled breath hydrogen measured at 0, 60 and 120 min
- *Results*: normal breath hydrogen is < 20 p.p.m. at 120 min. Positive breath hydrogen (consistent with hypolactasia) is > 20 p.p.m. at 120 min

Lactulose hydrogen breath test
- *Indication*: diagnosis of intestinal bacterial overgrowth
- *Principle*: lactulose is a synthetic disaccharide that is not absorbed, but is fermented to release hydrogen by intestinal bacteria. Release of hydrogen before 120 min in a person with normal orocaecal transit is consistent with bacteria in the small intestine. False-positives occur due to oral bacteria, intestinal hurry or elevated baseline breath hydrogen in cigarette smokers. False-negatives occur after intestinal resection or lack of hydrogen-producing bacteria
- *Method*: 10 g lactulose ingested after a fast and an antiseptic mouthwash. Exhaled breath hydrogen is measured at 0, 20, 40, 60, 80, 100, 120, 150 and 180 min (exact timings may vary)
- *Results*: normal breath hydrogen is > 20 p.p.m. at > 120 min (colonic peak, quite the opposite of the lactose breath test above). Positive (consistent with bacterial overgrowth) is a sustained increase in breath hydrogen > 10 p.p.m. above baseline value at a time < 120 min, but preferably < 60 min for a confident diagnosis

Other breath tests for bacterial overgrowth

- ^{14}C-xylose and ^{14}C-glycoholic acid (bile acid) breath tests
- *Principle*: xylose is metabolised and bile acids deconjugated by Gram-negative aerobes (always part of overgrowth flora). Carbon dioxide is released, then absorbed and exhaled. Unlike lactulose, the tests are positive in the absence of H_2-generating bacteria. Xylose is said to be the most specific and sensitive
- *Results*: elevated $^{14}CO_2$ levels (> 0.3%) detected at 2–3 h if bacteria present in small intestine

Gastric acid secretion

- *Indication*: investigation of elevated serum gastrin
- *Method*: patients should have stopped acid suppression for 2 weeks and be fasting. A nasogastric tube inserted and gastric juice aspirated every 15 min for 1 h for basal output. Pentagastrin 6 pg/kg (0.42 mg for 70 kg) is then given by intramuscular injection to stimulate gastric acid secretion. Further aspiration continues for 2 h. Cephalic stimulation to test vagal integrity by sham feeding, should be tested before administration of pentagastrin. Measurements of volume (mL), pH (units), titratable acidity (mmol/L), acid output (mmol/h, calculated as volume (L) × titratable acidity) are made for each collection period, by prior arrangement with the biochemistry department
- *Results*: normal basal acid secretion (the sum of four 15 min collections) is 0–5 mmol/h; peak acid output (sum of the two highest collections after pentagastrin) ranges from 1 to 45 (mean 22) mmol/h; maximal acid output is titratable acidity in the single highest 15 min collection
- *Interpretation*: high basal output and no response to pentagastrin is consistent with Zollinger–Ellison syndrome. Absent basal output and no response to pentagastrin indicates achlorhydria or ingestion of PPIs

Intestinal absorption and permeability tests

These tests have limited clinical application despite decades of development and largely remain research tools. Enthusiasts at some hospitals use them for discriminating between functional bowel disorders and organic disease. Unfortunately, they still have a tendency to crop up as questions in post-graduate exams, so limited details are given.

Xylose absorption

- *Indication*: investigation of suspected carbohydrate malabsorption
- *Method*: ingestion of 5 g D-xylose (non-metabolised monosaccharide), followed by a 5 h urine collection or 60 min blood xylose
- *Results*: normal urinary excretion is > 22%, or blood xylose > 0.56 mmol/L at 60 min
- *Interpretation*: excretion < 22% is consistent with poor mucosal absorption, but 20% untreated coeliacs have normal values, and rapid gastric emptying, fast intestinal transit, renal dysfunction or incomplete urine collection give false-positive results. The test is non-specific and insufficiently sensitive to act as a screening test for small intestinal disease, so is rarely used

Intestinal permeability

- Isotonic 5 g lactulose and 0.1 g L-rhamnose in 250 mL water, followed by a 5 h urine collection and calculation of the lactulose/rhamnose ratio, detects abnormal intestinal permeability. The test is sensitive but not specific
- Normal ratio < 0.04. Higher values indicate small intestinal disease (coeliac, Crohn's). High permeability in Crohn's disease predicts a risk of early relapse
- Other dual sugar tests (lactulose/mannitol) depend on local assay techniques and utilise the same principle as the lactulose/rhamnose test. Single marker tests (polyethylene glycol or ^{51}Cr-EDTA) may give false results for the same reasons as the xylose absorption test

^{14}C-triolein breath test

- *Indication*: diagnosis of fat malabsorption
- *Principle*: triolein is a triglyceride that normally undergoes lipid hydrolysis and absorption as oleic acid, before metabolism to release carbon dioxide. After ingestion of ^{14}C-labelled triolein (glycerol ^{14}C-trioleic acid), ^{14}CO$_2$ can be detected in the breath. In fat malabsorption, less oleic acid is absorbed. False-positives occur when triolein metabolism is impaired for reasons other than pancreatic insufficiency (diabetes, liver disease, lung disease). The test lacks sensitivity
- *Results*: normal breath ^{14}CO$_2$ rises above baseline (> 0.0005%). When positive (consistent with fat malabsorption), breath ^{14}CO$_2$ remains low (< 0.0005%). It is not specific for the cause of fat malabsorption (pancreatic insufficiency, coeliac disease, gastric surgery)

Faecal fat excretion

- *Indication*: originally a test to confirm a suspicion of malabsorption, but the lack of sensitivity and specificity means that it is rarely appropriate
- *Method*: 3-day faecal collection during a controlled diet (100 g fat/day)
- *Results*: > 6 g/day fat excretion is abnormal
- *Interpretation*: a high value simply confirms a clinical suspicion and does not avoid the need for further investigation. A normal result does not exclude malabsorption (e.g. coeliac disease), so the test has limited value

Malabsorption is better evaluated via history, signs, blood tests, intestinal biopsy, small bowel radiology and pancreatic ultrasound (p. 218). Stool inspection (coproscopy) for steatorrhoea has a variable sensitivity, low specificity and poor positive predictive value

Ileal absorption SeHCAT test

- *Indication*: investigation of chronic watery diarrhoea (bile salt malabsorption, p. 213)
- *Interpretation*: requested, if available, through the nuclear medicine department, who will supply the local normal range. A normal test reliably excludes ileal disease and a positive test predicts a good response of diarrhoea to cholestyramine. Many results are equivocal. Some prefer a therapeutic trial of cholestyramine

Pancreatic function

The principal indication is to investigate symptoms of exocrine insufficiency (p. 116), with minimal or no changes on ultrasound or MRCP. Pancreatic supplements should be stopped 5 days before the test. Direct intubation tests have no clinical role. Faecal elastase (p. 119) is a sensitive marker of pancreatic insufficiency with a high negative predictive value (reliably confirms normal function), but is not widely available. Use of the fluorescein dilaurate test is decreasing, because it is complex and lacks sensitivity.

Fluorescein dilaurate ('Pancreolauryl') test

- *Principle*: pancreatic enzymes normally split fluorescein from dilaurate. Urinary excretion of fluorescein is measured using a spectrophotometer
- *Method*: the test takes 2–3 days. On the first day, 2 capsules of fluorescein dilaurate are ingested and urine collected for 10 h (accurately timed). The percentage of dye excretion is calculated. On the second day, fluorescein alone (sodium salt) is ingested and urine collected for 10 h. The fluorescein excretion ratio on days 1 and 2 is calculated
- *Results*: normal excretion index is > 30, but > 90% pancreatic function needs to be lost to be detectable. A positive result < 20 usually indicates pancreatic insufficiency, but false-positives occur

14.5 Other tests

Oesophageal manometry

Manometry is a specialist procedure that is best performed at a referral centre. The procedure is not difficult, but considerable expertise is needed for useful interpretation of the results.

- *Indications*: all patients prior to antireflux surgery or with suspected achalasia. Also for chest pain of uncertain cause (p. 73), but only patients with disabling symptoms should be referred
- *Method*: acid suppression and drugs affecting oesophageal motility (prokinetics, nitrates, calcium antagonists, tricyclic agents) should be stopped for 1 week before the test, which is performed on fasting patients. A tiny nasogastric catheter is passed and pressure recorded by intraluminal transducers. A sleeve sensor is best for measuring lower oesophageal sphincter pressure, because focal sensors become displaced during swallowing. Provocative stimuli (acid perfusion) are sometimes used to trigger oesophageal contraction and elucidate unusual causes of chest pain
- *Results*: a normal recording shows sequential progression of the peristaltic wave (pressure is measured at 5 cm intervals) and relaxation of the lower oesophageal sphincter. Abnormalities occur in either the pressure generated (amplitude can be > 80 mmHg in oesophageal spasm) or the wave progression (failure of relaxation of the lower oesophageal sphincter in achalasia, Fig 2.5, p. 66)

Oesophageal pH monitoring

As with manometry, 24 h pH monitoring is best done at a referral centre, because interpretation can be complex.

- *Indications*: refractory symptoms of gastro-oesophageal reflux or undiagnosed chest pain, in the absence of visible oesophagitis (p. 73)

- *Method*: drugs for the treatment of gastro–oesophageal reflux should be stopped 1 week before testing. A nasal catheter with a pH-sensitive transducer is introduced and placed 5 cm above the oesophagogastric junction, attached to an electronic recorder carried at the waist. Frequency, time and duration that pH < 4 are measured. Alkaline reflux is defined as pH > 7. Symptoms and position (lying or standing) are recorded by the patient
- *Results*: expressed as a percentage of the total recording time that oesophageal pH is below a certain level (usually <4). Normal individuals have about 20 episodes when pH <4 during 24 h, totalling <2% of the recording time, and rarely at night. Symptoms due to reflux must correlate with abnormal oesophageal pH, but biliary reflux can confound results since pH may be high during symptoms

Helicobacter pylori: ^{14}C- or ^{13}C-urea breath test

- *Indication*: confirmation that *H. pylori* infection has been eradicated (especially after treatment in patients with complicated peptic ulcer disease), or those who continue to have symptoms (p. 86)
- *Principle*: *H. pylori* produces urease. ^{14}C-labelled urea is metabolised by urease to release $^{14}CO_2$ (and NH_4). $^{14}CO_2$ is detected in the breath
- *Method*: acid-suppressing drugs, antibiotics and bismuth compounds must have been stopped for 4 weeks to avoid false-negative results. After a 6 h fast, breath is exhaled through a straw into a test tube and the top capped, to act as baseline. Labelled urea is drunk and breath collected at 20 and 40 min (exact timings vary). ^{14}C isotope is measured by a scintillation counter, or ^{13}C assayed by mass spectrometry
- *Results*: normal breath $^{13/14}CO_2$ does not rise above baseline. In positive results, consistent with current *H. pylori* infection, $^{13/14}CO_2$ at 20 min is more than fivefold baseline

Gastric motility

Gastroparesis due to autonomic neuropathy (diabetes, amyloidosis) occasionally causes recurrent vomiting (p. 401). A barium meal provides subjective information about gastric emptying, but isotope studies provide a quantitative measurement

- Drugs that affect motility (metoclopramide, domperidone, cisapride, anticholinergics, opiates) are avoided for 72 h. Fluids only for 12 h and nil by mouth for 4 h is usual before the test
- A radiolabelled meal (such as 100 g scrambled egg) is eaten, followed by gamma camera counting for about 90 min. Normal emptying is 20–30% solids and 40–50% liquids within 60 min, but ranges vary between laboratories

Anorectal manometry

- *Indications*: defaecation disorders or faecal incontinence (p. 294). Some colorectal surgeons perform anorectal manometry before ileoanal pouch surgery. It is only available at specialist centres
- *Method*: a multilumen tube, with a distal balloon and three side ports connected to pressure transducers, is inserted 10 cm into the rectum. The rectum is distended by

inflating the distal balloon (50–200 mL air). Myoelectric recordings from the external anal sphincter or puborectalis can be measured simultaneously through needle electrodes. Perineal sensation is best assessed by measuring the current threshold at which a tingling sensation is felt between two cutaneous electrodes

- *Results*: normal recordings show relaxation of the internal sphincter during rectal distension and a rebound increase in pressure during deflation. Absent sphincter relaxation may be detected during rectal distension (aganglionosis, p. 289), abnormal sphincteric tone (in faecal incontinence), or abnormal rectal sensation (desire to defecate at high or low rectal volumes)

Gut hormones

- All tests are performed after an overnight fast, most easily when the patient attends for endoscopy (p. 104), or during the assessment of secretory diarrhoea (Fig. 7.2, p. 212)
- Acid-suppressing drugs must be stopped for 2 weeks before gastrin levels are measured. High gastrin levels are otherwise impossible to interpret, although patients most likely to have Zollinger–Ellison syndrome (p. 105) are also those most likely to be taking these drugs. Symptomatic treatment with antacids for these 2 weeks is trying for the patient and doctors
- 10 mL blood is taken into an ice-cold heparinised tube with 200 pL aprotinin (Trasylol 4000 iu/mL). The sample is immediately taken to biochemistry for separation and freezing
- A supraregional assay service (Appendix 1, p. 439) measures gastrin, glucagon, VIP, somatostatin or pancreatic polypeptide. Calcitonin should be measured in patients with unexplained diarrhoea, to exclude extremely rare cases of medullary thyroid carcinoma

Appendices

433

1 Useful addresses

Local organisations are listed in the telephone directory under Social Service and Welfare Organisations, or Charitable and Benevolent Organisations. These are especially helpful for alcohol abuse, services for the elderly or disabled, drug abuse, hospices, or the bereaved. The Internet has transformed access and information, so web addresses are given where possible, together with brief details of the service. Readers must forgive the UK bias!

Adverse drug reactions
See Committee on Safety of Medicines or Drug Information.

Al-Anon
http://www.al-anonuk.org.uk. 61 Great Dover Street, London SE1 4YF (Tel.: 020 7403 0888; Fax: 020 7378 9910); 24 h telephone service. Offers support for friends and relatives of problem drinkers. Groups in Eire and North America (Al-Anon/Alateen North America)

Alcoholics Anonymous
General Service Office, PO Box 1, Stonebow House, Stonebow, York YO1 7NJ (Tel.: 01904 644026) or 11 Redcliffe Gardens, London SW10 (Helpline 10 AM to 10 PM; Tel.: 020 7352 3001; Fax: 01904 629091). Provides anonymous groups for the assistance of alcoholics and problem drinkers. Local numbers in the telephone directory: over 3200 groups in the UK.

Alcohol Concern (National Agency on Alcohol Misuse)
http://www.alcoholconcern.org.uk; email: contact@alcoholconcern.org.uk. Waterbridge House, 32–36 Loman Street, London SE1 0EE (Tel.: 020 7928 7377). Fax: 020 7928 4644. Concerned with prevention and treatment of alcohol misuse.

Anorexia and Bulimia Nervosa Association
Harringey Women and Health Centre, Annexe C, Tottenham Town Hall, Approach Rd, London N15 4RB (Tel.: 020 8885 3936). Provides a confidential helpline, support and information. Helpline Wed. 6–9 PM.

Association of Glycogen Storage Disease
email: president@agsd.org.uk. 9 Lindop Road, Hale, Altrincham, Cheshire WA15 9DZ (Tel.: 0161 980 7303 after 6 PM); Fax: 0161 226 3813. Provides information and support for all persons affected by glycogen storage disease and their families. Acts as a focus for educational, scientific and charitable activities for this disorder.

British Association for Parenteral and Enteral Nutrition (BAPEN)

http://www.bapen.org.uk. BAPEN Office, Secure Hold Business Centre, Studley Road, Redditch, Worcs BN98 7LG (Tel.: 01527 457850). Principal nutrition group for professionals involved in nutritional care, related research and development in the UK.

British Colostomy Association

http://www.bcass.org.uk. 15 Station Road, Reading RG1 1LG (Tel.: 0118 939 1537). Comprised of volunteers who are colostomists who will visit in hospital or at home, pre- and postoperatively. Advisory leaflets are available free on request.

British Liver Trust

http://www.britishlivertrust.org.uk. British Liver Trust, Portman House, 44 High Street, Ringwood, BH2 (Tel.: 01425 463080). Raises funds for research, provides patient information leaflets and advice for patients with chronic liver disease.

British Nutrition Foundation

http://www.nutrition.org.uk. email: postbox@nutrition.org.uk. High Holborn House, 52–54 High Holborn, London WC1V 6RQ (Tel.: 020 7404 6504, Fax: 020 74046747). Provides information and scientifically based advice to help consumers understand the relationship between nutrition, diet and lifestyle.

British Society of Gastroenterology

http://www.bsg.org.uk. 3 St Andrews Place, Regent's Park, London NW1 4LB (Tel.: 020 7387 3534). Encourages education, training and audit in gastroenterology and gastrointestinal endoscopy.

CancerBACUP

http://www.cancerbacup.org.uk. 3 Bath Place, Rivington Street, London EC2A 3JR (Cancer Information Service: Tel.: 0800 181199; Cancer Counselling Service Tel.: 020 7696 9003 M–F 9 AM–5.30 PM; Fax: 020 7696 9002). Provides information and support for patients and relatives using a telephone and written answer service by experienced cancer nurses. One-to-one counselling is available from some offices.

Carers National Association

http://www.londonhealth.co.uk. 20–25 Glasshouse Yard, London EC1A 4JS (Tel.: 020 7490 8818; Fax: 020 7490 8824). Offers information and support for all people caring for relatives and friends at home.

Children's Liver Disease Foundation

http://www.cildliverdisease.org.uk email: info@childliverdisease.org. 36 Great Charles Street, Birmingham B3 3JY (Tel.: 0121 212 3839). Supports research and provides advice or emotional support for families with a child suffering from liver disease.

CICRA (Crohn's in Childhood Research Association)
http://www.cicra.org. CICRA, Parkgate House, 356 West Barnes Lane, Motspur Park, Surrey KT3 6NB. (Tel.: 020 8949 6209). Supports research and provides advice and support for children with Crohn's or colitis and their families.

Coeliac Society of the UK
http://www.coeliac.co.uk. PO Box 220, High Wycombe, Bucks HP11 2HY (Tel.: 01494 437278; Helpline 0870 444 8804). Provides advice and counselling concerning the disease and diet, together with holidays and social activities.

Committee on Safety of Medicines
http://www.mca.gov.uk; email: leslie.Whitbread@mhra.gsi.gov.uk. Market Towers, 1 Nine Elms Lane, London SW8 5NQ (Tel.: 020 7084 2451). Notification of adverse drug reactions and regulatory matters.

CORE/Digestive Disorders Foundation
email: ddf@digestive disorders.org.uk. 3 St Andrews Place, Regent's Park, London NW1 4LB (Tel.: 020 7486 0341). Produces patient-orientated information leaflets and supports research.

Crohn's and Colitis Foundation of America
http://www.ccfa.org; email: info@ccfa.org. 386 Park Avenue South, 17th Floor, New York, NY 10016 (Tel.: 800-932-2423). Research-orientated organisation with a useful website, also provides information leaflets for patients.

Cystic Fibrosis Trust
http://www.cftrust.org.uk. 11 London Road, Bromley, Kent BR1 1BY (Tel.: 020 8464 7211). Provides support for parents, their children and adults suffering from cystic fibrosis.

DIAL UK (Disablement Information and Advice Lines)
http://www.dialuk.org.uk. Park Lodge, 1 St Catherine's, Tickhill Road, Doncaster, South Yorkshire DN4 8QN (Tel.: 01302 310123, Fax: 01302 310404). Provides free, impartial and confidential advice on all aspects of disablement to help the disabled live independently in the community. Provides home helps and meals on wheels.

Drug Abuse ('Release')
email: ask@release.org.uk. 388 Old Street, London EC1V 9LT (Tel.: 020 7729 5255; Fax: 020 7729 2599). Offers advice and information for individuals or their relatives charged with drug offences. It deals with the social, medical and legal problems arising from drug abuse.

Drug Abuse (Families Anonymous UK)
email: office@famanon.org.uk. The Doddington and Rollo Community Association, Charlotte Despard Avenue, London SW11 5JE (Tel.: 020 7498 4680; helpline: 0845

1200 660). Helps families and friends of drug abusers to relieve stress and aid recovery. Groups worldwide.

ECCO (European Crohn's and Colitis Organisation)
http://www.ecco-ibd.org. Facilitates research across Europe, runs courses for IBD specialist trainees, contributes to the programme for UEGW and has one or two representatives from most European countries.

EDA (Eating Disorders Association)
http://www.edauk.com; email: info@edauk.com. 103 Prince of Wales road, Norwich NR1 1DW (Tel.: 0870 770 3256; international tel.: +44 1603 619090). Offers mutual support and sharing of information. Concerned to promote education and understanding about the illness.

Employment Medical Advisory Services (EMAS)
http://www.hse.gov.uk/fod/fodhome.htm. The EMAS is part of the UK Government's Field Operations Directorate; it supports all Health & Safety Executive's frontline activities and provides occupational health advice direct to employers. The website contains addresses and street maps to find local offices.

Environmental Health—Medical Officer
UK names and addresses available from Strategic Health Authority, local Microbiology Department, or Public Health Laboratory (PHLS).

The European Federation of Crohn's and Ulcerative Colitis Associations (EFCCA)
http://www.efcca.org; email: sandee@freestamp.com. Provides links and addresses to Crohn's disease patient organisations all over the world, both national and international.

Familial Adenomatous Polyposis
http://www.polyposisregistry.org.uk The Polyposis Registry, St Mark's Hospital, Northwick Park, London Tel.: 020 76017958 (direct line). Primarily research-based, data collection and follow-up, also provides information and support for families with FAP in the UK.

Family Cancer Clinic
http://www.stmarkshospital.org.uk/pdf/familycancerclinic.pdf The Family Cancer Clinic, St Mark's Hospital, Northwick Park, London. Guidelines for referral to The Family Cancer Clinic

Food and Chemical Allergy Association
27 Ferringham Lane, Ferring-by-Sea, West Sussex BN12 5NB (letters only). Supplies names of doctors specialising in this field. Gives help and advice to sufferers of allergy-induced illness.

Gastrointestinal Hormone Supraregional Assay Service

Hammersmith Hospital, DuCane Road, London W12 0HS (Tel.: 020 8740 3044). Specialist gut hormone assays available. Discuss the problem before sending samples.

Genetic Counselling

Tel.: the department of medical/clinical genetics at most teaching hospitals.

Haemochromatosis Society

email: info@ghsoc.org. Hollybush House, Hadley Green Road, Barnet, Herts EN5 5PR. (Tel.: 020 8449 1363). Provides information and advice for patients with this condition.

Helen House Hospice

http://www.helen-house.org.uk; email: admin@helen-house.org.uk. 37 Leopold Street, Oxford, Oxon OX4 1QT (Tel.: 01865 728251). A hospice for children, providing terminal and short-term relief care.

Hospice Information Service

http://www.hospiceinformation.info. St Christopher's Hospice, 51–59 Lawrie Park Road, Sydenham, London SE26 6DZ (Tel.: 0870 903 3903). A resource link producing directories of hospices in the UK and around the world.

Ileostomy Association (ia)

http://www.the-ia.org.uk; email: infor@the-ia.org.uk. Peverill House, 1–5 Mill Road, Ballyclare, Co. Antrim, BT39 9DR (Tel.: 028 9334 4043 or freephone: 0800 0184 724). Advisory service for people with ileostomies by way of hospital and home visits. Many of the volunteers are ileostomists themselves.

Irritable Bowel Syndrome Network (IBS Network)

http://www.ibsnetwork.org.uk; email: info@ibsnetwork.org.uk. Northern general Hospital, Sheffield S5 7AU (Tel.: 0114 261 1531; Helpline: 01543 492 192, 6 PM–8 PM M-F). Provides advice and help to alleviate the distress and isolation felt by people suffering from IBS.

Kingston Trust

http://www.guide-information.org.uk; email: secretary@ktrust.org.uk. Mrs. Michele Cory-Smith, PO Box 6457, Basingstoke, Hants, RG24 8LG. Provides help for elderly ileostomists (aged over 50) in need of short stay or permanent accommodation.

Macmillan Cancer Relief

http://www.macmillan.org.uk; Macmillan Cancer Relief, 89 Albert Embankment, London SE1 7UQ. (Freephone: 0808 808 2020). Provides nursing services and support for patients with cancer.

Marie Curie Cancer Care

http://www.mariecurie.org.uk; 89 Albert Embankment, London SE1 7TP (Tel.: 020 7599 7777). Runs 11 UK nursing homes and a nationwide domicilliary nursing service, especially night nursing. Provides urgent welfare needs in kind, advice and general information.

National Advisory Service for Parents of Children with a Stoma (NASPCS)

http://www.naspcs.org.uk; email:john@stoma.freeserve.co.uk. 51 Anderson Drive, Valley View Park, Darvel KA17 0DE (Tel.: 01560 220 24). Provides support and advice for parents of children who have a stoma, ileostomy, colostomy or urostomy.

National Association for Colitis and Crohn's Disease

http://www.nacc.org.uk (link to IBD Associations around the world); 98A London Road, St Albans, Hertfordshire AL1 1NX (Information line: 0845 130 2233 (including disability living allowance support); Press and membership: 01727 830038. Offers support and information for patients with inflammatory bowel disease and their families. Local groups throughout the country.

National Society for Phenylketonuria

http://www.nsphu.org; PO Box 26642, London N14 4ZF (Tel.: 0845 603 9136). Offers support for parents of children suffering from phenylketonuria concerning their medical, social and educational welfare.

Oesophageal Patients Association (OPA)

http://www.opa.org uk; 22 Vulcan House, Vulcan Road, Solihul, West Midlands B91 2JY (Tel.: 0121 704 9860). Provides leaflets and support for patients with oesophageal cancer and other oesophageal disorders.

Primary Biliary Cirrhosis Foundation

http://www.pbcfoundation.com; email: info@pbcfoundation.com. The PBC Foundation, 54 Queen Street, Edinburgh EH2 3NS (Tel.: 0131 225 8586). Raises funds for research and provides patient information, advice and support.

Primary Care Society for Gastroenterology

http://www.pcsg.org.uk. Provides a forum for doctors to address the issues of education and research in gastroenterology in primary care.

Public Health Laboratory Service

http://www.phls.co.uk; 61 Colindale Avenue, London NW9 5DF (Tel.: 020 8200 1295). Central reference laboratory with local laboratories covering all areas, providing investigations and advice.

Share-a-Care (National Register for Rare Diseases)

19 Coxwell Road, Faringdon, Oxfordshire, SN7 7EB. Puts people with rare diseases in contact with others with the same disorder, as well as compiling a national register.

Tropical diseases

London: Hospital for Tropical Diseases, 4 St Pancras Way, London NW1 0PE (Tel.: 020 7387 4411); Liverpool: Liverpool School of Tropical Medicine, Pembroke Place, Liverpool L3 5QA (Tel.: 0151 708 9393). Offers clinical advice and information on immunisation for foreign travel.

Tracheo-oesophageal Support Group

http://www.tofs.org.uk; St George's Centre, 91 Victoria Road, Netherfield, Nottingham NG4 2NN (Tel.: 0115 961 3092). Run by parents for parents of children born with an oesophageal disorder.

2 Further reading

A bibliography in a rapid reference book cannot be comprehensive. This section suggests general reference texts and refers to papers or reviews covering areas of controversy or particular complexity.

Gastroenterology on the Internet
There are numerous gastroenterology websites on the Internet, many of which are excellent and also cross-refer to others. The following are useful starting points.

Guidelines
- Avicenna—http://www.avicenna.com (includes NIH's AHCPR guidelines)
- BSG—http://www.bsg.org.uk
- Healthgate—http://www.healthgate.com (a proactive site)
- Medscape—http://www.medscape.com (with limited free access to Medline)
- NICE-http://www.nice.org.uk

Journals
- *Alimentary Pharmacology & Therapeutics*—http://www.blackwellpublishing.com/journal.asp?ref=0269-2813
- *American Journal of Gastroenterology*—http://www.amjgastro.com
- *Canadian Journal of Gastroenterology*—http://www.pulsus.com/Gastro/home2.htm
- *European Journal of Gastroenterology*—http://www.eurojgh.com
- *Gastroenterology*—http://www.gastrojournal.org
- *Gut*—http://www.bmjpg.com/data/gut.htm
- *Hepatology*—http://www.hepatology.aasldjournals. org
- *Journal of Hepatology*—http://www.jhep.elsevier.com

Organisations
- American Association for the Study of the Liver (AASLD)—http://www.aasld.org (includes practice guidelines)
- British Society for The Study of the Liver (BASL)—http://www.basl.org.uk
- British Society of Gastroenterology—http://www.bsg.org.uk (includes clinical guidelines)
- Digestive Diseases Foundation—http://www.ddf.org.uk (provides patient information)
- European Society for The Study of the Liver (EASL)—http://www.easl.ch
- GastroHep.com—http://www.gastrohep.com (links to journals, guidelines)
- OMGE—http://www.excerptamedica.com/ OMGE (sources)

Alimentary emergencies
Dargan PI, Jones AL. Acetaminophen poisoning: an update for the intensivist. *Crit Care* 2002; **6**: 108–10.

Imrie CW. Prognostic indicators in acute pancreatitis. *Can J Gastroenterol* 2003; **17**: 325–8.

Kovacs TO, Jensen DM. Recent advances in the endoscopic diagnosis and therapy of upper gastrointestinal, small intestinal and colonic bleeding. *Med Clin North Am* 2002; **86**: 1319–56.

Liu JP, Gluud LL, Als-Nielsen B, Gluud C. Artificial and bioartificial support systems for liver failure. *Cochrane Database Syst Rev* 2004; **1**: CD003628.

Ryan BM, Stockbrugger RW, Ryan JM. A pathophysiologic, gastroenterologic and radiologic approach to the management of gastric varices. *Gastroenterology* 2004; **126**: 1175–89.

Schiodt FV, Lee WM. Fulminant liver disease. *Clin Liver Dis* 2003; **7**: 331–49.

Stack LB, Munter DW. Foreign bodies in the gastrointestinal tract. *Emerg Clin North Am* 1996; **94**: 493–521.

Yousaf M, McCallion K, Diamond T. Management of severe acute pancreatitis. *Br J Surg* 2003; **90**: 407–20.

Oesophagus

Dent J, Armstrong D, Delaney B, Moayyedi P, Talley NJ, Vakil N. Symptom evaluation in reflux disease: workshop background, processes, terminology, recommendations, and discussion outputs. *Gut* 2004; **53(Suppl 4)**: iv1–24.

Fennerty MB. Endoscopic therapy for gastroesophageal reflux disease: what have we learned and what needs to be done. *Gastrointest Endosc Clin North Am* 2003; **13**: 201–9.

Gerson LB, Shetler K, Triadafilopoulos G. Prevalence of Barrett's esophagus in asymptomatic individuals. *Gastroenterology* 2002; **123**: 461–7.

Jankowski J, Sharma P. Review article: approaches to Barrett's oesophagus treatment—the role of proton pump inhibitors and other interventions. *Aliment Pharmacol Ther* 2004; **19(Suppl 1)**: 54–9.

Lagergren J, Bergstrom R, Lindgren A, Nyren O. Symptomatic gastro–oesophageal reflux as a risk factor for esophageal adenocarcinoma. *N Engl J Med* 1999; **340**: 825–31.

Mattioli S, Lugaresi ML, Pierluigi M, Di Simone MP, D'Ovidio F. Review article: indications for antireflux surgery in gastro–oesophageal reflux disease. *Aliment Pharmacol Ther* 2003; **17(Suppl 2)**: 60–7.

Moss SF, Armstrong D, Arnold R, Ferenci P, Fock KM, Holtmann G, McCarthy DM, Moraes-Filho JP, Mutschler E, Playford R, Spechler SJ, Stanghellini V, Modlin IM. GERD 2003—A consensus on the way ahead. *Digestion* 2003; **67**: 111–17.

Petruzziello L, Costamagna G. Stenting in esophageal strictures. *Dig Dis* 2002; **20**: 154–66.

Sharma P, Vakil N. Review article: *Helicobacter pylori* and reflux disease. *Aliment Pharmacol Ther* 2003; **17**: 297–305.

Spechler SJ. Barrett's esophagus and esophageal adenocarcinoma: pathogenesis, diagnosis and therapy. *Med Clin North Am* 2002; **86**: 1423–45.

Stomach and duodenum

Ahmad A, Govil Y, Frank BB. Gastric mucosa-associated lymphoid tissue lymphoma. *Am J Gastroenterol* 2003; **98**: 975–86.

Allum WH, Griffin SM, Watson A, Colin-Jones D. Guidelines for the management of oesophageal and gastric cancer. *Gut* 2002; **50(Suppl 5):** v1–23.

American Gastroenterological Association medical position statement: nausea and vomiting. *Gastroenterology* 2001; **120:** 261–3

Duffaud F, Blay JY. Gastrointestinal stromal tumors: biology and treatment. *Oncology* 2003; **65:** 187–97.

Evans LS, Hancock BW. Non-Hodgkin lymphoma. *Lancet* 2003; **362:** 139–46.

Gonzalez CA, Sala N, Capella G. Genetic susceptibility and gastric cancer risk. *Int J Cancer* 2002; **100:** 249–60.

Kabir S. Review article: clinic-based testing for *Helicobacter pylori* infection by enzyme immunoassay of faeces, urine and saliva. *Aliment Pharmacol Ther* 2003; **17:** 1345–54.

Kelley JR, Duggan JM. Gastric cancer epidemiology and risk factors. *J Clin Epidemiol* 2003; **56:** 1–9.

Megraud F, Lamouliatte H. Review article: the treatment of refractory *Helicobacter pylori* infection. *Aliment Pharmacol Ther* 2003; **17:** 1333–43.

Micklewright R, Lane S, Linley W *et al.* Review article: NSAIDs, gastroprotection and cyclo-oxygenase-II-selective inhibitors. *Aliment Pharmacol Ther* 2003; **17:** 321–32.

Quan C, Talley NJ. Management of peptic ulcer disease not related to *Helicobacter pylori* or NSAIDs. *Am J Gastroenterol* 2002; **97:** 2950–61.

Suerbaum S, Michetti P. *Helicobacter pylori* infection. *N Engl J Med* 2002; **347:** 1175–86.

Talley NJ. Diabetic gastropathy and prokinetics. *Am J Gastroenterol* 2003; **98:** 264–71.

Talley NJ. Update on the role of drug therapy in non-ulcer dyspepsia. *Rev Gastroenterol Disord* 2003; **3:** 25–30.

Talley NJ, Quan C. Review article: *Helicobacter pylori* and nonulcer dyspepsia. *Aliment Pharmacol Ther* 2002; **16(Suppl 1):** 58–65.

Pancreatic disease

Abbruzzese JL. Past and present treatment of pancreatic adenocarcinoma: chemotherapy as a standard treatment modality. *Semin Oncol* 2002; **29:** 2–8.

Chin BB, Wahl RL. 18F-fluoro-deoxyglucose positron emission tomography in the evaluation of gastrointestinal malignancies. *Gut* 2003; **52(Suppl 4):** 23–9.

Clarke DL, Thomson SR, Madiba TE, Sanyika C. Pre-operative imaging of pancreatic cancer: a management-orientated approach. *J Am Coll Surg* 2003; **196:** 119–29.

Grendell JH. Genetic factors in pancreatitis. *Curr Gastroenterol Rep* 2003; **5:** 105–9.

Lankisch PG, Droge M, Gottesleben F. Drug-induced acute pancreatitis: incidence and severity. *Gut* 1995, **37:** 565–7.

Mitchell RM, Byrne MF, Baillie J. Pancreatitis. *Lancet* 2003; **361:** 1447–55.

Rocha Lima CM, Centeno B. Update on pancreatic cancer. *Curr Opin Oncol* 2002; **14:** 424–30.

Liver disease

Aithal GP, Rawlins MD, Day CP. Clinical diagnostic scale: a useful tool in the evaluation of suspected hepatotoxic adverse drug reactions. *J Hepatol* 2000; **33:** 949–52.

Alvarez F, Berg PA, Bianchi FB *et al*. International Autoimmune Hepatitis Group Report: review of criteria for diagnosis of autoimmune hepatitis. *J Hepatol* 1999; **31**: 929–38.

Angulo P. Nonalcoholic fatty liver disease. *N Engl J Med* 2002; **18**: 1221–31.

Botta F, Giannini E, Romagnoli P *et al*. MELD scoring system is useful for predicting prognosis in patients with liver cirrhosis and is correlated with residual liver function: a European study. *Gut* 2003; **52**: 134–9.

Collier J, Bassendine M. How to respond to abnormal liver function tests. *Clin Med* 2002; **2**: 406–9.

Garcia-Tsao G. Current management of the complications of cirrhosis and portal hypertension: variceal haemorrhage, ascites and bacterial peritonitis. *Gastroenterology* 2001; **120**: 726–48.

Gitlin JD. Wilson disease. *Gastroenterology* 2003; **125**: 1868–77.

Lee WM. Drug-induced hepatotoxicity. *N Engl J Med* 2003; **349**: 474–85.

National Institute of Health. Consensus Development Conference Management of Hepatitis C: 2002. *Hepatology* 2002; **36(Suppl 1)**.

Neuberger J. Developments in liver transplantation. *Gut* 2004; **53**: 759–68.

Talwalkar JA, Lindor KD. Primary biliary cirrhosis. *Lancet* 2003; **362**: 53–61.

Biliary disease

Bjornsson E, Boberg KM, Cullen S *et al*. Patients with small duct primary sclerosing cholangitis have a favourable long-term prognosis. *Gut* 2002; **51**: 731–5.

Boyer J L. Advancing the bileology of cholestatic liver disease. *Hepatology* 2001; **33**: 633–46.

Cullen S, Chapman R. Primary sclerosing cholangitis. *Autoimmun Rev* 2003; **2**: 305–12.

Prajapati DN, Hogan WJ. Sphincter of Oddi dysfunction and other functional biliary disorders: evaluation and treatment. *Gastroenterol Clin North Am* 2003; **32**: 601–18.

Tranter SE, Thompson MH. Comparison of endoscopic sphincterotomy and laparoscopic exploration of the common bile duct. *Br J Surg* 2002; **89**: 1495–504.

Small intestine

Camilleri M. Chronic diarrhea: a review of pathophysiology and management for the clinical gastroenterologist. *Clin Gastroenterol Hepatol* 2004; **2**: 198–206.

Dieterich W, Ehnis T, Bauer M *et al*. Identification of tissue transglutaminase as the autoantigen of coeliac disease. *Nat Med* 1997, **3**: 797–801.

Green PH, Jabri B. Coeliac disease. *Lancet* 2003; **362**: 383–91.

Howdle PD, Jalal PK, Holmes GK, Houlston RS. Primary small-bowel malignancy in the UK and its association with coeliac disease. *QJM* 2003; **96**: 345–53.

Langnas AN. Advances in small-intestine transplantation. *Transplantation* 2004; **77(Suppl 9)**: S75–8.

Nightingale JM. The medical management of intestinal failure: methods to reduce the severity. *Proc Nutr Soc* 2003; **62**: 703–10.

Singh VV, Toskes PP. Small bowel bacterial overgrowth: presentation, diagnosis, and treatment. *Curr Gastroenterol Rep* 2003; **5**: 365–72.

Ulcerative colitis and Crohn's disease

Ahmad T, Satsangi J, McGovern D, Bunce M, Jewell DP. Review article: the genetics of inflammatory bowel disease. *Aliment Pharmacol Ther* 2001; **15**: 731–48.

Caprilli R, Viscido A, Guagnozzi D. Review article: biological agents in the treatment of Crohn's disease. *Aliment Pharmacol Ther* 2002; **16**: 1579–90.

Dunckley P, Jewell DP. Management of severe ulcerative colitis. *Best Pract Res Clin Gastroenterol* 2003; **17**: 89–103.

Edwards CM, George BD, Jewell DP, Warren BF, Mortensen NJ, Kettlewell MG. Role of a defunctioning stoma in the management of large bowel Crohn's disease. *Br J Surg* 2000; **87**: 1063–6.

Francella A, Dyan A, Bodian C *et al.* The safety of 6-mercaptopurine for childbearing patients with inflammatory bowel disease: a retrospective cohort study. *Gastroenterology* 2003; **124**: 9–17.

Gasche C, Scholmerich J, Brynskov J *et al.* A simple classification of Crohn's disease: report of the Working Party for the World Congresses of Gastroenterology, Vienna 1998. *Inflamm Bowel Dis* 2000; **6**: 8–15.

Goh J, O'Morain CA. Review article: nutrition and adult inflammatory bowel disease. *Aliment Pharmacol Ther* 2003; **17**: 307–20.

Loftus EV. Clinical epidemiology of inflammatory bowel disease: incidence, prevalence and environmental influences. *Gastroenterology* 2004; **126**: 1504–17.

Sandborn W, McLeod R, Jewell DP. Pharmacotherapy for inducing and maintaining remission in pouchitis. *Cochrane Database Syst Rev* 2001; **2**: CD001176.

Satsangi J, Sutherland LR, eds. *Inflammatory Bowel Diseases*. Churchill Livingstone, London, 2003.

Sutherland LR, Roth D, Beck P *et al.* Oral 5-aminosalicylic acid for maintaining remission in ulcerative colitis. *Cochrane Database Syst Rev* 2002; **4**: CD000544.

Travis SPL ed. Recent advances in immunomodulation in the treatment of inflammatory bowel disease: review in depth. *Eur J Gastroenterol Hepatol* 2003; **15**: 215–48.

Warren BF, Edwards CM, Travis SPL. Microscopic colitis—classification and terminology. *Histopathology* 2002; **40**: 374–6.

Zachos M, Tondeur M, Griffiths AM. Enteral nutritional therapy for inducing remission of Crohn's disease. *Cochrane Database Syst Rev* 2001; **3**: CD000542.

Large intestine

Baron TH, Kozarek RA. Endoscopic stenting of colonic tumours. *Best Pract Res Clin Gastroenterol* 2004; **18**: 209–29.

Braun AH, Achterrath W, Wilke H *et al.* New systemic frontline treatment for metastatic colorectal carcinoma. *Cancer* 2004; **100**: 1558–77.

Cheung O, Wald A. Review article: the management of pelvic floor disorders. *Aliment Pharmacol Ther* 2004; **19**: 481–95.

Leddin D, Hunt R, Champion M *et al.* Canadian Association of Gastroenterology and the Canadian Digestive Health Foundation: guidelines on colon cancer screening. *Can J Gastroenterol* 2004; **18**: 93–9.

Lewis B, Goldfarb N. Review article: the advent of capsule endoscopy—a not-so-futuristic approach to obscure gastrointestinal bleeding. *Aliment Pharmacol Ther* 2003; **17**: 1085–96.

Lieberman DA, Atkin W. Review article: balancing the ideal versus the practical considerations of colorectal cancer prevention and screening. *Aliment Pharmacol Ther* 2004; **19 (Suppl 1)**: 71–6.

Lucas CA, Logan ECM, Logan RFA. Audit of the investigation and outcome of iron deficiency anaemia in one health district. *Journal of the Royal College of Physicians of London* 1996; **30**: 33–5.

Selvachandran SN, Hodder RJ, Ballal MS, Jones P, Cade D. Prediction of colorectal cancer by a patient consultation questionnaire and scoring system: a prospective study. *Lancet* 2002; **360**: 278–83.

Winawer S, Fletcher R, Rex D *et al*. Colorectal cancer screening and surveillance: clinical guidelines and rationale—Update based on new evidence. *Gastroenterology* 2003; **124**: 544–60.

Wu JS, Fazio VW. Management of rectal cancer. *J Gastrointest Surg* 2004; **8**: 139–49.

Irritable bowel syndrome

Bass C. Somatization. *Med Intern* 1996; **24**: 58–61.

Bijkerk CJ, Muris JW, Knottnerus JA, Hoes AW, de Wit NJ. Systematic review: the role of different types of fibre in the treatment of irritable bowel syndrome. *Aliment Pharmacol Ther* 2004; **19**: 245–51.

Brandt LJ, Bjorkman D, Fennerty MB *et al*. Systematic review on the management of irritable bowel syndrome in North America. *Am J Gastroenterol* 2002; **97**: S7–S26.

Cremonini F, Delgado-Aros S, Camilleri M. Efficacy of alosetron in irritable bowel syndrome: a meta-analysis of randomized controlled trials. *Neurogastroenterol Motil* 2003; **15**: 79–86.

Dapoigny M, Stockbrugger RW, Azpiroz F *et al*. Role of alimentation in irritable bowel syndrome. *Digestion* 2003; **67**: 225–33.

Hammer J, Eslick GD, Howell SC, Altiparmak E, Talley NJ. Diagnostic yield of alarm features in irritable bowel syndrome. *Gut* 2004; **53**: 666–72.

Olden KW. Diagnosis of irritable bowel syndrome. *Gastroenterology* 2002; **122**: 1701–14.

Spanier JA, Howden CW, Jones MP. A systematic review of alternative therapies in the irritable bowel syndrome. *Arch Intern Med* 2003; **163**: 265–74.

Thompson DG. The treatment of irritable bowel syndrome. *Aliment Pharmacol Ther* 2002; **16**: 1395–1406.

Gastrointestinal infections

Casburn-Jones AC, Farthing MJG. Management of infectious diarrhoea. *Gut* 2004; **53**: 296–305.

Kirkwood C. Viral gastroenteritis in Europe: a new norovirus variant? *Lancet* 2004; **363**: 671–2.

Oldfield EC. Evaluation of chronic diarrhea in patients with human immunodeficiency virus infection. *Rev Gastroenterol Disord* 2002; **2**: 176–88.

Petri WA Jr. Therapy of intestinal protozoa. *Trends Parasitol* 2003; **19**: 523–6.

Ross AG, Bartley PB, Sleigh AC *et al.* Schistosomiasis. *N Engl J Med* 2002; **346**: 1212–20.

Nutrition

Carlson GL. Surgical management of intestinal failure. *Proc Nutr Soc* 2003; **62**: 711–18.

Colquitt J, Clegg A, Sidhu M, Royle P. Surgery for morbid obesity. *Cochrane Database Syst Rev* 2003; **2**: CD003641.

Kopelman PG, Grace C. New thoughts on managing obesity. *Gut* 2004; **53**: 1044–53.

Stroud M, Duncan H, Nightingale J. Guidelines for enteral feeding in adult hospital patients. *Gut* 2003; **52(Suppl VII)**: vii1–12.

Vanderhoof JA, Young RJ. Enteral and parenteral nutrition in the care of patients with short-bowel syndrome. *Best Pract Res Clin Gastroenterol* 2003; **17**: 997–1015.

The gut in systemic disease

Ch'ng CL, Morgan M, Hainsworth I *et al.* Prospective study of liver dysfunction in pregnancy in Southwest Wales. *Gut* 2002; **51**: 876–80.

Doshi S, Zucker SD. Liver emergencies during pregnancy. *Gastroenterol Clin North Am* 2003; **32**: 1213–27.

Lock G. Physiology and pathology of the oesophagus in the elderly patient. *Best Pract Res Clin Gastroenterol* 2001; **15**: 919–41.

Makins R, Ballinger A. Gastrointestinal side-effects of drugs. *Expert Opin Drug Saf* 2003; **2**: 421–9.

Pengiran Tengah DS, Wills AJ, Holmes GK. Neurological complications of coeliac disease. *Postgrad Med J* 2002; **78**: 393–8.

Ramsey DJ, Smithard DG, Kalra L. Early assessments of dysphagia and aspiration risk in acute stroke patients. *Stroke* 2003; **34**: 1252–7.

Raoul JM, Verma M, Tan E, Peterson TC. Cytokines as therapeutic targets for the gastrointestinal manifestations of scleroderma. *Can J Gastroenterol* 2004; **18**: 22–4.

Smith DS, Williams CS, Ferris CD. Diagnosis and treatment of chronic gastroparesis and chronic intestinal pseudo-obstruction. *Gastroenterol Clin North Am* 2003; **32**: 619–58.

Procedures and investigations

Baillie J, Paulson EK, Vitellas KM. Biliary imaging: a review. *Gastroenterology* 2003; **124**: 1686–99.

Buckley A, Petrunia D. Practice guidelines for liver biopsy. Canadian Association of Gastroenterology. *Can J Gastroenterol* 2000; **14**: 481–2.

Chowdhury RS, Forsmark CE. Pancreatitic function testing. *Aliment Pharmacol Ther* 2003; **36**: 733–50.

Cotton PB, Williams CB. *Practical Gastrointestinal Endoscopy*, 5th edn. Blackwell Science, Oxford, 2002.

Debnam ES, Grimble GK. Methods for assessing intestinal absorptive function in relation to enteral nutrition. *Curr Opin Clin Nutr Metab Care* 2001; **4**: 355–67.

Hirota WK, Petersen K, Baron TH *et al.* Guidelines for antibiotic prophylaxis for GI endoscopy. *Gastrointest Endosc* 2003; **58**: 475–82.

Rex DK, Rahmani EY, Haseman JH, Lemmel GT, Kaster S, Buckley JS. Relative sensitivity of colonoscopy and barium enema for detection of colorectal cancer in clinical practice. *Gastroenterology* 1997; **112**: 17–23.

Santucci R, Rondonotti E *et al.* Outcome of patients with obscure gastrointestinal bleeding after capsule endoscopy: report of 100 consecutive cases. *Gastroenterology* 2004; **126**: 643–53.

Sosna J, Morrin MM, Kruskal JB, Lavin PT, Rosen MP, Raptopoulos V. CT colonography of colorectal polyps: a meta-analysis. *AJR Am J Roentgenol* 2003; **181**: 1593–8.

Young GP, St John DJ, Winawer SJ *et al.* Choice of fecal occult blood tests for colorectal cancer screening: recommendations based on performance characteristics in population studies: a WHO (World Health Organization) and OMED (World Organization for Digestive Endoscopy) report. *Am J Gastroenterol* 2002; **97**: 2499–507.

3 Height and weight charts

- 'Overweight' is defined as 10–19% above the upper limit for either men or women
- 'Obesity' is $\geq$ 20% above the upper limit

The desirable weight for height shown in Table A3.1 is based on actuarial data for longevity and good health and should form the basis of advice on body weight

- BMI (weight (kg)/height^2 (m^2)), normal range 20–25 kg/m^2) is explained on p. 402. See Fig. 12.1, p. 403

BMI is a more sensitive index of the relationship between body weight and disease and is becoming the accepted standard of reference. Table A3.2 shows values of BMI according to height and weight data.

Table A3.1(a) Height and weight chart for men

Height		Weight								
		Small frame			Medium frame			Large frame		
cm	ft in	kg	st.	lb	kg	st.	lb	kg	st.	lb
158	5.2	57.6–60.3	9.2–9.8	128–134	59.0–63.5	9.5–10.1	131–141	62.1–67.5	9.12–10.10	138–150
160	5.3	58.5–61.2	9.4–9.10	130–136	59.9–64.4	9.7–10.3	133–143	63.0–68.9	10.0–10.13	140–153
163	5.4	59.4–62.1	9.6–9.12	132–138	60.8–65.3	9.9–10.5	135–145	63.9–70.2	10.2–11.2	142–156
165	5.5	60.3–63.0	9.8–10.0	134–140	61.7–66.6	9.11–10.8	137–148	64.8–72.0	10.4–11.6	144–160
168	5.6	61.2–63.9	9.10–10.2	136–142	62.6–68.0	9.13–10.11	139–151	65.7–73.8	10.6–11.10	146–164
170	5.7	62.1–65.3	9.12–10.5	138–145	63.9–69.3	10.2–11.0	142–154	67.1–75.6	10.9–12.0	149–168
173	5.8	63.0–66.6	10.0–10.8	140–148	65.3–70.7	10.5–11.3	145–157	68.4–77.4	10.12–12.4	152–172
175	5.9	63.9–68.0	10.2–10.11	142–151	66.6–72.0	10.8–11.6	148–160	69.8–79.2	11.1–12.8	155–176
178	5.10	64.8–69.3	10.4–11.0	144–154	68.0–73.4	10.11–11.9	151–163	71.1–81.0	11.4–12.12	158–180
180	5.11	65.7–70.7	10.6–11.3	146–157	69.3–74.7	11.0–11.12	154–166	72.5–82.8	11.7–13.2	161–184
183	6.0	67.1–72.0	10.9–11.6	149–160	70.7–76.5	11.3–12.2	157–170	73.8–84.6	11.10–13.6	164–188
185	6.1	68.4–73.8	10.12–11.10	152–164	72.0–78.3	11.6–12.6	160–174	75.6–86.4	12.0–13.10	168–192
188	6.2	69.8–75.6	11.1–12.0	155–168	73.8–80.1	11.10–12.10	164–178	77.4–88.7	12.4–14.1	172–197
191	6.3	71.1–77.4	11.4–12.4	158–172	75.2–81.9	11.13–13.0	167–182	79.2–90.9	12.8–14.6	176–202
193	6.4	72.9–79.2	11.8–12.8	162–176	77.0–84.2	12.3–13.3	171–185	81.5–93.2	12.13–14.11	181–207

Source: From 1983 Metropolitan Life Insurance Company height and weight tables, for men aged 25–59 in shoes and wearing indoor clothing.

Table A3.1(b) Height and weight chart for women

Height		Weight								
		Small frame			Medium frame			Large frame		
cm	ft in	kg	st.	lb	kg	st.	lb	kg	st.	lb
147	4.10	45.9–50.5	7.4–7.13	102–111	49.1–54.5	7.11–8.9	109–121	53.1–59.0	8.6–9.5	111–131
150	4.11	46.4–50.9	7.5–8.1	103–113	50.0–55.4	7.13–8.12	111–124	54.0–60.3	8.8–9.8	120–134
152	5.0	46.8–51.8	7.6–8.3	104–115	50.9–56.7	8.1–9.0	113–126	54.9–61.7	8.10–9.11	122–137
155	5.1	47.7–53.1	7.8–8.6	106–118	51.8–58.1	8.3–9.3	115–129	56.3–63.0	8.13–10.0	125–140
158	5.2	48.6–54.5	7.10–8.9	108–121	53.1–59.4	8.6–9.6	118–132	57.6–64.4	9.2–10.3	128–143
160	5.3	50.0–55.8	7.13–8.12	111–124	54.5–60.8	8.9–9.9	121–135	59.0–66.2	9.5–10.7	131–147
163	5.4	51.3–57.2	8.2–9.1	114–127	55.8–62.1	8.12–9.12	124–138	60.3–68.0	9.8–10.11	134–151
165	5.5	52.7–58.5	8.5–9.4	117–130	57.2–63.5	9.1–10.1	127–141	61.7–69.8	9.11–11.1	137–155
168	5.6	54.0–59.9	8.8–9.7	120–133	58.5–64.8	9.4–10.4	130–144	63.0–71.6	10.0–11.5	140–159
170	5.7	55.4–61.2	8.11–9.10	123–136	59.9–66.2	9.7–10.7	133–147	64.4–73.4	10.3–11.9	143–163
173	5.8	56.7–62.6	9.0–9.13	126–139	61.2–67.5	9.10–10.10	136–150	65.7–75.2	10.6–11.13	146–167
175	5.9	58.1–63.9	9.3–10.2	129–142	62.6–68.9	9.13–10.13	139–153	67.1–76.5	10.9–12.2	149–170
178	5.10	59.4–65.3	9.5–10.5	131–145	63.9–70.2	10.2–11.2	142–156	68.4–77.9	10.12–12.5	152–173
180	5.11	60.8–66.6	9.8–10.8	134–148	65.3–71.6	10.5–11.5	145–159	69.8–79.2	11.1–12.8	154–176
183	6.0	62.1–68.0	9.11–10.11	137–151	66.6–72.9	10.8–11.8	148–162	71.1–80.6	11.4–12.11	158–179

Table A3.2 Body mass index ready-reckoner

Category	BMI				Weight (to the nearest kg)					
Dangerously overweight	45	101	104	107	110	112	115	118	121	124	127
	44	99	102	104	107	110	113	115	118	121	124
	43	97	99	102	105	107	110	113	116	118	121
	42	95	97	100	102	105	108	110	113	116	119
	41	92	95	97	100	102	105	108	110	113	116
Seriously overweight	40	90	92	95	97	100	102	105	108	110	113
	39	88	90	93	95	97	100	102	105	108	110
	38	86	88	90	93	95	97	100	102	105	107
	37	83	86	88	90	92	95	97	100	102	104
	36	81	83	85	88	90	92	95	97	99	102
	35	79	81	83	85	87	90	92	94	96	99
	34	77	79	81	83	85	87	89	91	94	96
	33	74	76	78	80	82	85	87	89	91	93
	32	72	74	76	78	80	82	84	86	88	90
	31	70	72	74	75	77	79	81	83	85	88
Overweight	30	68	69	71	73	75	77	79	81	83	85
	29	65	67	69	71	72	74	76	78	80	82
	28	63	65	66	68	70	72	74	75	77	79
	27	61	62	64	66	67	69	71	73	74	76
	26	59	60	62	63	65	67	68	70	72	73
Acceptable	25	56	58	59	61	62	64	66	67	69	71
	24	54	55	57	58	60	61	63	65	66	68
	23	52	53	55	56	57	59	60	62	63	65
	22	50	51	52	54	55	56	58	59	61	62
	21	47	49	50	51	52	54	55	57	58	59
	20	45	46	47	49	50	51	53	54	55	56
Underweight	19	43	44	45	46	47	49	50	51	52	54
	18	41	42	43	44	45	46	47	48	50	51
	17	38	39	40	41	42	44	45	46	47	48
Height	m	1.50	1.52	1.54	1.56	1.58	1.60	1.62	1.64	1.66	1.68
	ft in.	4.11	5.0	5.0¾	5.1½	5.2¼	5.3	5.3¾	5.4½	5.5½	5.6

Table A3.2 *(continued)*

BMI	Category	Weight (to the nearest kg)													
45	Dangerously overweight	130	133	136	139	143	146	149	152	156	159	162	166	169	173
44		127	130	133	136	139	143	146	149	152	156	159	162	166	169
43		124	127	130	133	136	139	142	146	149	152	155	159	162	165
42		121	124	127	130	133	136	139	142	145	148	152	155	158	161
41		119	121	124	127	130	133	136	139	142	145	148	151	154	158
40	Seriously overweight	116	118	121	124	127	130	133	135	138	141	144	148	151	154
39		113	115	118	121	124	126	129	132	135	138	141	144	147	150
38		110	112	115	118	120	123	126	129	132	134	137	140	143	146
37		107	110	112	115	117	120	123	125	128	131	134	136	139	142
36		104	107	109	112	114	117	119	122	125	127	130	133	136	138
35		101	104	106	108	111	113	116	119	121	124	126	129	132	134
34		98	101	103	105	108	110	113	115	118	120	123	125	128	131
33		95	98	100	102	105	107	109	112	114	117	119	122	124	127
32		93	95	97	99	101	104	106	108	111	113	116	118	120	123
31		90	92	94	96	98	100	103	105	107	110	112	114	117	119
30	Overweight	87	89	91	93	95	97	99	102	104	106	108	111	113	115
29		84	86	88	90	92	94	96	98	100	103	105	107	109	111
28		81	83	85	87	89	91	93	95	97	99	101	103	105	108
27		78	80	82	84	86	88	89	91	93	95	98	100	102	104
26		75	77	79	81	82	84	86	88	90	92	94	96	98	100
25	Acceptable	72	74	76	77	79	81	83	85	87	88	90	92	94	96
24		69	71	73	74	76	78	80	81	83	85	87	89	90	92
23		67	68	70	71	73	75	76	78	80	81	83	85	87	88
22		64	65	67	68	70	71	73	75	76	78	79	81	83	85
21		61	62	64	65	67	68	70	71	73	74	76	77	79	81
20		58	59	61	62	63	65	66	68	69	71	72	74	75	77
19	Underweight	55	56	58	59	60	62	63	64	66	67	69	70	72	73
18		52	53	55	56	57	58	60	61	62	64	65	66	68	69
17		49	50	52	53	54	55	56	58	59	60	61	63	64	65
Height	m	1.70	1.72	1.74	1.76	1.78	1.80	1.82	1.84	1.86	1.88	1.90	1.92	1.94	1.96
	ft in	5.6¾	5.7¾	5.8½	5.9¼	5.10	5.10¾	5.11¾	6.0½	6.1¼	6.2	6.2½	6.3½	6.4½	6.5½

4 Diagnostic dilemmas

When the diagnosis is in doubt, or investigations contribute to, rather than resolve, the confusion, the following approach is recommended:
- Take a careful history again, paying attention to what the patient says
- Re-examine the patient, paying special attention to lymph nodes, external genitalia and rectal examination, because these areas are often overlooked on the initial examination
- List the investigations and results, in chronological order
- Seek advice if the way ahead remains unclear
- Do not order another test and hope that someone else sees the patient next time!

Index

Index

Index

Index

Index

Index

Index

Index

Index

Index

Index

Index

Index

Index

Index

Index

Index

Index

Index

Index

Index